AF133693

Marine-Derived Products for Biomedicine

Marine-Derived Products for Biomedicine

Editor

Marco Giovine

MDPI • Basel • Beijing • Wuhan • Barcelona • Belgrade • Manchester • Tokyo • Cluj • Tianjin

Editor
Marco Giovine
University of Genova
Italy

Editorial Office
MDPI
St. Alban-Anlage 66
4052 Basel, Switzerland

This is a reprint of articles from the Special Issue published online in the open access journal *Marine Drugs* (ISSN 1660-3397) (available at: https://www.mdpi.com/journal/marinedrugs/special_issues/Biomedicine).

For citation purposes, cite each article independently as indicated on the article page online and as indicated below:

LastName, A.A.; LastName, B.B.; LastName, C.C. Article Title. *Journal Name* **Year**, *Article Number*, Page Range.

ISBN 978-3-03943-130-4 (Hbk)
ISBN 978-3-03943-131-1 (PDF)

Cover image courtesy of Tal Idan.

© 2020 by the authors. Articles in this book are Open Access and distributed under the Creative Commons Attribution (CC BY) license, which allows users to download, copy and build upon published articles, as long as the author and publisher are properly credited, which ensures maximum dissemination and a wider impact of our publications.
The book as a whole is distributed by MDPI under the terms and conditions of the Creative Commons license CC BY-NC-ND.

Contents

About the Editor vii

Preface to "Marine-Derived Products for Biomedicine" ix

Simone S. Silva, Joana M. Gomes, Luísa C. Rodrigues and Rui L. Reis
Marine-Derived Polymers in Ionic Liquids: Architectures Development and Biomedical Applications
Reprinted from: *Mar. Drugs* **2020**, *18*, 346, doi:10.3390/md18070346 1

Juan Eduardo Sosa-Hernández, Kenya D. Romero-Castillo, Lizeth Parra-Arroyo, Mauricio A. Aguilar-Aguila-Isaías, Isaac E. García-Reyes, Ishtiaq Ahmed, Roberto Parra-Saldivar, Muhammad Bilal and Hafiz M. N. Iqbal
Mexican Microalgae Biodiversity and State-Of-The-Art Extraction Strategies to Meet Sustainable Circular Economy Challenges: High-Value Compounds and Their Applied Perspectives
Reprinted from: *Mar. Drugs* **2019**, *17*, 174, doi:10.3390/md17030174 31

Lamiaa A. Shaala, Hani Z. Asfour, Diaa T. A. Youssef, Sonia Żółtowska-Aksamitowska, Marcin Wysokowski, Mikhail Tsurkan, Roberta Galli, Heike Meissner, Iaroslav Petrenko, Konstantin Tabachnick, Viatcheslav N. Ivanenko, Nicole Bechmann, Lyubov V. Muzychka, Oleg B. Smolii, Rajko Martinović, Yvonne Joseph, Teofil Jesionowski and Hermann Ehrlich
New Source of 3D Chitin Scaffolds: The Red Sea Demosponge *Pseudoceratina arabica* (Pseudoceratinidae, Verongiida)
Reprinted from: *Mar. Drugs* **2019**, *17*, 92, doi:10.3390/md17020092 55

Kseniia N. Bardakova, Tatiana A. Akopova, Alexander V. Kurkov, Galina P. Goncharuk, Denis V. Butnaru, Vitaliy F. Burdukovskii, Artem A. Antoshin, Ivan A. Farion, Tatiana M. Zharikova, Anatoliy B. Shekhter, Vladimir I. Yusupov, Peter S. Timashev and Yury A. Rochev
From Aggregates to Porous Three-Dimensional Scaffolds through a Mechanochemical Approach to Design Photosensitive Chitosan Derivatives
Reprinted from: *Mar. Drugs* **2019**, *17*, 48, doi:10.3390/md17010048 73

Van Bon Nguyen, Shan-Ping Chen, Thi Hanh Nguyen, Minh Trung Nguyen, Thi Thanh Thao Tran, Chien Thang Doan, Thi Ngoc Tran, Anh Dzung Nguyen, Yao-Haur Kuo and San-Lang Wang
Novel Efficient Bioprocessing of Marine Chitins into Active Anticancer Prodigiosin
Reprinted from: *Mar. Drugs* **2020**, *18*, 15, doi:10.3390/md18010015 91

Sonia Scarfì, Marina Pozzolini, Caterina Oliveri, Serena Mirata, Annalisa Salis, Gianluca Damonte, Daniela Fenoglio, Tiziana Altosole, Micha Ilan, Marco Bertolino and Marco Giovine
Identification, Purification and Molecular Characterization of Chondrosin, a New Protein with Anti-tumoral Activity from the Marine Sponge *Chondrosia Reniformis* Nardo 1847
Reprinted from: *Mar. Drugs* **2020**, *18*, 409, doi:10.3390/md18080409 105

Ji Min Kim, Jeong Hun Kim, Sung-Chan Shin, Gi Cheol Park, Hyung Sik Kim, Keunyoung Kim, Hyoung Kyu Kim, Jin Han, Natalia P. Mishchenko, Elena A. Vasileva, Sergey A. Fedoreyev, Valentin A. Stonik and Byung-Joo Lee
The Protective Effect of Echinochrome A on Extracellular Matrix of Vocal Folds in Ovariectomized Rats
Reprinted from: *Mar. Drugs* **2020**, *18*, 77, doi:10.3390/md18020077 131

Catherine Malaplate, Aurelia Poerio, Marion Huguet, Claire Soligot, Elodie Passeri, Cyril J. F. Kahn, Michel Linder, Elmira Arab-Tehrany and Frances T. Yen
Neurotrophic Effect of Fish-Lecithin Based Nanoliposomes on Cortical Neurons
Reprinted from: *Mar. Drugs* **2019**, *17*, 406, doi:10.3390/md17070406 . . . . **147**

Fazlurrahman Khan, Panchanathan Manivasagan, Jang-Won Lee, Dung Thuy Nguyen Pham, Junghwan Oh and Young-Mog Kim
Fucoidan-Stabilized Gold Nanoparticle-Mediated Biofilm Inhibition, Attenuation of Virulence and Motility Properties in *Pseudomonas aeruginosa* PAO1
Reprinted from: *Mar. Drugs* **2019**, *17*, 208, doi:10.3390/md17040208 . . . . **161**

Erika Bellini, Matteo Ciocci, Saverio Savio, Simonetta Antonaroli, Dror Seliktar, Sonia Melino and Roberta Congestri
Trichormus variabilis (Cyanobacteria) Biomass: From the Nutraceutical Products to Novel EPS-Cell/Protein Carrier Systems
Reprinted from: *Mar. Drugs* **2018**, *16*, 298, doi:10.3390/md16090298 . . . . **181**

About the Editor

Marco Giovine holds a degree in Biological Sciences and PhD in Biochemistry. He served as Scientific Director of the Marine Biotechnology laboratory of the Advanced Biotechnology Center of Genoa until 2012. He is currently Associate Professor of Molecular Biology, a position he has held since December 2005. He carries out his scientific activity at DISTAV, University of Genova, mainly focused on the molecular biology of marine organisms and marine biotechnology. His specific research topics are i) biomineralization mechanisms in marine invertebrates; ii) the study of extracellular matrix proteins of Porifera and their biotechnological applications, iii) the study of cellular models of Porifera. These studies also involve examination of the evolutive molecular mechanisms underlying the interaction between animal cells and mineral structure from sponges to human beings. He was National Coordinator of PRIN Ministerial Projects and research unit PI of European Union projects under the 6th and 7th framework programs. He is currently responsible for a research project in Italy under the bilateral scientific and technological cooperation agreement between Italy and Israel. He has authored more than 60 publications in international journals, some contributions in book chapters with a biotechnological theme, a report as invited speaker to the International Marine Biotechnology Conference in 2016, and six patents in the biotechnology sector. He founded two university spin-offs in the fields of marine biotechnology (MUDS SRL) and environmental biotechnology and food safety (MICAMO SRL). He is a member of the scientific board of the PhD in Sea Science and Technology at the University of Genoa. Since 2014, he has been the Rector's Delegate for guidance and career counselling. From 2020, he is serving as Vice President of the "Centro del mare" at the University of Genova. He carries out teaching activities for the Biology and Biology and Marine Ecology courses.

Preface to "Marine-Derived Products for Biomedicine"

Marine biodiversity is a planetary resource, and its sustainable exploitation is one pillar of the so-called "blue economy". Among the treasures guarded by Poseidon, the great variety of organisms living in the seas is an invaluable source of natural compounds and biomaterials that are potentially useful for biomedicines. New biologically active compounds, exploited for the design and production of new drugs, biomaterials, tissue engineering, and highly ordered biomineralized structural organizations, inspiring biomimicry approaches, are typical examples of applications of marine-derived products. Marine invertebrates are the best candidates for new natural compound discovery and for the characterization of new biomaterials. Similar opportunities are also found in algae and microorganisms. All these living beings undoubtedly represent a field for the mining of novelties by biotechnologists and material scientists.

The strong surge, worldwide, in research for the exploitation of marine resources to be used for biomedical purposes is clearly documented by the high numbers of grants and increasing numbers of new publications and patents on these topics. This fact denotes a remarkable incentive by political and industrial decision-makers to work on marine biotechnology as applied to biomedicine, and this Special Issue was developed on the basis of this evidence.

The volume comprises two reviews and eight regular articles whose topics provide a good representation of the richness of opportunities offered to biomedicine by the living beings of the sea. The reviews focus on novel green techniques of extraction of compounds from marine algae or from fishery waste, two significant sources of bioactive compounds, the exploitation of which, however, is strictly dependent on sustainable production procedures. The regular articles show the original results of research on new materials and compounds of marine origin used in different fields of biomedicine. More specifically, they describe 1) the potential employment of peculiar marine sponge-derived chitin scaffolds in biomedicine; 2) the use of laser stereolithography for the production of advanced 3D scaffolds from crustacean-derived chitosan; 3) the exploitation of marine α chitin as a carbon source for the production of the anticancer compound prodigiosin by means of *Serratia marcescens* fermentation; 4) the identification of a new type of marine toxin (chondrosin) with anticancer potentialities from the marine sponge *Chondrosia reniformis*; 5) the therapeutic effects of echinochrome A on extracellular matrix reconstitution after estrogen deficiency in ovariectomized rats; 6) the neurotrophic effect of fish lecithin-based nanoliposomes on cortical neurons; 7) the use of fucoidan-stabilized gold nanoparticles to inhibit biofilm formation and to attenuate the virulence of *Pseudomonas aeruginosa*; and 8) the protocols for low-cost cultivation of a native strain of the cyanobacteria *Trichormus variabilis* in a photobioreactor for the production of polyunsaturated fatty acids and exopolymeric substances. This collection of selected scientific publications gives an exhaustive overview of the different up-to-date approaches used by marine biotechnologists to exploit marine biodiversity in a sustainable way.

Marco Giovine
Editor

marine drugs

Review

Marine-Derived Polymers in Ionic Liquids: Architectures Development and Biomedical Applications

Simone S. Silva [1,2,*], Joana M. Gomes [1,2], Luísa C. Rodrigues [1,2] and Rui L. Reis [1,2,3]

1 3B´s Research Group, I3Bs- Research Institute on Biomaterials, Biodegradables and Biomimetics, University of Minho, Headquarters of the European Institute of Excellence on Tissue Engineering and Regenerative Medicine, Avepark, 4805-017 Barco, Guimarães, Portugal; joana.gomes@i3bs.uminho.pt (J.M.G.); luisa.rodrigues@i3bs.uminho.pt (L.C.R.); rgreis@i3bs.uminho.pt (R.L.R.)

2 ICVS/3B´s – PT Government Associate Laboratory, 4805-017 Braga/Guimarães, Portugal

3 The Discoveries Centre for Regenerative and Precision Medicine, Headquarters at University of Minho, Avepark, 4805-017 Barco, Guimarães, Portugal

* Correspondence: simonesilva@i3bs.uminho.pt; Tel.: +351-253-510-900

Received: 27 May 2020; Accepted: 27 June 2020; Published: 30 June 2020

Abstract: Marine resources have considerable potential to develop high-value materials for applications in different fields, namely pharmaceutical, environmental, and biomedical. Despite that, the lack of solubility of marine-derived polymers in water and common organic solvents could restrict their applications. In the last years, ionic liquids (ILs) have emerged as platforms able to overcome those drawbacks, opening many routes to enlarge the use of marine-derived polymers as biomaterials, among other applications. From this perspective, ILs can be used as an efficient extraction media for polysaccharides from marine microalgae and wastes (e.g., crab shells, squid, and skeletons) or as solvents to process them in different shapes, such as films, hydrogels, nano/microparticles, and scaffolds. The resulting architectures can be applied in wound repair, bone regeneration, or gene and drug delivery systems. This review is focused on the recent research on the applications of ILs as processing platforms of biomaterials derived from marine polymers.

Keywords: marine polymers; ionic liquids; tissue engineering; membranes; hydrogels; sponges

1. Introduction

Natural polymers from marine resources have increasingly attracted attention in recent years, as they are abundant and biologically active when compared to polymers from other resources. In fact, marine sources such as crustaceans, seaweeds, and algae are enriched with polysaccharides such as agar, chitin/chitosan, alginate, and glycosaminoglycans, exhibiting interesting features and properties [1–3]. For instance, chitin acts as a structural material in the exoskeletons of crustaceans and insects. Such marine-derived biomaterials constitute a platform for the development of value chains with environmental and economic advantages. In fact, several marine polymers are entering the biomedical market due to their abundance and their intrinsic features, namely biocompatibility, biodegradability, and biological activity. Despite these advantages, some mentioned polysaccharides have limitations of solubility in water and most organic solvents, due to the strong intra- and intermolecular hydrogen bonds in their polymeric chains, which limit their processing and conversion into value-added matrices, e.g., membranes, fibers, nanomaterials, and scaffolds. Hence, searching for effective, ecofriendly, and feasible solvents is very important.

Ionic liquids (ILs) are organic salts and an important green media [4], mainly explored in biopolymers processing, but also able to be extracted directly from their sources [5–8]. The interest in ILs occurs due to their excellent properties, such as very high thermal stability, recyclability, noninflammability, negligible vapor pressure, and miscibility in various solvents [4]. A vast range of available ILs can be tuned, combining different cations and anions, which would tailor their intrinsic features, such as viscosity, ionic conductivity, density, polarity, solvation power, hydrophilicity, and hydrophobicity [9–11]. Different researchers proposed distinct strategies that combine green chemistry principles with the use of biorenewable feedstocks, e.g., natural macromolecules envisioning the formation of 2D/3D matrices as innovative biomaterials [12–17]. Pioneering work on the use of 1-butyl-3-methylimidazolium chloride (Bmim)(Cl), an IL as a solvent for cellulose in relatively high concentrations (30–40% wt), was developed by Swatloski et al. in 2002 [18]. Their success in the dissolution of cellulose in ILs opened new avenues for the processing of other biopolymers [6,19,20].

Despite the advantages of ILs, their high cost is a major issue in large-scale applications, making their recycling an important issue to assure economic sustainability. Taking into account that ILs cannot be purified by distillation due to their low volatility, the recycling of ILs could be challenging. For their part, simple protocols based on the solubility of ILs in organic solvents have been developed [21].

Particularly, the use of ILs to extract marine polysaccharides like agarose, chitin, carrageenan from their sources, residues, or even waste is a sustainable approach that has been indicated as easy and highly efficient, as compared to the conventional methods of extraction [7,22]. Besides polymer extraction, many studies have also shown the potential of ILs as suitable platforms for the production of 2D and 3D-based marine polymers, namely gels, films, micro/nanoparticles, and sponges. Given the performance of these matrices, they have been proposed as wound dressing, drug delivery, bone repair, and gene delivery systems. Therefore, this review is focused on the overview of the properties, strategies, and biomedical applications of marine-derived polysaccharides processed in different ILs (see Figure 1).

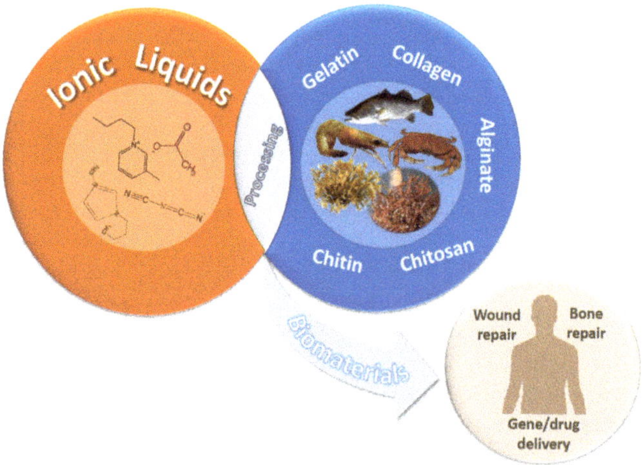

Figure 1. Strategies and biomedical applications of chitin/chitosan-based biomaterials prepared in ionic liquids (ILs).

2. Dissolution of Marine-Derived Polymers Using Ionic Liquids

The unique physicochemical properties and improved solvating power of ILs allow to dissolve a variety of polysaccharides through the disruption of hydrogen bonding. In particular, many ILs, such as 1-ethyl-3-methylimidazolium acetate ((Emim)OAc)) [23,24], 1-butyl-3-methylimidazolium acetate((Bmim)(OAc)) [25], N-butylpyridinium hexafluorophosphate (BPPF6) [26], 1-butyl-3-methylimidazolium chloride ((Bmim)(Cl)) [27], 1-ethyl-3-methylimidazolium ethylsulfate ((Emim)(C_2OSO_3)), 1-hydrogen-3-methylimidazolium hydrogen sulfate ((Hmim)(HSO_4)) [28], 1-Butyl-3-

methylimidazolium tetrafluoroborate ((Bmim)(BF_4)) [29], 1-ethyl-3-methylimidazolium chloride ((Emim)(Cl)) [30], and 1-ethyl-3-methyl-imidazolium ethyl sulfate ((Emim)($EtSO_4$)) [31] have been reported in the literature as capable of dissolving many marine polysaccharides, such as alginate, chitin, chitosan, collagen, and gelatin, among others.

The abundance of marine microalgae and the skeletons of crustaceans is large, but its poor solubility in conventional solvents restricts the efficient extraction of its value compounds. Nevertheless, there are some reports on ILs as extraction mediums for polysaccharides from marine residues [5,7,22,32,33]. Details about the structures, properties, and strategies involving the use of ILs on the dissolution and processing of selected marine polymers are made in the following sections.

Moreover, the interaction of the matrices, especially of proteins with ILs, has been assessed with various ILs, being the dominance of anionic interactions considered mostly responsible for governing stabilization [34–38]. Considering collagen, ILs based on imidazolium, phosphonium, and ammonium had destabilizing effects because of the chaotropic of anions resulting in collagen structural degradation rather than the strengthening of interactions, although choline dihydrogen phosphate (Ch)(DHP) stabilized the collagen structure [37,39–41]. In another work, choline amino acid-based ILs also demonstrated a destabilizing effect at the molecular and fibrillar levels, due to competitive hydrogen bonding between its molecules [37]. Either (Ch)(DHP) and choline amino acid-based ILs belong to the biocompatible ILs (bio-ILs) family. Bio-ILs emerged due to the need to develop more biological and environmental-friendly compounds that will allow extending the use of ILs to a broader range of fields, preventing the associated toxicity issues. The synthesis of bio-ILs is mainly performed using the choline cation as the cationic counterpart; however, in recent years, more synthetic strategies have been developed [42]. Furthermore, the role played by the cation can not be neglected; according to Mehta et al., significant physicochemical impacts, including on thermal denaturation, were observed for different aqueous solutions of imidazolium chlorides ((Emim)(Cl), (Bmim)(Cl)), and 1-decyl-3-methylimidazolium chloride ((Dmim)(Cl])) [40].

2.1. Alginate

Alginate is a linear polymer with a high abundance in nature [21]. It is present in the cell wall of brown algae, playing not only a structural function but also being involved in ionic exchange mechanisms. Alginate is an unbranched polysaccharide composed of β(1-4)-linked D-mannuronic acid (M) and α(1-4)-linked L-guluronic acid (G) (Figure 2), which are stereoisomers and differ in the composition of the carboxyl group [1,43]. M and G units can be present in blocks of (M and G) or mixed (MG) [1].

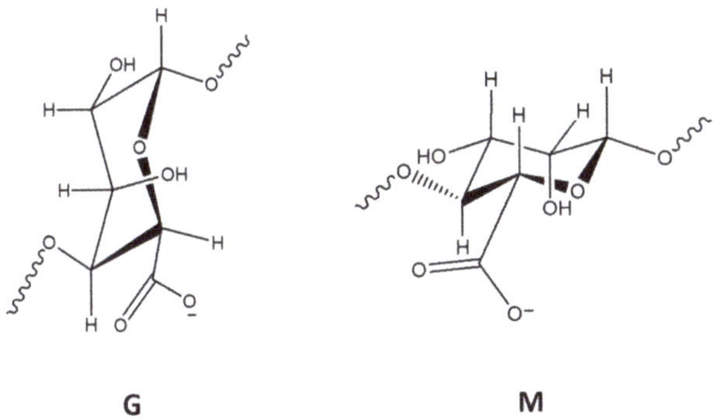

Figure 2. Chemical structure representation of alginate's α(1-4)-linked L-guluronic acid (G) and β(1-4)-linked D-mannuronic acid (M) units.

Alginate is water-soluble, being well-known for its gelling capacity [21]. The physicochemical properties of alginate, as well as its gelling ability, are strongly influenced by its structure, which is dependent on the variability in the ratio and sequence of the M and G units. Other factors influencing the alginate's gelling capacity are the experimental conditions, including the solutions viscosity and the used gelation agent concentration, as well as the molecular weight. The most commonly used gelation agents are calcium and other divalent ions [1]. G monomers play a vital role in the ionic gelation mechanisms, forming ionic bonds induced by the presence of divalent ions [44]. G-rich alginate promotes the formation of more stiff and transparent gels, while M-rich alginate originates more flexible gels [45]. Alginate's biocompatibility, low toxicity, and low cost have been boosting its wide use in areas, including food, cosmetics, pharmaceutical, and biomedical industries [1,21].

Despite alginate's remarkable and exclusive features, depending on the target application, it generally lacks the desired physicochemical properties. Therefore, ILs are often used in combination with alginate to improve these properties. Some works have reported the development of electrolytes using alginate and ILs, with applications in electrochemistry and catalysis [21,26]. Ding and coworkers were able to develop a biosensor and biocatalyst of horseradish peroxidase using the IL N-butylpyridinium hexafluorophosphate ($BPPF_6$) and sodium alginate [26]. These biosensing systems took advantage of the intrinsic ILs' electrochemical properties, which allow a direct electron transfer. The produced film revealed to have good detection precision, bioactivity, storage stability, and reproducibility, suggesting the extension of its application to other enzymes. This is relevant, since the direct electrochemistry of redox proteins may help to understand the electron transfer mechanisms in the biological systems. Since ILs are great solvents for a wide range of other natural polymers, they also have been used for the preparation of composites consisting of alginate and other polymers, such as chitin [25]. In 2014, Shamshina et al. produced wound care dressings using chitin-calcium alginate composite fibers spun from an IL (Emim)(OAc) solution [25]. The produced fibers presented strength and water absorption, which met the technical specifications for wound care and allowed to accelerate the wound recovery, even though optimizations were needed.

2.2. Chitin

Chitin is the second most abundant natural polymer, just after cellulose [46]. It is found in the shell of crustaceans, squid pens, fungi, and cuticles of insects [46,47]. Structurally, chitin is composed of a long chain made up of β (1→4)-linked primary units of N-acetyl D-glucosamine [48–50] (Figure 3). Chitin is characterized by its degree of acetylation (DA), which is defined as the ratio of 2-acetamido-2-deoxy-d-glucopyranose to 2-amino-2-deoxy-d-glucopyranose structural units, which is typically 0.90, indicating the presence of about 5-15% of amino groups due to deacetylation that might occur during chitin extraction [50].

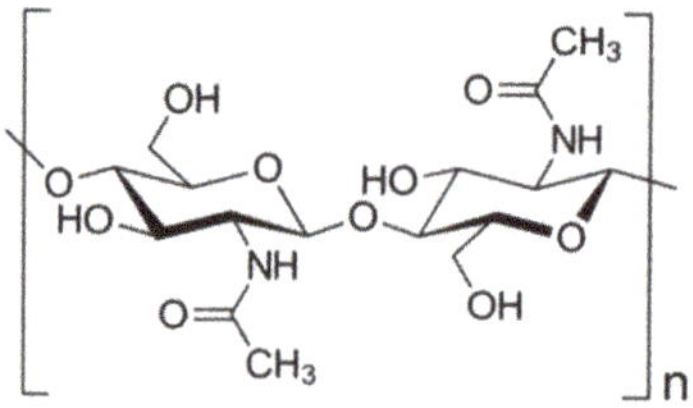

Figure 3. Chitin chemical structure representation.

Depending on the source, chitin can be characterized mainly by α- and β-forms [49,51]. In both types of chitins, the chains are organized in sheets and held together by intrasheet hydrogen bonds. However, β-chitin (e.g., from squid pens) presents weaker intermolecular bonds as compared to the α-chitin structure (e.g., from crabs and shrimp shells), which may explain its higher affinity for solvents and higher reactivity. Chitin is a highly crystalline polysaccharide due to the strong intra- and intermolecular interactions, namely hydrogen bonds derived from acetamido groups—more specifically, between C = O and NH groups of the adjacent chitin chains, established between the polymeric chains, which makes difficult its dissolution and, consequently, its processing.

The biomedical potential of chitin is enormous, not only due to its abundance but, also, due to its biocompatibility, nontoxicity, and suitability for wound and burn healing. Despite the annual production of the biomass, the utilization of chitin as a raw material is limited due to its lack of isolation and solubility. In fact, chitin has shown difficulties using traditional solvents. A large volume of research has demonstrated the isolation and efficient dissolution of chitin, followed by the production of chitin-based matrices for many applications. Rogers et al. have shown that high molecular regenerated chitin can be extracted directly from shellfish waste (yield of 46%), and it could easily be processed into nanomats through electrospinning and ILs ((Emim)(OAc)) [5,23,24]. In another study, chitin was directly extracted from crab shells by using an ionic liquid, 1-allyl-3-methylimidazolium bromide ((Amim)(Br)) [52]. They indicated that ILs tend to extract chitin without addition to strong acid and/or base. Although there are promising findings on the use of ILs to dissolve chitin, little research has been performed on the influence of IL composition and polarity into the chitin dissolution mechanism. It seems that the requirement is of a higher polarity and more basic anions, e.g., acetate, probably due to the higher number of hydrogen bond donors and acceptors [23,53,54]. The studies suggested that acetate ions gave origin to weak conjugate acids able to interact with H-bonds of chitin, destroying them and leading to chitin crystal dissolution. Therefore, acetate ions can be more effective than chloride or dimethylphosphate anions. Studies involving a molecular dynamics (MD) approach to evaluate the dissolution of chitin crystals in imidazolium-based ILs revealed that the solubility of chitin can be correlated with the number of intermolecular hydrogen bonds by acetamido groups in the chitin crystal [55]. The data also proved that mixing a small amount of 2-bromoethyl acetate, as a bromide generator, with (Amim)(Br)can enhance chitin solubility. Besides the chosen solvent, parameters such as the degree of acetylation, pH, and chain molecular weight of chitin can affect its solubility, and it should be considered to understand the ability of this polymer to solubilize with ILs.

Moreover, different chitin-based materials processed through ILs have been prepared, such as chitin ion gels made with (Amim)(Br) (9.1–10.7 wt%) [56] that were used to produce highly entangled nanofibers with added functional components and modulated material morphology, which may find potential applicability in membrane preparation [57], biomedical and tissue engineering applications [58, 59], biosensors [60], or carbon capture sorbents [61].

2.3. Chitosan

Chitosan is a deacetylated derivative of chitin, and it has also been extensively studied for several purposes in food science, agriculture, environmental, textile, and biomedical fields [48,49]. It is composed of β-(1-4)-linked D-glucosamine (deacetylated monomer) and *N*-acetyl-d-glucosamine (acetylated monomer) units (Figure 4), in which the glucosamine backbone holds a high number of available amino groups that can be protonated. It is commercially available in a broad range of molecular weights and degrees of deacetylation. Moreover, amino groups of chitosan have a pKa value close to 6.5, which confers it with solubility in weak acid solutions, namely dilute acidic solutions of acetic, citric, and lactic acids [48]. Therefore, its charge density is dependent on the pH and the degree of deacetylation. Both the degree of deacetylation and molecular weight determine the properties of chitosan, e.g., biodegradability, biocompatibility, and solubility.

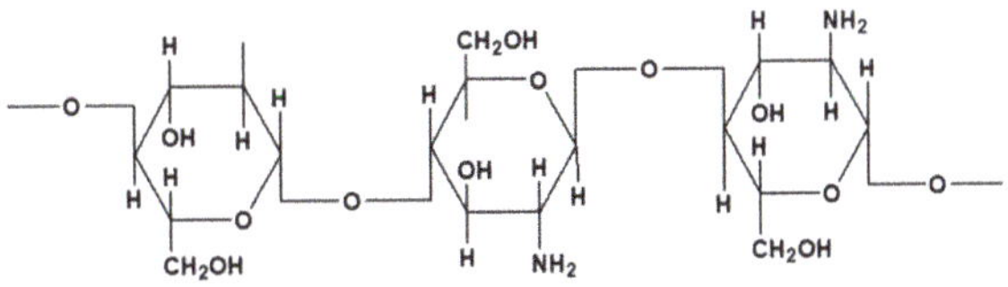

Figure 4. Chitosan chemical structure representation.

Similar to chitin, chitosan is extremely difficult to dissolve in water and most of the conventional organic solvents due to its strong intra- and intermolecular hydrogen bonds. Therefore, the search for sustainable solvents of chitosan has drawn wide attention to overcome the environmental issues related to acid-base treatments. Specifically, the role of ILs for the dissolution of chitosan has been evidenced with different degrees of success. So far, the existent similarity between cellulose and chitosan and the acquired know-how achieved for cellulose processing in IL have acted as a starting point for many strategies for chitosan processing in ILs. The research performed involved the elucidation of the effect of the IL composition, dissolution conditions (temperature and polymer concentrations), and water content in the chitosan hydrogen bonds' disruption promoted by ILs. Based on many studies, some ILs, including those with chloride, formate, and acetate as anions and 1-allyl-3-methylimidazolium ((Amim)), 1,3-dimethylimidazolium ((Dmim)), 1-hydrogen-3-methylimidazolium ((mim)), and 1-butyl-3-methylimidazolium ((Bmim)) as cations, as well as their mixtures, have been investigated as solvent and reaction mediums for chitosan [17,19,62–64]. The performance of a series of imidazolium-based ILs on chitosan dissolution demonstrated that (Bmim)(OAc) IL is the most efficient one [62]. Following the findings, the ability to dissolve chitosan follows the order: (Bmim)(OAc) > (Emim)(OAc), (Bmim)(OAc) > 1-hydrogen-3-methylimidazolium hydrogen acetate ((Hmim)(OAc)) > 1-octyl-3-methylimidazolium acetate (Omim)(OAc), and (Bmim)(Ac) > 1-butyl-2,3-dimethylimidazolium acetate (Bmmim)(OAc). The solubility of chitosan decreased with the increase of the water content at temperatures below 110 °C—after which, the values were resembled, probably due to water evaporation, while other studies observed an enhanced chitosan solubility with the increase of the dissolution temperature, e.g., from 50 °C up to 150 °C [64,65]. This effect is mainly associated with a change of the transport properties of the ILs and, simultaneously, to the evaporation of residual water from the system that is considered as antisolvent. Considering all the mentioned variables, the imidazolium-based ILs are advantageous for chitosan dissolution [65].

(Bmim)(Cl) has been used as an environmentally friendly solvent to prepare chitosan/cellulose biocomposites sorbents for industrial effluent treatments [22]. Moreover, due to its strong interactions with negatively charged entities, including lipids and proteins, IL/chitosan-based aerogels are used to stabilize the complexes, with DNA fragments being good choices for gene delivery systems [66].

2.4. Collagen

Collagen is the major supportive component of connective tissue, making up about 25–35% of the whole-body protein, being present in bone, tendon, teeth, skin, ligaments, and cartilage [67–71]. Collagen-based products, with high added values and low environmental impacts, have gained interest from the research community, as they can be obtained through the conversion of low-cost by-products. The preferential sources for collagen extractions are terrestrial mammals like cows, pigs, and sheep, due to the high-sequence homology with human collagen [72]. However, different concerns are associated with mammalian collagen, such as the trigger of an immune reaction (around 3% of the population), the transfer of zoonosis, and cultural or religious concerns associated with the use of porcine and bovine collagen, which further restrict its application [73]. The use of marine-derived collagen significantly restrings those concerns, being free from religious concerns and intrinsically showing a lower threat of transmissible diseases. Therefore, the possibility to valorize the fish byproducts (e.g. fish skin and scales) derived from the largely available polluting by-products from the fish processing industry as collagen sources makes marine-derived collagen ecofriendly and particularly attractive in terms of profitability and cost-effectiveness [72,74,75].

Considering the collagen molecule chemical composition, it can be described as a protein containing three polypeptide chains, each of which is composed of one or more regions containing an uninterrupted repeat of Gly-X-Y sequences, where X and Y can be any other amino acid residue. The sterical constraints due to proline and hydroxyproline cause the collagen regions with this tripeptide repeat to adopt three left-handed polypeptide chains (called α helices), which self-assemble to form at least one right-handed triple-helical domain [72,76,77], providing not only structural support for cells but, also, acting as an important regulator of cell behavior [78]. Collagen can be isolated from natural products, being relatively nonimmunogenic and, consequently biocompatible, opening the possibility to use it in a wide range of applications in commercial fields, including food [79,80], cosmetics [80–82], and medicine [72,83–86]. However, collagen application is tremendously limited by the strong inter- and intramolecular hydrogen and ionic bonds, van der Waals' forces, and hydrophobic bonds between the polar and nonpolar groups, which have extremely difficult collagen dissolution and consequent processing [71]. The hydrogen bonds formed by proline and hydroxyproline have a fundamental role in stabilizing the triple helical structure in physiological conditions, preventing chain free rotation [87]. Those bonds can be broken upon denaturation through thermal or chemical treatments, significantly impacting the collagen properties as it transforms collagen into a random coil form known as gelatin [72]. Several efforts have been made to disperse or dissolve collagen, preserving its native structure and simultaneously improving the content of collagen in the solution, as it is insoluble in organic solvents and only a low percentage is soluble in dilute acids and alkalis [88]. Different strategies have been employed to improve collagen dissolution. Poluboyarov et al. [89] reported values reaching 19.5g/L after five days for the combined effects of mechanical (ultrasonic and laboratory mixer) and enzymatic treatments, and Qi et al. [78] reported the achievement of a 10% (1 g/10 mL) collagen dissolution in a NaAc/HAc buffer solution. Another successful approach is the dissolution of collagen using ionic liquids (ILs) as a solvent. In this approach, the IL interacts with collagen by a hydrogen bond, promoting its dissolution [38,71,86]. Imidazolium-based ILs have brought about significant changes at the higher structural hierarchical level of collagen, developing a different hierarchical ordering [40]. Phosphonium and ammonium-based ionic liquids have a destabilizing effect on collagen [35,36]. On the other hand, (Ch)(DHP) IL stabilized collagen by exerting an electrostatic force on collagen, and due to its biocompatibility, has potential as biocompatible crosslinkers [90]. Collagen-based biomaterials prepared using choline salt, as crosslinkers, exhibited good cell viability and adhesion properties, as required for biomedical implantable applications [91].

2.5. Gelatin

Gelatin is the partially hydrolyzed form of collagen. Although their sources are bovine and porcine skin, some studies demonstrated their extraction from marine sources such as sponges and fish skin [43]. The chemical composition of gelatin depends on the source, but hydrophobic amino acids like proline (Pro), hydroxyproline (Hyp), and glycine (Gly) are more likely to be present in gelatin. The general primary sequence is given by (Gly-X-Pro) and (Gly-X-Hyp), in which X represents other amino acids [92]. In Figure 5 is presented the model structure of gelatin.

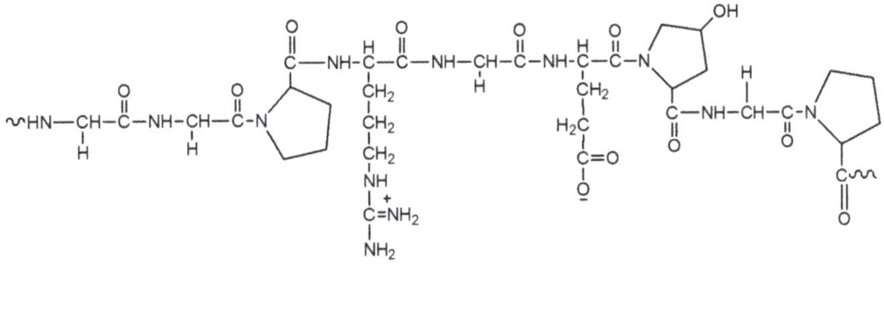

Figure 5. Basic chemical structure of gelatin (Ala—alanine, Arg—arginine, and Glu—glutamate).

Gelatin has a high solubility in water, as well as in many ILs [31]. The dissolution of gelatin in water occurs after the polypeptide strands in its structure undergo a coil-helix transition, and it happens at 30–35 °C [93]. Gelatin's amino acid content, which includes positively charged (lysine and Arg, 7.5%); negatively charged (Glu and aspartic acid, 12%); neutral (Gly, Pro, and Hyp, 58%); and hydrophobic (leucine, isoleucine, methionine, and valine, 6%) amino acid residues, promotes a different set of interactions with solvents or electrolytes [31]. This polymer is inexpensive, biocompatible, and biodegradable and interacts strongly with molecules that are soluble in aqueous media [93].

The gelatin and ILs combination strongly contributes to a broader use of this polymer. ILs can provide different physical-chemical properties and, also, change the gelatin microenvironment, being able to address one of gelatin's limitations, which concerns the entrapment of poorly water-soluble molecules [93]. The combination of ILs with gelatin is often used for the production of ion gels (IGs) [31,93,94]. This is mainly possible due to the expected set of electrostatic, hydrophobic, and H-boding interactions between the biopolymer and ILs, which lead to the formation of IGs [31]. This gelation process is based on a good compromise between the retention of the IL and its fluidity inside the polymeric network [93]. This technology allows the production of versatile and conductive gels that can be molded into different shapes using different methodologies. The produced IGs are usually simpler than the common solid polymer electrolytes and exhibit improved conductivities, which boosts its use as substitutes for the existing solid-state polyelectrolytes in energy devices [94]. Moreover, these electrolytes may often be used as printable "inks" [31,94]. Several authors have been using these IGs for the development of biosensing devices, namely for the immobilization of oxidoreductases, such as glucose oxidase (GOD) and horseradish peroxidase (HRP) [93,95,96]. Lourenço et al. prepared glucose paper test strips by the physical deposition of gelatin-1-ethyl-3-methyl-imidazolium ethyl sulfate ((Emim)EtSO4) containing GOD and HRP, as well as color-generating precursors [95]. The entrapment of GOD and HRP in the IGs show lower activity than for the free enzyme—in both cases, however, with excellent storage stability at 4 °C for a period of two weeks. Moreover, the immobilization of color-generating precursors in combination with the enzymes in the composite materials demonstrates that it can be used for the development of cheap and straightforward glucose paper test strips, with a quick response in less than one minute. Furthermore, these systems are used as drug delivery systems either by the functionalization of IL-based polymer gels by the incorporation of the active principle or by exploring the IL as the active principle ingredient [93,97]. Moreover, the use of ILs as the substituent of the chemical crosslinkers may allow to form relatively nonsoluble networks and significantly expand gelatin applications, since some of these polymers' limitations are extensive swelling, rapid dissolution, and drug release [93]. In 2019, Maneewattanapinyo and coworkers were able to develop a lidocaine–diclofenac-IL drug–loaded transdermal patch using the polymers gelatin/poly(vinyl alcohol), where the IL worked as the active pharmaceutical ingredient [97]. The developed biomaterial presented good physicochemical properties and showed to be viable to be used in pharmaceutics, mainly due to the control release of both lidocaine and diclofenac. Moreover, the developed patch presented good stability over the study period of three months when kept at 4 °C or under ambient temperature.

2.6. Other Marine-Derived Polymers

Besides the mentioned polymers above, the use of ILs to solubilize or even extract the medium for other marine-derived polymers such as carrageenan [33,98], agarose [6,7,30], and chondroitin sulfate [28] have also been investigated. Some authors explored the ability of ILs as a medium for the efficient extraction of agarose, the main agar constituent, from red algae (Rhodophyta). For that purpose, different ILs (1-ethyl-3-methylimidazolium acetate, (Emim)(OAc), choline acetate, (Ch)(OAc), and 1-ethyl-3-methyl imidazolium diethyl phosphate, (Emim)(Dep)) and heating or microwave irradiation were applied in the process [7]. As compared to conventional methods, a very high extraction yield of good quality agarose (as high as 39 wt%) was obtained. In other studies, the versatility of ILs combined with the morphological adaptability of the agarose was investigated to the formation of agarose-based highly soft ion gels [6]. In other approaches, the extraction of k-carrageenan from the red marine macroalgae Kappaphycus alvarezii was studied, applying an ionic liquid-assisted subcritical water (SWE) [33]. The findings showed that the SWE with a (Bmim)(OAc) IL catalyst exhibited the highest percentage yield, probably due to its high depolymerization and dissolution ability. Additionally, the formation of carrageenan (k-, ι-, and λ) combined with cellulose was achieved using (Bmim)(Cl), where λ-carrageenan gave a better miscible composite gel with the IL [98]. In a similar approach, chondroitin sulphate, a macromolecule classified as glycosaminoglycan, was blended with chitosan, using (Hmim)(HSO_4) as an appropriate solvent to create blended hydrogels. Those hydrogels showed excellent stabilities in a wide pH range (1.2–10) and excellent biocompatibility with epithelial cells.

3. Development of Marine-Polymeric Architectures via Ionic Liquids

Many 2D and 3D-based architectures have been produced using the dissolution of marine polymers with different ILs at moderated high temperatures, followed by cooling the polymer/IL solution to low temperatures (4–25 °C), promoting the formation of weak gel-like materials (ion gels), films, and hydrogels (see examples in Tables 1 and 2). By soaking those gels in water or ethanol and/or applying a suitable processing technique, e.g., freeze-drying, solvent casting, or electrospinning on the polymer/IL-based solutions, sponges, films, hydrogels, or nano/microspheres can be produced. Considering that some toxicity studies on ILs suggested that they exhibit a certain level of toxicity, their total or partial removal from the structures should be made. More details about the production of different matrices involving marine polymers and ILs are described in the following sections.

3.1. Films and Hydrogels

The ability of ILs in dissolving marine-derived polymers have been used to create films and hydrogels. The general procedure involves the dissolution of the polymers at a high temperature and gelation at room temperature with or without the use of specific molds, followed by immersion of the polymer/IL gels in solvents such as ethanol, acetone, or isopropanol. The choice of those solvents is related to their miscibility with the ILs, which, in turn, promotes the IL removal from the structures. Chitin films with tunable strength and morphology were designed by different drying methods, e.g., a simple casting method from a solution from (Emim)(OAc) or sc-CO_2-drying [99]. The chitin films were able to load and release caffeine, which was used as a model drug, indicating that they may have potential as drug-releasing membranes. It was shown that combinations of marine polymers with other polysaccharides, proteins, or even inorganic particles, using a common IL as the solvent, can be used to mimic the naturally occurring environment of certain tissues. Chitosan/silk fibroin (CSF) hydrogels were prepared in (Bmim)(OAc) as a common solvent and a soxhlet extraction with ethanol for IL removal [14]. The CSF exhibited viscoelastic behavior, lamellar structure, and rubbery consistency and, also, supported the adhesion and growth of primary human dermal fibroblasts. In another study, chitosan/chondroitin sulfate hydrogels were prepared in (Hmim)(HSO_4). Figure 6A depicts the IL structure, as well as the polymer dissolution mechanism proposed. The (Hmim)(HSO_4) solvent displayed a pH of 2.5 at 25 °C, and thus, the NH_2 ionization of chitosan can occur according to the following reaction: $R - NH_2 + H^+ \rightarrow R - NH_3^+$, whereas the pKa amino site is roughly 6.5. The coulombic, H-bond, ion-dipole, and London forces between CHT/IL foster CHT-dissolving (Figure 6A, right panel). Regarding the CS solution, there is an equilibrium of charges [-OSO_3H] ≈ [-OSO_3^-] under IL (pH 2.5) due to the pKa for −OSO3H being approximately 2.6. The CS dissolving was similar to that designated for CHT (6A, right panel). Thus, polyelectrolyte complexes (PECs) are inherently established by coulombic, H-bonds, and ion-dipole forces (Figure 6B, right panel). The chitosan/chondroitin sulfate hydrogels achieved excellent stability in the 1.2-10 pH range, considerable swelling abilities, and were devoid of toxicity towards the normal healthy kidney epithelial and epithelial colorectal adenocarcinoma cells [28]. Moreover, chitosan films with the potential to be used as drug delivery systems were developed using the bio-IL (Ch)(DHP) and the cholinium salt choline chloride [100]. The use of the bio-ILs provided the films with enhanced drug-release profiles, which associated with their conductivities/impedances, as well as pH sensitivities, allowing the development of biodegradable and biocompatible responsive drug delivery systems. In another study, choline nitrate (Ch)(NO_3) was used in combination with chitosan to produce a thin-film polymer gel electrolyte [101]. Besides their biocompatible and biodegradable features, the developed films presented robust mechanical properties and high ionic conductivity, leading the authors to suggest their application as implantable medical devices, including cardiac pacemakers or biomonitoring systems.

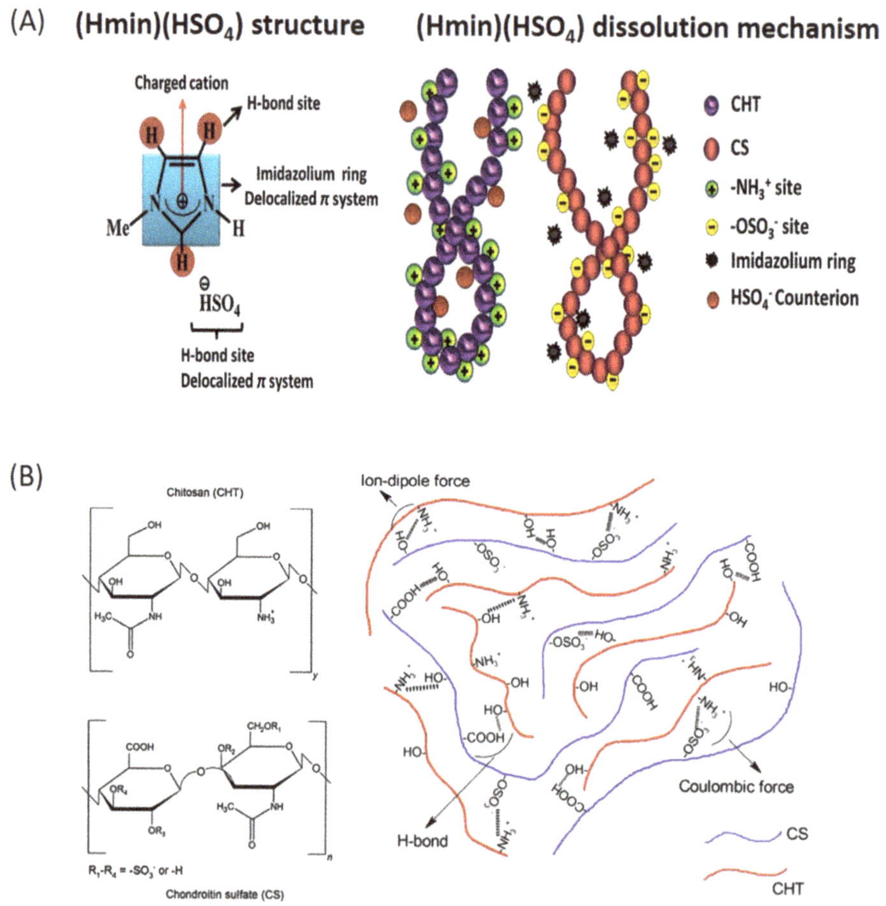

Figure 6. (**A**) (Hmim)(HSO_4) structure and its solvation capacity over the biopolymers and (**B**) the polysaccharide structures (left panel) and chitosan/chondroitin sulfate (CHT/CS) arrangement (right panel). Reprinted from [28], Copyright 2017, with permission from Elsevier.

3.2. Nanomicrofibers and Nanomicroparticles

Over the past decades, we have witnessed significant progress in marine-derived nanostructured materials. Nanofibrous materials have a remarkable potential, being useful in different applications such as drug delivery systems, tissue engineering scaffolds, wound dressing materials, antimicrobial agents, and biosensors. Due to their appealing physical and biological features, chitin and chitosan nanofibers have attracted the scientific community's attention [19]. Pure high molecular weight chitin nanofibers were electrospun through a one-pot process in an [Emim][OAc] solution of chitin extracted from dried shrimp shells [23,24,102]. This strategy allowed achieving smooth, continuous chitin nanofibers directly from an extract that provided the optimal viscosity, concentration, and necessary entanglement density for electrospinning. Chitin-calcium alginate composite fibers were also prepared from a solution of high molecular weight chitin and alginic acid in (Emim)(OAc) by dry-jet wet-spinning into an aqueous bath saturated with $CaCO_3$ [25]. Composite fibers presented consistent reproducibility and blend-homogeneity, meting the technical specifications (strength and water sorption) needed for wound care fiber applications; however, with the potential to be enhanced, envisioning different applications. High-tenacity chitosan fibers with excellent strength and initial modulus were generated with a dry-wet spinning technology from dissolved chitosan in binary IL mixtures of acidic and neutral IL of glycine hydrochloride (Gly·H)Cl and (Bmim)(Cl) [103]. The same procedures were used to produce chitosan-cellulose composite fibers with 9.4 wt% chitosan, which presented good mechanical strength and excellent thermal stability [104]. The same polymeric mixture was electrospun from an IL solution ((Emim)(Ac)) [105] to produce fiber films with the potential to be applied as antibacterial and antimicrobial agents to treat skin ulcers.

Collagen solutions were prepared in PBS containing different ration of ILs—respectively, 1-ethyl-3-methylimidazolium bromide ((Emim)(Br), 1-ethyl-3-methylimidazolium chloride ((Emim)(Cl)), or (Emim)(OAc) [106]. The thermal stability of the designed collagen fibril was significantly enhanced when the self-assembling was carried out in the presence of ILs, promoting as well the improvement of the viscoelastic properties of the collagen gel.

Microdroplets in ILs as unique interfaces led to the development of simple and rational methods for preparing biopolymer-encapsulated protein microcapsules [63]. The conventionally used methods for protein-based particle preparations have been employed (emulsification, desolvation, coacervation, and electrospray drying); however, other alternative strategies (template method, microfluidic technology, etc.) have been used to overcome the limitations associated with conventional approaches as low yields, low control of particles features (size distribution and shape), and collagen denaturation. Protein-based micro- and nanoparticles present high biodegradability and low thermal and mechanical stability, which lead to collagen chemical modification (maintaining its native structure) or the combination with other biopolymers or synthetic polymers or even inorganic materials, also allowing to increase the system functionality [107,108] and to modulate their properties according to the desired application. Thus, several collagen-based micro- and nanoparticles were developed with different biomedical applications (tissue engineering, imagistic/diagnosis, and drug/gene delivery) [109].

Oil-in-water microemulsions were used to prepare protein microcapsules (3-40 μm) [63,110]; however, the inner oil droplets are not suitable to dissolve water-soluble guest biopolymers. This issue can be overcome through the use of ILs, with the advantage that the microcapsules formed in the IL phase can be easily extracted to the aqueous phase after consecutive crosslinking and surface modification reactions [63,111–113]. Modifications were introduced into the emulsification method to improve the delivery kinetics, maintaining the collagen meshwork biocompatibility as the replacement of chemicals for photochemical crosslinking or the use of self-assembling collagen fiber reconstitution [114]. However, the emulsion method remains to present poor control of the particle shape and size, as well as a reduced loading level [109], which leads to the exploitation of other strategies to produce micro- or nanoparticles.

Metal nanoparticles attract significant attention based on their properties, as they are reported to be monodispersed and non-agglomerated as a result of ionic liquid stabilization [112]. Polymers added to the nanoparticle–ionic liquid dispersion promotes a partial coverage of the nanoparticle surfaces where polymer coils extend between the particle surface, acting as bridges between nanoparticles through molecular contact. In higher amounts, the polymers can fully cover the nanoparticle surface to form an adsorbed polymer layer, which is responsible for steric repulsions between neighboring nanoparticles, "pushing" nanoparticles away from each other [112]. The generation of Ag_2O nanoparticles in DSIL-gelatin sols showed uniform decorations of 50–100-nm size Ag_2O

nanoparticles over gelatin, wherein the imidazolium cation acted as a reducing agent [34]. This system presented good bactericidal activity on Gram-negative bacteria showing the potential to be used for food packaging, wound dressings, and other biomedical applications [34]. Hollow spheres were also fabricated according to template methodology, allowing to achieve gelatin particles with defined sizes and improved drug/protein loading and encapsulation efficiency, resulting in reservoir systems for the sustained delivery of proteins useful for different therapies [115].

Various self-organized structures based on nanoparticles are generated as a result of a balance of the intermolecular interactions between ionic liquids constituents and marine-derived polymers and proteins. Chitosan nanoparticles by ionic crosslinking with IL, which consist in self-assembling methods of adding (Bmim)(C_8OSO_3) or (Omim)(Cl) above the critical micelle concentration to an aqueous solution of chitosan, aggregate in a gelated complex [116]. The nanoparticles with diameters ranging from 300–560 nm and Zeta potential above +58.5 mV were formed due to the electrostatic and hydrophobic interactions established between chitosan and IL, being the IL aggregates used as templates for the structure build-up.

3.3. Scaffolds, Sponges, and Beads

The combination of marine origin materials, in conjunction with green-processing technologies and solvents, has been proven to be effective for the development of scaffolds, sponges, and beads, with broad applications. Silva et al. [117] have successfully produced porous chitin aerogels by dissolving the polymer using the IL (Bmim)(OAc) by employing high-temperature stirring. After the mixture was gelified at room temperature and removed, and the IL was removed by supercritical fluid drying using a soxhlet extraction and SCF extraction using carbon dioxide/ethanol ratios. This procedure promoted the production of chitin aerogels with a porous and interconnected structure, large surface area, and low density. Moreover, chitin microparticles prepared in ILs were produced using a similar method to produce 3D constructs with the flexibility to adapt according to defect sites, osteoinductive behavior, and the potential use as controlled drug-release devices [58]. The sol-gel methodology was used to promote the formation of a silica network as a coating in the chitin beads, as well as a means to promote the IL removal from the beads, followed by the supercritical agglomeration method.

The production of multifunctional composites using ILs, achieved by blends of different polymers or even inorganic particles (hydroxyapatite, HA), has also been a focus of study. In a work from 2013, Silva et al. [118] produced chitin–hydroxyapatite composites using (Bmim)(OAc) to dissolve chitin, followed by the addition of salt particles (salt leaching methodology) to promote pore formation and/or HA to induce osteoinductive behavior and drying by supercritical fluid drying. In a recent work from the same group, both chitin and *Antheraea pernyi* silk fibroin were dissolved using the same IL and used for the production of sponges from blends [13]. The produced sponges revealed to have good porosity, interconnectivity, and pore sizes values, presenting considerable swelling and adequate viscoelastic properties, making them promising candidates in cartilage regeneration. Composites with potential applications in bone tissue engineering were also formed by the dissolution of chitosan and cellulose in ILs with the addition of HA [27]. The produced structures presented good antimicrobial activity, the ability to deliver growth factors/drugs (from chitosan), and mechanical strength (from cellulose).

4. Environmental and Biological Impact of ILs Used in the Development of Marine Polymer-Based Architectures

4.1. IL's Recycling and Reuse

The recycling and reuse of the ILs increase the sustainability of the implemented processes while reducing the economical burdens sometimes related to ILs' use, increasing the opportunity for the large-scale application of the developed methodologies [42]. The techniques used to recover and reuse ILs strongly depend on its application, considering that, usually, it involves a recovering or regeneration step, followed by a purification stage, to avoid the deterioration of the ILs [119,120].

The recycling of ILs used for the processing of marine-based biopolymers are regularly made by using an antisolvent (such as water and ethanol) that works as a coagulant to the dissolved polymer by solvating the ILs, constituting the recovering step. The purification step is usually performed by the distillation of the antisolvents from the ILs [120,121]. The use of water to recover the ILs after the polymer's pretreatment is the most straightforward purification strategy [5,102,120]. Iqbal et al. prepared collagen-alginate-hydroxyapatite beds to be used as bone fillers, using (Emim)(Cl) as a solvent [122]. The IL was recovered from the water and $CaCl_2$ mixture, used for the beads preparation, by rotary evaporation for water removal, followed by mixing with cold acetone to dissolve IL and precipitate out the $CaCl_2$. After filtration, (Emim)(Cl) was obtained by the rotary evaporation of acetone, a process repeated many times, aiming to obtain a high yield of IL (95 ± 1). As well,(Bmim)(Cl), used as a green solvent to dissolve and synthesize the [CEL/CHT] composites, was removed from the composites by washing them with water. The IL was recovered by distilling the washing solution, from which the IL remained due to its high melting (>400 °C), with a recovery rate of at least 88% of the IL, being the proposed method considered as recyclable [123]. In another work, (Emim)(OAc) was used to directly recover high molecular weight chitin from raw crustacean shells [5]. Fibers were spun directly from the extract solution, and the IL recycling was carried out by evaporation of the aqueous wash.

The use of aqueous biphasic systems in this process may contribute to a reduction of the energy needed for water evaporation since the kosmotropic salts pull some of the water present in the mixture. However, a further dewatering step using evaporation techniques is mandatory [5]. The dewatering strategies used for the purification of the ILs usually involve the use of deep vacuum (0.02mbar to 10mbar). Moreover, the use of heat or microwave-assisted eating proved to be helpful in that process, with the latter being 52 times more efficient than conventional heating [5]. When small molecules are formed, the product is usually recovered with a suitable volatile organic solvent (VOC) such as ethyl acetate, diethyl ether, or dichloromethane. This process is followed by the IL, and the additive or catalyst is used for recovery, and the water is removed through evaporation under high vacuum, and the products are used in the following catalytic steps [124]. Barber et al. extracted chitin from dried shrimp shells using (Emim)(OAc), followed by the chemisorption of CO_2 in (Emim)(OAc) through the chemical reaction [121]. The use of CO_2 proved to be an economical and energy-efficient method for the potential recycling of the IL by reducing the use of antisolvents and eliminating the need for using higher boiling coagulation solvents.

Nevertheless, the choice and application of the recycling and purification method is always dependent on the starting material and contaminant level, as well as the chemical nature of the components. Moreover, and despite our knowledge not being reported in the literature for chitin or other marine polymers conversions, there are other methodologies that are independent of the mixture components [120]. One of the methods, which is patented by a Chemical Company, BASF, comprises the recovery of the IL through the formation of the distillable carbene, involving the imidazolium IL treatment with a strong base, which deprotonates the imidazolium cation at the C-2 position, forming 1,3-dimethyl-imidazol-2-ylidene carbene [125]. The formed carbene could be distillable out, and its reaction with the acid of the desired anion reforms the imidazolium IL. The described process can be applied after the desired products have been extracted from the IL, as well as after the dewatering of the IL/residues mixture. The use of membrane separation can also be considered as an effective strategy, including the commercially available pervaporation systems (PV). However, the efficiency of these systems is strongly dependent on the size and molecular weight of the mixture constituents, and it involves quite extensive work [102,120]. Every IL has different properties, which include different decomposition temperatures, hydrophilicity, and an optimal number of reuses [102]. Nonetheless, the persistent challenge is to find the best balance between the energy involved in the processes and its economical burdens.

4.2. Biocompatibility

Although the IL platform suggests different pathways for the dissolution and processing of marine biomaterials into many matrices, as mentioned above, studies involving their in vitro/in vivo biocompatibility have not yet been fully explored. In fact, the application of 2D/3D-based marine biomaterials produced using ILs in the biomedical field is facing many challenges, since the implanted material could be influenced by the composition, architecture, and biocompatibility of the material. Considering that, ILs have been used in different approaches, such as a common solvent for combinations of marine polymers [25,123,126], proteins [14], or hydroxyapatites [122] as crosslinker agents [91] and modifiers [127] to render biomaterials with improved biocompatibility. An earlier report showed that the application of synthesized choline salts as crosslinkers on collagen-based biomaterials resulted in crosslinked materials with better cell growths compared to the sample crosslinked with glutaraldehyde [91], where the cells were found to be healthy and able to proliferate. In another approach [14], the use of ILs—particularly, (Emim)(OAc)—was useful as a common solvent in the combination of polysaccharides (chitosan) and proteins (silk fibroin) into hydrogels. Those hydrogels supported the adhesion and growth of primary human dermal fibroblasts, suggesting that they could be useful in skin regeneration approaches. In a similar study [86], an IL—namely, 1-methylimidazolium acetate ([Mim)(OAc))—facilitated the formation of alginate/collagen hydrogels with high hemocompatibility and satisfactory biocompatibility assessed by rat mesenchymal stem cells (rMSC), which rendered them as promising for skin dressings. Beyond that, another report showed that an IL, (Emim)(OAc), promoted the production of an electrically conducting chitin scaffold permissive for mesenchymal stem cell functions [127].

Table 1. Marine-derived polymers prepared using different ionic liquids.

Polymer/Matrix	Ionic Liquid/other Reagents	Process	Improved Properties	Potential Applications	References
Chitin	(Emim)(OAc)	Extraction/dissolution/ electrospinning	✓ smooth, continuous chitin nanofibers	Not defined	[23,24,102]
Chitosan	(Gly·H)Cl and (Bmim)Cl	Dissolution/dry-wet spinning	✓ nanofibers with excellent strength and initial modulus	Not defined	[103]
	(Bmim)(EtSO$_4$) or (Omim)(Cl)	Ionic crosslinking	✓ NPs (diameters 300–560 nm) have controlled shape and size	Not defined	[116]
Collagen	(Emim)(Br)/ (Emim)(Cl)/ (Emim)(OAc)	Self-assembling	✓ fibril enhanced thermal stability; ✓ improvement of the viscoelastic properties of the collagen gel	Not defined	[106]
Collagen-based hydrogels	(Emim)(OAc)	Sol-gel transition	✓ [Emim][OAc] promoted high mechanical strength, degradation, resistance, and anti-inflammation effects.	Tissue engineering and cancer therapy.	[128]
Gelatin Microcapsules	(Bmim)(BF$_4$)	Microemulsion	✓ excellent in vitro compatibility in physiological environment, and efficacy in cancer cells killing when exposed to MW;	MR imaging-guided MW thermotherapy.	[29]
Gelatin Ion Gels	(Emim)(EtSO$_4$)	Dissolution/ Photoreduction	✓ induction of antimicrobial activity by *in situ* preparation and $AgNO_3$ Nps inclusion by photoreduction; ✓ IGs have self-healing properties, multiadhesive nature, reversible stretching efficiency, and high conductivity.	Not defined	[31]
	(Emim)(Cl)	Gelation	✓ more IL leads to a lower gel modulus due to the tendency of hydrophobic linkages; however, these IGs are able to recover their network structures to a higher degree during the healing process.	biomedical engineering	[92]
	(Emim)(EtSO$_4$)	Dissolution/Gelation	✓ [Emim][EtSO$_4$] was found to be the entrapment of GOD and HRP in gelatin type A with subsequent maturation; ✓ GOD retain up to 70% of the initial activity after storing at 4 °C for 2 weeks, while HRP retained 91% of its initial activity.	colorimetric glucose detection	[95]

Table 1. *Cont.*

Polymer/Matrix	Ionic Liquid/other Reagents	Process	Improved Properties	Potential Applications	References
Gelatin films	(Emim)(OAc)	Doping	✓ PE stable until 220 °C; ✓ PE are good ionic conductors.	smart windows and other ECD-based devices	[129]
Gelatin hydrogels	Omim·PF6	Ultrasonication	✓ immobilized HRP have higher thermal stability; ✓ better enzyme electrode performance using more hydrophobic ILs; ✓ sensitive response in the presence of H_2O_2.	immobilization of enzymes and fabrication of biosensors	[96]

Abbreviations: ((Bmim))((BF4))—1-Butyl-3-methylimidazolium tetrafluoroborate, ECD—electrochromic devices, (Emim)(Cl)—1-ethyl-3-methylimidazolium chloride, (Emim)(OAc)—1-ethyl-3-methylimidazolium acetate, (Emim)(Br)—1-ethyl-3-methylimidazolium bromide, (Emim) ($EtSO_4$)—1-ethyl-3-methyl-imidazolium ethyl sulfate, (Omim)(Cl)—1-octyl-3-methylimidazolium chloride, OMIM·PF_6—1-Octyl-3- methylimidazolium hexafluorophsohate, (Gly·H)Cl—glycine hydrochloride, GOD—glucose oxidase, HRP—horseradish peroxidase, IGs—ionogels, IL—ionic liquid, MW—microwave, MR—magnetic resonance, NPs—nanoparticles, PBS—phosphate-buffered saline, PE—polymer electrolyte, $AgNO_3$—silver nitrate, and H_2O_2—hydrogen peroxide.

Table 2. Marine-derived blended polymers processed in different ionic liquids.

Polymer Blends	Ionic Liquid/other Reagents	Process	Improved Properties	Potential Applications	References
Chitin/ Antheraea pernyi silk fibroin based sponges	(Bmim))(OAc))	Co-dissolution/ Freeze-drying	✓ sponges presented good porosity and interconnectivity values, and a considerably high swelling degree in PBS	Cartilage regeneration	[13]
Chitin-sodium alginate film	BPPF6	Solutions mixing	✓ good detection precision of H_2O_2 detection; ✓ sensor with improved bioactivity, storage stability, and reproducibility	biosensor	[26]
Chitin-calcium alginate fibers	(Emim)(OAc)	Microwave IL-assisted extraction/dissolution/ electrospinning	✓ great in vivo outcomes, with re-epithelialization and complete coverage of the dermal fibrosis with hyperplastic epidermis after only 7 days of treatment	wound care dressings	[25]
Chitin–Cellulose Nanofibers	(Emim)(OAc)	Electrospinning	✓ Incorporation of MCC allows the preparation of materials with improved strength.	Not defined	[24]

Table 2. *Cont.*

Polymer Blends	Ionic Liquid/other Reagents	Process	Improved Properties	Potential Applications	References
Chitin and hydroxyapatite	(Bmim)(OAc)	Dissolution	✓ 3D porous microstructure positively influence osteoblast-like cells viability and proliferation (65%–85% porosity and of 100–300 µm pore sizes).	bone tissue engineering	[19,118]
Chitin–poly(lactic acid) Fibers	(Emim)(OAc)	Co-dissolution/wet-jet spun	✓ tensile strength and plasticity of the fibers depended on the chitin to PLA ratio;	Not defined	[130]
Chitin/SAIB scaffolds	(Bmim)(OAc)	Co-dissolution/freeze-drying	✓ different values of porosity (ranging from 52 to 85%); ✓ no cytotoxicity when culturing in vitro human adipose-derived stem cells onto the surface of the scaffolds for 72 h	tissue engineering scaffolding	[131]
Agarose/chitosan ionogels	(Bmim)(Cl)	Blending/Gelation	✓ good stability and enhanced material properties compared with individual biopolymers	quasisolid dye sensitized solar cells, actuators, sensors or electrochromic displays	[30]
Carrageenan/cellulose gels	(Bmim)(Cl)	Co-dissolution	✓ three types of carrageenans (k-, ι- and λ) were blended with cellulose; ✓ λ-carrageenan gave a better miscible composite gel		[98]
Chitosan/cellulose	(Gly·H)(Cl) and (Bmim)(Cl)	Dissolution/dry-wet spinning	✓ good mechanical strength and excellent thermal stability		[104]
	(Emim)(OAc)	Dissolution/electrospinning	✓ produce fiber films with the potential to be applied as an antibacterial and antimicrobial agent to treat skin ulcers	Wound treatment	[105]
	(Bmim)(Cl)	Co-dissolution/cast into substrate	✓ Produce composite films with the combined advantages of their components: superior mechanical strength (from CEL) and excellent adsorption capacity from CHT. ✓ They can be reused with similar adsorption efficiency.	Adsorption of microcystin LR, produced by cyanobacteria present in drinking waterWound dressings	[126,132]

Table 2. *Cont.*

Polymer Blends	Ionic Liquid/other Reagents	Process	Improved Properties	Potential Applications	References
Chitosan/cellulose/ hydroxyapatite	(Bmim)(Cl)	Dissolution	✓ synergy of the individual properties of the used components (mechanical strength from cellulose, antimicrobial activity, and an ability to deliver active agents from chitosan)	bone tissue engineering	[27]
Chitosan/cellulose/ keratin	(Bmim)(Cl)	Co-dissolution/cast into substrate	✓ Improved mechanical and thermal physical properties.	treatment of chronic and ulcerous wounds	[133]
Chitosan/chondroitin sulfate hydrogels	(Hmim)(HSO_4)	Blending/gelation	✓ excellent stabilities (in the 1.2–10 pH range); ✓ larger swelling capacities; ✓ excellent biocompatibility upon both VERO and HT29 cells	treatment of water and wastewater	[28]
Chitosan/silk fibroin hydrogels	(Bmim)(OAc)	Blending/Gelation	✓ hydrogels have microporous, lamellar structure and viscoelastic behavior; ✓ supported the adhesion and growth of primary human dermal fibroblasts	skin tissue engineering approaches	[14]
Collagen-alginate-hydroxyapatite beads	(TEA)(OAc)	$CaCl_2$-based crosslinking	✓ higher water uptake ability due to collagen addition that decreases after 5 days; ✓ successful drug loading and good antimicrobial properties; ✓ hemolysis rates below the permissible limit (5%) thereby showed hemocompatibility	bone regeneration	[122]
Collagen/ Hydroxyapatite/ Alginate	(TEA)(OAc)	Dissolution	✓ hemocompatibility, promising antibacterial properties and drug load efficacy; ✓ used as potential bone filler	treatment of deep intraosseous defects	[134]

Table 2. *Cont.*

Polymer Blends	Ionic Liquid/other Reagents	Process	Improved Properties	Potential Applications	References
Collagen/PVA hydrogels	(Bmim)(OAc)	Blending	✓ tensile strength in the range of 2.4 to 8.5 MPa; ✓ hemocompatible (less than 5%) without toxic effects to the blood	osteochondral patches	[135]
Gelatin/Poly(Vinyl Alcohol) films	Lidocaine–Diclofenac IL	Freeze-thawing	✓ successful physical transformation of the lidocaine–diclofenac ionic liquid drug; ✓ controlled drug release patch	transdermal patches	[97]

Abbreviations: (Bmim)(OAc)—1-Butyl-3-methylimidazolium acetate, (Bmim)(Cl)—1-Butyl-3-methylimidazolium chloride, $BPPF_6$—N-butylpyridinium hexafluorophosphate, (Emim)(OAc)—1-ethyl-3-methylimidazolium acetate, (Gly·HCl)—glycine hydrochloride, (Hmim)(HSO_4)—1-hydrogen-3-methylimidazolium hydrogen sulfate, HT29—epithelial colorectal adenocarcinoma cells, IL—ionic liquid, MCC—microcrystalline cellulose, PBS—phosphate-buffered saline, PLA—poly(lactic acid), PVA—poly(vinyl alcohol), (TEA)(OAc)—triethanolamine acetate, VERO—healthy kidney epithelial cells originated from African green monkey, 3D—three-dimensional, H_2O_2—hydrogen peroxide, κ—kappa, λ—lambda, and ι—iota.

5. Biomedical Applications of Marine-derived Polymers in Ionic Liquids

5.1. Wound Repair

The beneficial features of marine polymers for wound healing have stimulated many studies involving the use of marine polymers/IL solutions in the production of biomaterials to be applied as support to enhance the wound-healing process [14,133]. In those approaches, the biomacromolecules combination such as chitosan/silk fibroin in (Bmim)(OAc) [14] or chitosan/cellulose/keratin in (Bmim)(Cl) [133] played a positive influence on the development of structures that showed suitable adhesion and the proliferation of human dermal fibroblasts (hDFb) and superior mechanical strength, bactericide action, and the controlled release of drugs, respectively. Roger RD et al. proposed the co-dissolution of chitin and alginate in (Bmim)(OAc), followed by extrusion of the solution into a coagulation bath to form chitin-based fibers as wound dressings [25]. Those fibers were applied on a full-dermal-thickness wound model (rat model, histological evaluation) and maintained on the wounds for up to 14 days. The wound-healing studies indicated that the chitin-calcium alginate-covered wound sites underwent normal wound healing with re-epithelization and that the coverage of the dermal fibrosis with the hyperplastic epidermis was consistently complete after seven days of treatment (Figure 7).

The (CEL/CHT) composite films prepared using a green and totally recyclable method were also developed for wound-dressing applications, helping to promote wound healing by creating a moist microenvironment for proper tissue regeneration [132]. According to the authors, (Bmim)(Cl) was used as a single solvent to produce composites that are antibacterial, hemostatic, biocompatible, nontoxic to fibroblasts, and a good absorbent for anticoagulated whole blood and are able to maintain moisture balance for wound healing. The composites absorbed blood at the same rate and volume as commercially available wound dressings [132].

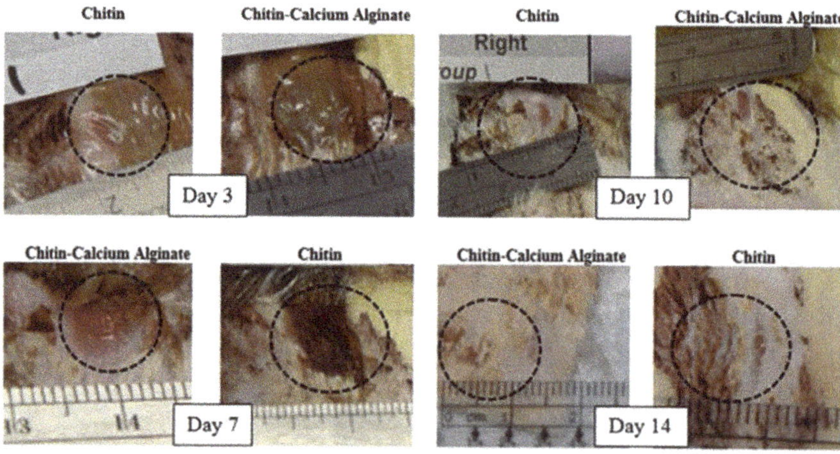

Figure 7. Representative images of the wound sites taken on days 3, 7, 10, and 14. Reprinted from [25]. Copyright 2017 with permission from Elsevier.

5.2. Bone Regeneration

Marine-derived polymers and proteins processed through IL have been used as excellent candidates for bone/cartilage tissue engineering applications, particularly when in composites containing hydroxyapatite (HA) [27,118,122,136,137]. These composites are mechanically superior when compared to the individual components—for example, the ductility of collagen or gelatin compensates for the poor fracture toughness of hydroxyapatite, and their biological functionality is improved, presenting antimicrobial activity due to chitosan and osteoconductivity derived from

HA. The addition of a ceramic compound (HA) promoted higher stability and better resistance to three-dimensional swelling and deformation.

Many clinical applications may benefit from the incorporation of collagen to hydroxyapatite due to shape command, spatial adaptation, enhanced wall adhesion, and the potential to promote clot formation and subsequent stabilization [134,138]. Bioactive beads composed of collagen, hydroxyapatite, and alginate were prepared using a triethanolamine acetate ionic liquid as a solvent and evaluated to be used as potential bone fillers. The prepared beads showed hemocompatibility, promising antibacterial properties and drug load efficacy [122].

Chitosan/cellulose/hydroxyapatite multifunctional composites using (Bmim)(Cl) as a solvent were proposed by Mututuvari et al. [27]. The proposed composite material presented the adequate features for bone tissue engineering derived from each of the individual components, mechanical strength from cellulose, antimicrobial activity, and an ability to deliver active agents (drugs or growth factors) from chitosan.

Chitin and hydroxyapatite composites were prepared by Silva et al. [118] using (Bmim)(OAc), achieving an enhanced dispersion of the hydroxyapatite (HA). μ-CT analysis of the chitin/HA composite showed a homogeneous distribution of the HA across the composite structure (Figure 8), where the HA content decreased with the increasing polymer concentration. The designed system has the potential to be applied for bone tissue engineering purposes, as it presented a porous microstructure (65%–85% porosity and pore sizes of 100–300 μm) able to influence osteoblast-like cells viability and proliferation [105] positively.

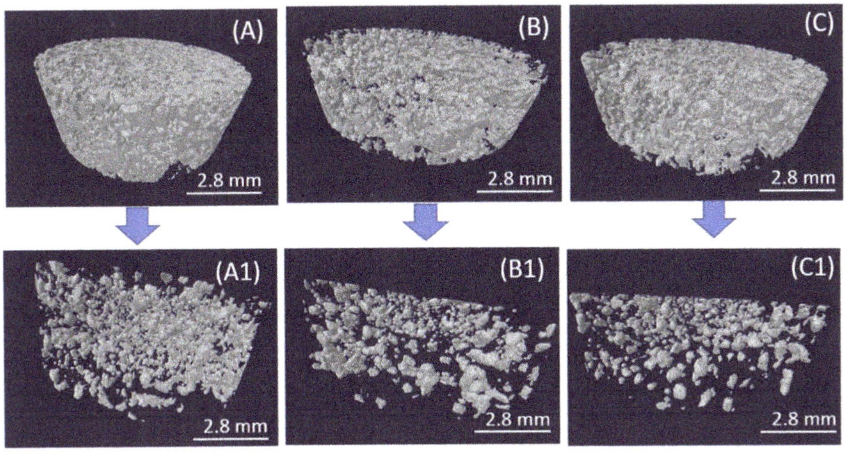

Figure 8. μ-microcomputed tomography of the chitin-based composite porous structure prepared using hydroxyapatite (HA): (**A**) Ch1HA, (**B**) Ch2HA, and (**C**) Ch3HA. (**A–C**) are complete structures, while (**A1–C1**) are HA-only. Modified from [118].

5.3. Drug and Gene Delivery

ILs have been extensively explored in the pharmaceutical field, mainly as stabilizer agents for biomolecules, as solvents, or as part of drug carrier systems for poorly soluble drugs, such as active pharmaceutical ingredients (APIs) in IL systems (APIs-IL) [42]. Chitosan has been studied for the development of stimuli-responsive chitosan-based biomaterials in combination with several ILs [100,139]. In 2011, Hua and coworkers developed an innovative method that promoted the stimuli-responsive intravenous administration of hydrophobic drugs by combining them with chitosan via a Schiff reaction, using IL 1-butyl-3-methylimidazolium chloride ((Bmim)(Cl)) [139].

Following a different approach, biocompatible ILs (bio-ILs) were used to develop multiresponsive chitosan biomaterials [100]. Ammonium-based bio-ILs—namely, choline chloride and choline dihydrogen phosphate—were used to dope chitosan-based biomaterials, and the release of the ionic drug, sodium phosphate dexamethasone, was studied. The results suggested that, depending on the different ionic interactions that can be established between chitosan, chitosan/IL, and dexamethasone, it was suggested that they can be used as an electrically modulated drug release systems for iontophoretic applications [139]. The modifications of chitosan using ILs through several strategies, including grafting with polyethylenimine (PEI) in (Bmim)(Ac) or the synthesis of O-alkylated chitosan derivatives in (Bmim)(Cl), were also attempted and proved to improve its gene transfection performance [140,141]. Chitosan-based vectors proved to be noncytotoxic and have the ability of transcellular transport, since the presence of positive charges from amine groups in chitosan enables it to transport plasmid DNA (pDNA) into cells via endocytosis and membrane destability [140]. The properties of ILs as solvent should promote the selective alkylation of hydroxyl groups of chitosan without protecting its amino groups, associated with an improvement of the solubility of the derivatives in the organic solvent. Moreover, a lidocaine–diclofenac ionic liquid drug was loaded into a gelatin/poly(vinyl alcohol) transdermal patch using a freeze/thaw method [97]. The developed patch allowed to control the high drug release values of both lidocaine and diclofenac, the gelatin/poly(vinyl alcohol) patch, which, in addition, showed good stability over the study period of three months when kept at 4 °C or under ambient temperatures. The presented methodology revealed promising outcomes for improving the physicochemical and biopharmaceutical characteristics of poorly water-soluble drugs.

6. Conclusions and Future Trends

Over the years, ILs have been used as an important tool with high significance from technological and academic perspectives. When used in combination with marine-derived polymers, ILs provide sustainable approaches not only to promote their isolation but, also, to produce derivatives with different shapes and applications. ILs have opened up a large window of possibilities for the processing of high—added—value biomaterials based on marine sources. Despite the clear advantages herein discussed, research on the use of ILs for the processing of marine polymers is still at an early stage. There are some persistent challenges to overcome—in particular, in the biomedical field, where the scale-up possibilities and in vitro/in vivo biocompatibility performances of the resulting matrices require additional research and investment.

Despite the considerable volume of research on ILs, its family has been growing along the years with the development of the biocompatibility of ionic liquids (bio-ILs) as an eco- and biofriendly alternative IL family. Exciting outcomes are expected as a result of the exploitation of bio-IL contributions in this field, since they retain the features of commonly used ILs while improving their biological activity with reduced toxicity. In consequence, new strategies will emerge, and a significant boost in the use of ILs is envisioned in a broader range of fields.

Author Contributions: S.S.S., J.M.G. and L.C.R. developed the concept for the manuscript, drafted and finalized the manuscript and figures. R.L.R. supervised the work and contributed to manuscript review. All authors have read and agreed to the published version of the manuscript.

Funding: The authors especially acknowledge financial support from Portuguese FCT (JMG, PD/BD/135247/2017 and LCR, SFRH/BPD/93697/2013). This work was also financially supported by a PhD programme in Advanced Therapies for Health (PATH) (PD/00169/2013); FCT R&D&I projects with references PTDC/BII-BIO/31570/2017, PTDC/CTM-CTM//29813/2017 and PTDC/CTM-BIO/4706/2014-(POCI-01-0145-FEDER-016716) and R&D&I Structured Projects with reference NORTE-01-0145-FDER-000021.

Conflicts of Interest: The authors declare no conflict of interest.

Abbreviations

$AgNO_3$	silver nitrate
(Amim)(Br)	1-allyl-3-methylimidazolium bromide
Amim	1-allyl-3-methylimidazolium
Ala	alanine

APIs	active pharmaceutical ingredients
APIs-IL	active pharmaceutical ingredients in ionic liquids systems
Arg	arginine
Bio-ILs	biocompatible IL
$BPPF_6$	N-butylpyridinium hexafluorophosphate
(Bmim)	1-butyl-3-methylimidazolium
(Bmim)(OAc)	1-butyl-3-methylimidazolium acetate
(Bmmim)(OAc)	1-butyl-2,3-dimethylimidazolium acetate
(Bmim)(BF4)	1-butyl-3-methylimidazolium tetrafluoroborate
(Bmim)](C_2OSO_3)	1-ethyl-3-methylimidazolium ethylsulfate
(Bmim)(Cl)	1-butyl-3-methylimidazolium chloride
(Ch)(DHP)	Choline dihydrogen phosphate
(Dmim)(Cl)	1-decyl-3-methylimidazolium chloride
(Emim)(Cl)	1-ethyl-3-methylimidazolium chloride
(Emim)(OAc)	1-ethyl-3-methylimidazolium acetate
(Emim)(Br)	1-ethyl-3-methylimidazolium bromide
(Dmim)	1,3-dimethylimidazolium
(Emim) ($EtSO_4$)	1-ethyl-3-methyl-imidazolium ethyl sulfate
Gly	glycine
(Gly·H)Cl	glycine hydrochloride
Glu	glutamate
GOD	glucose oxidase
HA	hydroxyapatite
H_2O_2	Hydrogen peroxide
HT29	epithelial colorectal adenocarcinoma cells
(Hmim)/ OAc)	1-hydrogen-3-methylimidazolium acetate
(Hmim)(HSO_4)	1-hydrogen-3-methylimidazolium hydrogen sulfate
HRP	horseradish peroxidase
Hyp	hydroxyproline
IGs	ion gels
IL	ionic liquid;
(Mim)(OAc)	1-methylimidazolium acetate
MCC	Microcrystalline cellulose
MW	microwave
MR	magnetic resonance
(mim)	1-hydrogen-3-methylimidazolium
NPs	nanoparticles
(Omim)(OAc)	1-octyl-3-methylimidazolium acetate
(Omim)(Cl)	1-octyl-3-methylimidazolium chloride
OMIM·PF_6	1-Octyl-3- methylimidazolium hexafluorophsohate
PBS	phosphate-buffered saline
PEI	polyethylenimine
PE	polymer electrolyte
Pro	proline
PLA	poly(lactic acid)
PVA	poly(vinyl alcohol)
(TEA)(Ac)	triethanolamine acetate
VERO	healthy kidney epithelial cells originated from African green monkey
3D	three-dimensional
Κ	kappa
λ	lambda

References

1. Silva, T.; Duarte, A.; Moreira-Silva, J.; Mano, J.F.; Reis, R.L. *Biomaterials from Marine-Origin Biopolymers*; Mano, J.F., Ed.; Wiley-VCH Verlag: Weinheim, Germany, 2012; pp. 3–24.
2. Silva, T.H.; Alves, A.; Ferreira, B.M.; Oliveira, J.M.; Reys, L.L.; Ferreira, R.J.F.; Sousa, R.A.; Silva, S.S.; Mano, J.F.; Reis, R.L. Materials of marine origin: A review on polymers and ceramics of biomedical interest. *Int. Mater. Rev.* **2012**, *57*, 276–306. [CrossRef]
3. Hsiang-Jung, T.; Tai-Li, T.; Hsian-Jenn, W.; Shan-hui, H. Characterization of chitosan–gelatin scaffolds for dermal tissue engineering. *J. Tissue Eng. Regen. Med.* **2013**, *7*, 20–31.
4. Anthony, J.; Brennecke, J.; Holbrey, J.; Maginn, E.; Mantz, R.; Trulove, P.; Visser, A.; Welton, T. *Ionic Liquids in Synthesis*; Wasserscheid, P., Welton, T., Eds.; Wiley-VCH: Weinheim, Germany, 2002; pp. 41–55.
5. Qin, Y.; Lu, X.; Sun, N.; Rogers, R.D. Dissolution or extraction of crustacean shells using ionic liquids to obtain high molecular weight purified chitin and direct production of chitin films and fibers. *Green Chem.* **2010**, *12*, 968–971. [CrossRef]
6. Singh, T.; Trivedi, T.J.; Kumar, A. Dissolution, regeneration and ion-gel formation of agarose in room-temperature ionic liquids. *Green Chem.* **2010**, *12*, 1029–1035. [CrossRef]
7. Trivedi, T.; Kumar, A. Efficient extraction of agarose from red algae using ionic liquids. *Green Sustain. Chem.* **2014**, *4*, 190–201. [CrossRef]
8. Tolesa, L.D.; Gupta, B.S.; Lee, M.J. Chitin and chitosan production from shrimp shells using ammonium-based ionic liquids. *Int. J. Biol. Macromol.* **2019**, *130*, 818–826. [CrossRef]
9. Shi, R.; Wang, Y. Dual ionic and organic nature of ionic liquids. *Sci. Rep.* **2016**, *6*, 19644. [CrossRef]
10. Hulsbosch, J.; De Vos, D.E.; Binnemans, K.; Ameloot, R. Biobased ionic liquids: Solvents for a green processing industry? *ACS Sustain. Chem. Eng.* **2016**, *4*, 2917–2931. [CrossRef]
11. Silva, S.S.; Reis, R.L. CHAPTER 11 Ionic liquids as tools in the production of smart polymeric hydrogels. In *Polymerized Ionic Liquids*; The Royal Society of Chemistry: Burlington House : London, UK, 2018; pp. 304–318.
12. Silva, S.S.; Popa, E.G.; Gomes, M.E.; Oliveira, M.B.; Nayak, S.; Subia, B.; Mano, J.F.; Kundu, S.C.; Reis, R.L. Silk hydrogels from non-mulberry and mulberry silkworm cocoons processed with ionic liquids. *Acta Biomater.* **2013**, *9*, 8972–8982. [CrossRef]
13. Silva, S.S.; Gomes, J.; Vale, A.; Lu, S.; Reis, R.L.; Kundu, S. Green pathway for processing non-mulberry antheraea pernyi silk fibroin/chitin-based sponges: Biophysical and biochemical characterization. *Front. Mater.* **2020**, *7*, 1–9. [CrossRef]
14. Silva, S.S.; Santos, T.C.; Cerqueira, M.T.; Marques, A.P.; Reys, L.L.; Silva, T.H.; Caridade, S.G.; Mano, J.F.; Reis, R.L. The use of ionic liquids in the processing of chitosan/silk hydrogels for biomedical applications. *Green Chem.* **2012**, *14*, 1463–1470. [CrossRef]
15. Takegawa, A.; Murakami, M.; Kaneko, Y.; Kadokawa, J. Preparation of chitin/cellulose composite gels and films with ionic liquids. *Carbohyd. Polym.* **2010**, *79*, 85–90. [CrossRef]
16. Zhang, J.; Wu, J.; Yu, J.; Zhang, X.; He, J.; Zhang, J. Application of ionic liquids for dissolving cellulose and fabricating cellulose-based materials: State of the art and future trends. *Mater. Chem. Front.* **2017**, *1*, 1273–1290. [CrossRef]
17. Wu, Y.; Sasaki, T.; Irie, S.; Sakurai, K. A novel biomass-ionic liquid platform for the utilization of native chitin. *Polymer* **2008**, *49*, 2321–2327. [CrossRef]
18. Swatloski, R.P.; Spear, S.K.; Holbrey, J.D.; Rogers, R.D. Dissolution of cellulose with ionic liquids. *J. Am. Chem. Soc.* **2002**, *124*, 4974–4975. [CrossRef] [PubMed]
19. Silva, S.S.; Mano, J.F.; Reis, R.L. Ionic liquids in the processing and chemical modification of chitin and chitosan for biomedical applications. *Green Chem.* **2017**, *19*, 1208–1220. [CrossRef]
20. Singh, S.K. Solubility of lignin and chitin in ionic liquids and their biomedical applications. *Int. J. Biol. Macromol.* **2019**, *132*, 265–277. [CrossRef]
21. Mallik, A.K.; Shahruzzaman, M.; Zaman, A.; Biswas, S.; Ahmed, T.; Sakib, M.N.; Haque, P.; Rahman, M.M. 4-Fabrication of polysaccharide-based materials using ionic liquids and scope for biomedical use. In *Functional Polysaccharides for Biomedical Applications*; Maiti, S., Jana, S., Eds.; Woodhead Publishing: Duxford, UK, 2019; pp. 131–171.
22. Mahmood, H.; Moniruzzaman, M. Recent advances of using ionic liquids for biopolymer extraction and processing. *Biotechnol. J.* **2019**, *14*, e1900072. [CrossRef]

23. Barber, P.S.; Griggs, C.S.; Bonner, J.R.; Rogers, R.D. Electrospinning of chitin nanofibers directly from an ionic liquid extract of shrimp shells. *Green Chem.* **2013**, *15*, 601–607. [CrossRef]
24. Shamshina, J.L.; Zavgorodnya, O.; Choudhary, H.; Frye, B.; Newbury, N.; Rogers, R.D. In search of stronger/cheaper chitin nanofibers through electrospinning of chitin–cellulose composites using an ionic liquid platform. *ACS Sustain. Chem. Eng.* **2018**, *6*, 14713–14722. [CrossRef]
25. Shamshina, J.L.; Gurau, G.; Block, L.E.; Hansen, L.K.; Dingee, C.; Walters, A.; Rogers, R.D. Chitin–calcium alginate composite fibers for wound care dressings spun from ionic liquid solution. *J. Mater. Chem. B* **2014**, *2*, 3924–3936. [CrossRef] [PubMed]
26. Ding, C.; Zhang, M.; Zhao, F.; Zhang, S. Disposable biosensor and biocatalysis of horseradish peroxidase based on sodium alginate film and room temperature ionic liquid. *Anal. Biochem.* **2008**, *378*, 32–37. [CrossRef] [PubMed]
27. Mututuvari, T.M.; Harkins, A.L.; Tran, C.D. Facile synthesis, characterization, and antimicrobial activity of cellulose-chitosan-hydroxyapatite composite material: A potential material for bone tissue engineering. *J. Biomed. Mater. Res. A* **2013**, *101*, 3266–3277. [CrossRef] [PubMed]
28. Nunes, C.S.; Rufato, K.B.; Souza, P.R.; de Almeida, E.A.M.S.; da Silva, M.J.V.; Scariot, D.B.; Nakamura, C.V.; Rosa, F.A.; Martins, A.F.; Muniz, E.C. Chitosan/chondroitin sulfate hydrogels prepared in [Hmim][HSO4] ionic liquid. *Carbohyd. Polym.* **2017**, *170*, 99–106. [CrossRef]
29. Du, Q.; Ma, T.; Fu, C.; Liu, T.; Huang, Z.; Ren, J.; Shao, H.; Xu, K.; Tang, F.; Meng, X. Encapsulating ionic liquid and Fe3O4 nanoparticles in gelatin microcapsules as microwave susceptible agent for MR imaging-guided tumor thermotherapy. *ACS Appl. Mater. Interfaces* **2015**, *7*, 13612–13619. [CrossRef]
30. Trivedi, T.J.; Rao, K.S.; Kumar, A. Facile preparation of agarose-chitosan hybrid materials and nanocomposite ionogels using an ionic liquid via dissolution, regeneration and sol-gel transition. *Green Chem.* **2014**, *16*, 320–330. [CrossRef]
31. Singh, G.; Singh, G.; Damarla, K.; Sharma, P.K.; Kumar, A.; Kang, T.S. Gelatin-based highly stretchable, self-healing, conducting, multiadhesive, and antimicrobial ionogels embedded with Ag_2O nanoparticles. *ACS Sustain. Chem. Eng.* **2017**, *5*, 6568–6577. [CrossRef]
32. Łabowska, M.B.; Michalak, I.; Detyna, J. Methods of extraction, physicochemical properties of alginates and their applications in biomedical field—A review. *Open Chem.* **2019**, *17*, 738. [CrossRef]
33. Gereniu, C.R.N.; Saravana, P.S.; Chun, B.-S. Recovery of carrageenan from Solomon Islands red seaweed using ionic liquid-assisted subcritical water extraction. *Sep. Purif. Technol.* **2018**, *196*, 309–317. [CrossRef]
34. Mehta, M.; Bharmoria, P.; Bhayani, K.; Kumar, A. Gelatin solubility and processing in ionic liquids: An approach towards waste to utilization. *ChemistrySelect* **2017**, *2*, 9895–9900. [CrossRef]
35. Tarannum, A.; Muvva, C.; Mehta, A.; Rao, J.R.; Fathima, N.N. Phosphonium based ionic liquids-stabilizing or destabilizing agents for collagen? *RSC Adv.* **2016**, *6*, 4022–4033. [CrossRef]
36. Tarannum, A.; Muvva, C.; Mehta, A.; Raghava Rao, J.; Fathima, N.N. Role of preferential ions of ammonium ionic liquid in destabilization of collagen. *J. Phys. Chem. B* **2016**, *120*, 6515–6524. [CrossRef] [PubMed]
37. Tarannum, A.; Rao, J.R.; Fathima, N.N. Choline-based Amino Acid ILs–collagen interaction: Enunciating its role in stabilization/destabilization phenomena. *J. Phys. Chem. B* **2018**, *122*, 1145–1151. [CrossRef] [PubMed]
38. Tarannum, A.; Adams, A.; Blümich, B.; Fathima, N.N. Impact of ionic liquids on the structure and dynamics of collagen. *J. Phys. Chem. B* **2018**, *122*, 1060–1065. [CrossRef]
39. Schindl, A.; Hagen, M.L.; Muzammal, S.; Gunasekera, H.A.D.; Croft, A.K. Proteins in ionic liquids: Reactions, applications, and futures. *Front. Chem.* **2019**, *7*, 347. [CrossRef]
40. Mehta, A.; Rao, J.R.; Fathima, N.N. Effect of ionic liquids on the different hierarchical order of type I collagen. *Colloids Surf. B Biointerfaces* **2014**, *117*, 376–382. [CrossRef]
41. Tarannum, A.; Jonnalagadda, R.R.; Nishter, N.F. Stability of collagen in ionic liquids: Ion specific Hofmeister series effect. *Spectrochim. Acta A Mol. Biomol. Spectrosc.* **2019**, *212*, 343–348. [CrossRef]
42. Gomes, J.M.; Silva, S.S.; Reis, R.L. Biocompatible ionic liquids: Fundamental behaviours and applications. *Chem. Soc. Rev.* **2019**, *48*, 4317–4335. [CrossRef]
43. Silva, S.S.; Fernandes, E.M.; Pina, S.; Silva-Correia, J.; Vieira, S.; Oliveira, J.M.; Reis, R.L. Natural-origin materials for tissue engineering and regenerative medicine. In *Comprehensive Biomaterials II*; Ducheyne, P., Healy, K.E., Hutmacher, D.E., Grainger, D.W., Kirkpatrick, C.J., Eds.; Elsevier: Amsterdam, The Netherlands, 2017.
44. Siew, C.K.; Williams, P.A.; Young, N.W.G. New Insights into the mechanism of gelation of alginate and pectin: Charge annihilation and reversal mechanism. *Biomacromolecules* **2005**, *6*, 963–969. [CrossRef]

45. Drury, J.L.; Dennis, R.G.; Mooney, D.J. The tensile properties of alginate hydrogels. *Biomaterials* **2004**, *25*, 3187–3199. [CrossRef]
46. Kumar, M.N.V.R. A review of chitin and chitosan applications. *React. Funct. Polym.* **2000**, *46*, 1–27. [CrossRef]
47. Muzzarelli, R.A.A. Chitins and chitosans for the repair of wounded skin, nerve, cartilage and bone. *Carbohyd. Polym.* **2009**, *76*, 167–182. [CrossRef]
48. Younes, I.; Rinaudo, M. Chitin and chitosan preparation from marine sources. Structure, properties and applications. *Mar. Drugs* **2015**, *13*, 1133–1174. [CrossRef] [PubMed]
49. Rinaudo, M. Chitin and chitosan: Properties and applications. *Prog. Polym. Sci.* **2006**, *31*, 603–632. [CrossRef]
50. Pillai, C.K.S.; Paul, W.; Sharma, C.P. Chitin and chitosan polymers: Chemistry, solubility and fiber formation. *Prog. Polym. Sci.* **2009**, *34*, 641–678. [CrossRef]
51. Jang, M.-K.; Kong, B.-G.; Jeong, Y.-I.; Lee, C.H.; Nah, J.-W. Physicochemical characterization of α-chitin, β-chitin, and γ-chitin separated from natural resources. *J. Polym. Sci. Part A Polym. Chem.* **2004**, *42*, 3423–3432. [CrossRef]
52. Setoguchi, T.; Kato, T.; Yamamoto, K.; Kadokawa, J.-I. Facile production of chitin from crab shells using ionic liquid and citric acid. *Int. J. Biol. Macromol.* **2012**, *50*, 861–864. [CrossRef]
53. Wang, W.T.; Zhu, J.; Wang, X.L.; Huang, Y.; Wang, Y.Z. Dissolution behavior of chitin in ionic liquids. *J. Macromol. Sci. B* **2010**, *49*, 528–541. [CrossRef]
54. Li, J.; Huang, W.-C.; Gao, L.; Sun, J.; Liu, Z.; Mao, X. Efficient enzymatic hydrolysis of ionic liquid pretreated chitin and its dissolution mechanism. *Carbohyd. Polym.* **2019**, *211*, 329–335. [CrossRef]
55. Uto, T.; Idenoue, S.; Yamamoto, K.; Kadokawa, J.I. Understanding dissolution process of chitin crystal in ionic liquids: Theoretical study. *Phys. Chem. Chem. Phys. PCCP* **2018**, *20*, 20669–20677. [CrossRef]
56. Tajiri, R.; Setoguchi, T.; Wakizono, S.; Yamamoto, K.; Kadokawa, J.-I. Preparation of self-assembled chitin nanofibers by regeneration from ion gels using calcium halide · dihydrate/methanol solutions. *J. Biobased Mater. Bioenergy* **2013**, *7*, 655–659. [CrossRef]
57. Ifuku, S.; Saimoto, H. Chitin nanofibers: Preparations, modifications, and applications. *Nanoscale* **2012**, *4*, 3308–3318. [CrossRef] [PubMed]
58. Silva, S.S.; Duarte, A.R.C.; Mano, J.F.; Reis, R.L. Design and functionalization of chitin-based microsphere scaffolds. *Green Chem.* **2013**, *15*, 3252–3258. [CrossRef]
59. Jayakumar, R.; Prabaharan, M.; Nair, S.V.; Tamura, H. Novel chitin and chitosan nanofibers in biomedical applications. *Biotechnol. Adv.* **2010**, *28*, 142–150. [CrossRef] [PubMed]
60. Brondani, D.; Dupont, J.; Spinelli, A.; Vieira, I.C. Development of biosensor based on ionic liquid and corn peroxidase immobilized on chemically crosslinked chitin. *Sens. Actuators B Chem.* **2009**, *138*, 236–243. [CrossRef]
61. Xie, H.; Zhang, S.; Li, S. Chitin and chitosan dissolved in ionic liquids as reversible sorbents of CO_2. *Green Chem.* **2006**, *8*, 630–633. [CrossRef]
62. Sun, X.F.; Tian, Q.Q.; Xue, Z.M.; Zhang, Y.W.; Mu, T.C. The dissolution behaviour of chitosan in acetate-based ionic liquids and their interactions: From experimental evidence to density functional theory analysis. *Rsc. Adv.* **2014**, *4*, 30282–30291. [CrossRef]
63. Chen, J.; Xie, F.; Li, X.; Chen, L. Ionic liquids for the preparation of biopolymer materials for drug/gene delivery: A review. *Green Chem.* **2018**, *20*, 4169–4200. [CrossRef]
64. Chen, Q.; Xu, A.; Li, Z.; Wang, J.; Zhang, S. Influence of anionic structure on the dissolution of chitosan in 1-butyl-3-methylimidazolium-based ionic liquids. *Green Chem.* **2011**, *13*, 3446–3452. [CrossRef]
65. Feng, J.X.; Zang, H.J.; Yan, Q.; Li, M.G.; Jiang, X.Q.; Cheng, B.W. Dissolution and utilization of chitosan in a 1-carboxymethyl-3-methylimidazolium hydrochloride ionic salt aqueous solution. *J. Appl. Polym. Sci.* **2015**, *132*, 41965. [CrossRef]
66. Wei, S.; Ching, Y.C.; Chuah, C.H. Synthesis of chitosan aerogels as promising carriers for drug delivery: A review. *Carbohyd. Polym.* **2020**, *231*, 115744. [CrossRef] [PubMed]
67. Bozec, L.; de Groot, J.; Odlyha, M.; Nicholls, B.; Nesbitt, S.; Flanagan, A.; Horton, M. Atomic force microscopy of collagen structure in bone and dentine revealed by osteoclastic resorption. *Ultramicroscopy* **2005**, *105*, 79–89. [CrossRef]
68. Bailey, A.J.; Macmillan, J.; Shrewry, P.R.; Tatham, A.S.; Puxkandl, R.; Zizak, I.; Paris, O.; Keckes, J.; Tesch, W.; Bernstorff, S.; et al. Viscoelastic properties of collagen: Synchrotron radiation investigations and structural model. *Philos. Trans. R. Soc. Lond. Ser. B Biol. Sci.* **2002**, *357*, 191–197.

69. Bhattacharjee, A.; Bansal, M. Collagen structure: The madras triple helix and the current scenario. *IUBMB Life* **2005**, *57*, 161–172. [CrossRef] [PubMed]
70. Eyre, D. Articular cartilage and changes in Arthritis: Collagen of articular cartilage. *Arthritis Res. Ther.* **2001**, *3*, 107.
71. Meng, Z.; Zheng, X.; Tang, K.; Liu, J.; Ma, Z.; Zhao, Q. Dissolution and regeneration of collagen fibers using ionic liquid. *Int. J. Biol. Macromol.* **2012**, *51*, 440–448. [CrossRef]
72. Luca, S.; Nunzia, G.; Lucia, N.M.; Lorena, C.; Paola, L.; Marta, M.; Stella, B.F.; Angelo, C.; Loredana, C.; Alessandro, S. Marine collagen and its derivatives: Versatile and sustainable bio-resources for healthcare. *Mater. Sci. Eng. C* **2020**, *113*, 110963.
73. Silvipriya, K.; Kumar, K.; Bhat, A.; Kumar, B.D.; John, A.; Lakshmanan, P. Collagen: Animal sources and biomedical application. *J. Appl. Pharm. Sci.* **2015**, *5*, 123–127. [CrossRef]
74. Liu, D.; Zhang, X.; Li, T.; Yang, H.; Zhang, H.; Regenstein, J.M.; Zhou, P. Extraction and characterization of acid- and pepsin-soluble collagens from the scales, skins and swim-bladders of grass carp (Ctenopharyngodon idella). *Food Biosci.* **2015**, *9*, 68–74. [CrossRef]
75. Silva, T.H.; Moreira-Silva, J.; Marques, A.L.P.; Domingues, A.; Bayon, Y.; Reis, R.L. Marine origin collagens and its potential applications. *Mar. Drugs* **2014**, *12*, 5881–5901. [CrossRef]
76. Yadavalli, V.K.; Svintradze, D.V.; Pidaparti, R.M. Nanoscale measurements of the assembly of collagen to fibrils. *Int. J. Biol. Macromol.* **2010**, *46*, 458–464. [CrossRef] [PubMed]
77. Ideia, P.; Pinto, J.; Ferreira, R.; Figueiredo, L.; Spínola, V.; Castilho, P.C. Fish processing industry residues: A review of valuable products extraction and characterization methods. *Waste Biomass Valorization* **2019**. [CrossRef]
78. Yang, X.; Zhang, C.; Qiao, C.; Mu, X.; Li, T.; Xu, J.; Shi, L.; Zhang, D. A simple and convenient method to synthesize N-[(2-hydroxyl)-propyl-3-trimethylammonium] chitosan chloride in an ionic liquid. *Carbohydr. Polym.* **2015**, *130*, 325–332. [CrossRef] [PubMed]
79. Gómez-Guillén, M.C.; Giménez, B.; López-Caballero, M.E.; Montero, M.P. Functional and bioactive properties of collagen and gelatin from alternative sources: A review. *Food Hydrocoll.* **2011**, *25*, 1813–1827. [CrossRef]
80. Faria-Silva, C.; Ascenso, A.; Costa, A.M.; Marto, J.; Carvalheiro, M.; Ribeiro, H.M.; Simões, S. Feeding the skin: A new trend in food and cosmetics convergence. *Trends Food Sci. Technol.* **2020**, *95*, 21–32. [CrossRef]
81. Farage, M.A.; Miller, K.W.; Elsner, P.; Maibach, H.I. Intrinsic and extrinsic factors in skin ageing: A review. *Int. J. Cosmet. Sci.* **2008**, *30*, 87–95. [CrossRef] [PubMed]
82. Rodríguez, M.I.A.; Barroso, L.G.R.; Sánchez, M.L. Collagen: A review on its sources and potential cosmetic applications. *J. Cosmet. Dermatol.* **2018**, *17*, 20–26. [CrossRef]
83. Sionkowska, A.; Kozłowska, J. Characterization of collagen/hydroxyapatite composite sponges as a potential bone substitute. *Int. J. Biol. Macromol.* **2010**, *47*, 483–487. [CrossRef]
84. Mandal, A.; Panigrahi, S.; Zhang, C. Collagen as biomaterial for medical application—Drug delivery and scaffolds for tissue regeneration: A review. *Biol. Eng. Trans.* **2010**, *2*, 63–88. [CrossRef]
85. Mandal, A.; Meda, V.; Zhang, W.J.; Farhan, K.M.; Gnanamani, A. Synthesis, characterization and comparison of antimicrobial activity of PEG/TritonX-100 capped silver nanoparticles on collagen scaffold. *Colloids Surf. B Biointerfaces* **2012**, *90*, 191–196. [CrossRef]
86. Iqbal, B.; Muhammad, N.; Jamal, A.; Ahmad, P.; Khan, Z.U.H.; Rahim, A.; Khan, A.S.; Gonfa, G.; Iqbal, J.; Rehman, I.U. An application of ionic liquid for preparation of homogeneous collagen and alginate hydrogels for skin dressing. *J. Mol. Liq.* **2017**, *243*, 720–725. [CrossRef]
87. Bella, J. Collagen structure: New tricks from a very old dog. *Biochem. J.* **2016**, *473*, 1001–1025. [CrossRef] [PubMed]
88. Friess, W. Collagen–biomaterial for drug delivery1Dedicated to Professor Dr. Eberhard Nürnberg, Friedrich-Alexander-Universität Erlangen-Nürnberg, on the occasion of his 70th birthday.1. *Eur. J. Pharm. Biopharm.* **1998**, *45*, 113–136. [CrossRef]
89. Poluboyarov, V.; Voloskova, E.; Yankovaya, V.; Guryanova, T. Intensification of collagen dissolution process with the help of mechanochemical treatment. *Chem. Sustain. Dev.* **2009**, *17*, 177–183.
90. Mehta, A.; Raghava Rao, J.; Fathima, N.N. Electrostatic forces mediated by choline dihydrogen phosphate stabilize collagen. *J. Phys. Chem. B* **2015**, *119*, 12816–12827. [CrossRef]

91. Vijayaraghavan, R.; Thompson, B.C.; MacFarlane, D.R.; Kumar, R.; Surianarayanan, M.; Aishwarya, S.; Sehgal, P.K. Biocompatibility of choline salts as crosslinking agents for collagen based biomaterials. *Chem. Commun.* **2010**, *46*, 294–296. [CrossRef]
92. Sharma, A.; Rawat, K.; Solanki, P.R.; Bohidar, H.B. Self-healing gelatin ionogels. *Int. J. Biol. Macromol.* **2017**, *95*, 603–607. [CrossRef]
93. Lourenço, N.; Nunes, A.; Duarte, C.; Vidinha, P. Ionic liquids gelation with polymeric materials: The ion jelly approach. In *Applications of Ionic Liquids in Science and Technology*; Handy, P.S., Ed.; Scott Handy, IntechOpen: London, UK, 2011; pp. 155–172.
94. Carvalho, T.; Augusto, V.; Rocha, Â.; Lourenço, N.M.T.; Correia, N.T.; Barreiros, S.; Vidinha, P.; Cabrita, E.J.; Dionísio, M. Ion jelly conductive properties using dicyanamide-based ionic liquids. *J. Phys. Chem. B* **2014**, *118*, 9445–9459. [CrossRef]
95. Lourenço, N.M.T.; Österreicher, J.; Vidinha, P.; Barreiros, S.; Afonso, C.A.M.; Cabral, J.M.S.; Fonseca, L.P. Effect of gelatin–ionic liquid functional polymers on glucose oxidase and horseradish peroxidase kinetics. *React. Funct. Polym.* **2011**, *71*, 489–495. [CrossRef]
96. Yan, R.; Zhao, F.; Li, J.; Xiao, F.; Fan, S.; Zeng, B. Direct electrochemistry of horseradish peroxidase in gelatin-hydrophobic ionic liquid gel films. *Electrochim. Acta* **2007**, *52*, 7425–7431. [CrossRef]
97. Maneewattanapinyo, P.; Yeesamun, A.; Watthana, F.; Panrat, K.; Pichayakorn, W.; Suksaeree, J. Controlled release of lidocaine–diclofenac ionic liquid drug from freeze-thawed Gelatin/Poly(Vinyl Alcohol) transdermal patches. *AAPS PharmSciTech* **2019**, *20*, 322. [CrossRef] [PubMed]
98. Prasad, K.; Kaneko, Y.; Kadokawa, J.-I. Novel gelling systems of κ-, ι- and λ-Carrageenans and their composite gels with cellulose using ionic liquid. *Macromol. Biosci.* **2009**, *9*, 376–382. [CrossRef] [PubMed]
99. King, C.; Shamshina, J.L.; Gurau, G.; Berton, P.; Khan, N.F.A.F.; Rogers, R.D. A platform for more sustainable chitin films from an ionic liquid process. *Green Chem.* **2017**, *19*, 117–126. [CrossRef]
100. Dias, A.M.A.; Cortez, A.R.; Barsan, M.M.; Santos, J.B.; Brett, C.M.A.; de Sousa, H.C. Development of greener multi-responsive chitosan biomaterials doped with biocompatible ammonium ionic liquids. *Acs Sustain. Chem. Eng.* **2013**, *1*, 1480–1492. [CrossRef]
101. Jia, X.; Yang, Y.; Wang, C.; Zhao, C.; Vijayaraghavan, R.; MacFarlane, D.R.; Forsyth, M.; Wallace, G.G. Biocompatible ionic liquid–biopolymer electrolyte-enabled thin and compact magnesium–air batteries. *ACS Appl. Mater. Interfaces* **2014**, *6*, 21110–21117. [CrossRef] [PubMed]
102. Shamshina, J.L. Chitin in ionic liquids: Historical insights into the polymer's dissolution and isolation. A review. *Green Chem.* **2019**, *21*, 3974–3993. [CrossRef]
103. Ma, B.; Qin, A.; Li, X.; He, C. High tenacity regenerated chitosan fibers prepared by using the binary ionic liquid solvent (Gly·HCl)-[Bmim]Cl. *Carbohyd. Polym.* **2013**, *97*, 300–305. [CrossRef]
104. Ma, B.; Zhang, M.; He, C.; Sun, J. New binary ionic liquid system for the preparation of chitosan/cellulose composite fibers. *Carbohyd. Polym.* **2012**, *88*, 347–351. [CrossRef]
105. Park, T.-J.; Jung, Y.J.; Choi, S.-W.; Park, H.; Kim, H.; Kim, E.; Lee, S.H.; Kim, J.H. Native chitosan/cellulose composite fibers from an ionic liquid via electrospinning. *Macromol. Res.* **2011**, *19*, 213–215. [CrossRef]
106. Zhai, Z.; Wang, H.; Wei, B.; Yu, P.; Xu, C.; He, L.; Zhang, J.; Xu, Y. Effect of ionic liquids on the fibril-formation and gel properties of grass carp (Ctenopharyngodon idellus) skin collagen. *Macromol. Res.* **2018**, *26*, 609–615. [CrossRef]
107. Shi, D.; Mi, G.; Bhattacharya, S.; Nayar, S.; Webster, T.J. Optimizing superparamagnetic iron oxide nanoparticles as drug carriers using an in vitro blood-brain barrier model. *Int. J. Nanomed.* **2016**, *11*, 5371–5379. [CrossRef] [PubMed]
108. Sehgal, P.K.; Srinivasan, A. Collagen-coated microparticles in drug delivery. *Expert Opin. Drug Deliv.* **2009**, *6*, 687–695. [CrossRef] [PubMed]
109. David, G. Chapter 35—Collagen-based 3D structures—Versatile, efficient materials for biomedical applications. In *Biopolymer-Based Formulations*; Pal, K., Banerjee, I., Sarkar, P., Kim, D., Deng, W.-P., Dubey, N.K., Majumder, K., Eds.; Elsevier: Amsterdam, The Netherlands, 2020; pp. 881–906.
110. Maeda, Y.; Wei, Z.; Matsui, H. Biomimetic assembly of proteins into microcapsules on oil-in-water droplets with structural reinforcement via biomolecular-recognition-based cross-linking of surface peptides. *Small* **2012**, *8*, 1341–1344. [CrossRef] [PubMed]

111. Morikawa, M.-a.; Takano, A.; Tao, S.; Kimizuka, N. Biopolymer-Encapsulated Protein Microcapsules Spontaneously Formed at the Ionic Liquid–Water Interface. *Biomacromolecules* **2012**, *13*, 4075–4080. [CrossRef] [PubMed]
112. He, Z.; Alexandridis, P. Nanoparticles in ionic liquids: Interactions and organization. *Phys. Chem. Chem. Phys.* **2015**, *17*, 18238–18261. [CrossRef]
113. Montalbán, M.G.; Carissimi, G.; Lozano-Pérez, A.A.; Cenis, J.L.; Coburn, J.M.; Kaplan, D.L.; Víllora, G. *Biopolymeric Nanoparticle Synthesis in Ionic Liquids*; IntechOpen: London, UK, 2018; pp. 3–26.
114. Chan, O.C.M.; So, K.F.; Chan, B.P. Fabrication of nano-fibrous collagen microspheres for protein delivery and effects of photochemical crosslinking on release kinetics. *J. Control. Release* **2008**, *129*, 135–143. [CrossRef]
115. Solanki, P. Gelatin nanoparticles as a delivery system for proteins. *J. Nanomed. Res.* **2015**, *2*, 1–3. [CrossRef]
116. Bharmoria, P.; Singh, T.; Kumar, A. Complexation of chitosan with surfactant like ionic liquids: Molecular interactions and preparation of chitosan nanoparticles. *J. Colloid Interface Sci.* **2013**, *407*, 361–369. [CrossRef]
117. Silva, S.S.; Duarte, A.R.; Mano, J.F.; Reis, R.L. Development of a supercritical assisted particle-agglomeration method for the preparation of bioactive chitin-based matrices. In Proceedings of the 10th International Symposium on Supercritical Fluids San Franciscorices, San Francisco, CA, USA., 13–16 May 2012.
118. Silva, S.S.; Duarte, A.R.C.; Oliveira, J.M.; Mano, J.F.; Reis, R.L. Alternative methodology for chitin–Hydroxyapatite composites using ionic liquids and supercritical fluid technology. *J. Bioact. Compat. Polym.* **2013**, *28*, 481–491. [CrossRef]
119. Kuzmina, O. Chapter 5-methods of IL recovery and destruction. In *Application, Purification, and Recovery of Ionic Liquids*; Kuzmina, O., Hallett, J.P., Eds.; Elsevier: Amsterdam, The Netherlands, 2016; pp. 205–248.
120. Shamshina, J.L.; Berton, P. Use of ionic liquids in chitin biorefinery: A systematic review. *Front. Bioeng. Biotechnol.* **2020**, *8*, 11. [CrossRef]
121. Barber, P.S.; Griggs, C.S.; Gurau, G.; Liu, Z.; Li, S.; Li, Z.; Lu, X.; Zhang, S.; Rogers, R.D. Coagulation of chitin and cellulose from 1-ethyl-3-methylimidazolium acetate ionic-liquid solutions using carbon dioxide. *Angew. Chem.* **2013**, *52*, 12350–12353. [CrossRef] [PubMed]
122. Iqbal, B.; Sarfaraz, Z.; Muhammad, N.; Ahmad, P.; Iqbal, J.; Khan, Z.U.H.; Gonfa, G.; Iqbal, F.; Jamal, A.; Rahim, A. Ionic liquid as a potential solvent for preparation of collagen-alginate-hydroxyapatite beads as bone filler. *J. Biomater. Sci. Polym. Ed.* **2018**, *29*, 1168–1184. [CrossRef] [PubMed]
123. Tran, C.D.; Duri, S.; Harkins, A.L. Recyclable synthesis, characterization, and antimicrobial activity of chitosan-based polysaccharide composite materials. *J. Biomed. Mater. Res. Part A* **2013**, *101*, 2248–2257. [CrossRef] [PubMed]
124. Chen, X.; Gao, Y.; Wang, L.; Chen, H.; Yan, N. Effect of treatment methods on chitin structure and its transformation into nitrogen-containing chemicals. *ChemPlusChem* **2015**, *80*, 1565–1572. [CrossRef]
125. Earl, J.M.; Seddon, K.R. Preparation of imidazole carbene and the use thereof for the synthesis of ionic liquids. *WO* **2001**, *1*, 20.
126. Tran, C.D.; Duri, S.; Delneri, A.; Franko, M. Chitosan-cellulose composite materials: Preparation, Characterization and application for removal of microcystin. *J. Hazard. Mater.* **2013**, *252*, 355–366. [CrossRef]
127. Singh, N.; Koziol, K.K.K.; Chen, J.; Patil, A.J.; Gilman, J.W.; Trulove, P.C.; Kafienah, W.; Rahatekar, S.S. Ionic liquids-based processing of electrically conducting chitin nanocomposite scaffolds for stem cell growth. *Green Chem.* **2013**, *15*, 1192–1202. [CrossRef]
128. Li, X.; Fan, D. Smart collagen hydrogels based on 1-Ethyl-3-methylimidazolium acetate and microbial transglutaminase for potential applications in tissue engineering and cancer therapy. *ACS Biomater. Sci. Eng.* **2019**, *5*, 3523–3536. [CrossRef]
129. Leones, R.; Sentanin, F.; Rodrigues, L.C.; Ferreira, R.A.S.; Marrucho, I.M.; Esperança, J.M.S.S.; Pawlicka, A.; Carlos, L.D.; Silva, M.M. Novel polymer electrolytes based on gelatin and ionic liquids. *Opt. Mater.* **2012**, *35*, 187–195. [CrossRef]
130. Shamshina, J.L.; Zavgorodnya, O.; Berton, P.; Chhotaray, P.K.; Choudhary, H.; Rogers, R.D. Ionic liquid platform for spinning composite Chitin–Poly(lactic acid) fibers. *ACS Sustain. Chem. Eng.* **2018**, *6*, 10241–10251. [CrossRef]
131. Gonçalves, C.; Silva, S.S.; Gomes, J.M.; Oliveira, I.M.; Canadas, R.F.; Maia, F.R.; Radhouani, H.; Reis, R.L.; Oliveira, J.M. Ionic liquid-mediated processing of SAIB-Chitin scaffolds. *ACS Sustain. Chem. Eng.* **2020**, *8*, 3986–3994. [CrossRef]

132. Harkins, A.L.; Duri, S.; Kloth, L.C.; Tran, C.D. Chitosan-cellulose composite for wound dressing material. Part 2. Antimicrobial activity, blood absorption ability, and biocompatibility. *J. Biomed. Mater. Res. Part B Appl. Biomater.* **2014**, *102*, 1199–1206. [CrossRef] [PubMed]
133. Tran, C.D.; Mututuvari, T.M. Cellulose, chitosan, and keratin composite materials. controlled drug release. *Langmuir* **2015**, *31*, 1516–1526. [CrossRef] [PubMed]
134. Scabbia, A.; Trombelli, L. A comparative study on the use of a HA/collagen/chondroitin sulphate biomaterial (Biostite®) and a bovine-derived HA xenograft (Bio-Oss®) in the treatment of deep intra-osseous defects. *J. Clin. Periodontol.* **2004**, *31*, 348–355. [CrossRef] [PubMed]
135. Iqbal, B.; Muhammad, N.; Rahim, A.; Iqbal, F.; Sharif, F.; Safi, S.Z.; Khan, A.S.; Gonfa, G.; Uroos, M.; Rehman, I.U. Development of collagen/PVA composites patches for osteochondral defects using a green processing of ionic liquid. *Int. J. Polym. Mater. Polym. Biomater.* **2019**, *68*, 590–596. [CrossRef]
136. Ion, R.-M.; Poinescu, A.; Doncea, S. Novel three-component composite materials (Hydroxyapatite/Polymer mixtures) for bone regeneration. *Key Eng. Mater.* **2014**, *587*, 197–204. [CrossRef]
137. Wahl, D.; Sachlos, E.; Liu, C.; Czernuszka, J. Controlling the processing of collagen-hydroxyapatite scaffolds for bone tissue engineering. *J. Mater. Sci. Mater. Med.* **2007**, *18*, 201–209. [CrossRef]
138. Ryan, A.J.; Gleeson, J.P.; Matsiko, A.; Thompson, E.M.; O'Brien, F.J. Effect of different hydroxyapatite incorporation methods on the structural and biological properties of porous collagen scaffolds for bone repair. *J. Anat.* **2015**, *227*, 732–745. [CrossRef]
139. Hua, D.; Jiang, J.; Kuang, L.; Jiang, J.; Zheng, W.; Liang, H. Smart chitosan-based stimuli-responsive nanocarriers for the controlled delivery of hydrophobic pharmaceuticals. *Macromolecules* **2011**, *44*, 1298–1302. [CrossRef]
140. Chen, H.; Cui, S.; Zhao, Y.; Wang, B.; Zhang, S.; Peng, X. O-Alkylation of chitosan for gene delivery by using ionic liquid in an in- situ reactor. *Engineering* **2012**, *4*, 114–117. [CrossRef]
141. Chen, H.; Cui, S.; Zhao, Y.; Zhang, C.; Zhang, S.; Peng, X. Grafting chitosan with polyethylenimine in an ionic liquid for efficient gene delivery. *PLoS ONE* **2015**, *10*, e0121817. [CrossRef] [PubMed]

© 2020 by the authors. Licensee MDPI, Basel, Switzerland. This article is an open access article distributed under the terms and conditions of the Creative Commons Attribution (CC BY) license (http://creativecommons.org/licenses/by/4.0/).

marine drugs

MDPI

Review

Mexican Microalgae Biodiversity and State-Of-The-Art Extraction Strategies to Meet Sustainable Circular Economy Challenges: High-Value Compounds and Their Applied Perspectives

Juan Eduardo Sosa-Hernández [1], Kenya D. Romero-Castillo [1], Lizeth Parra-Arroyo [1], Mauricio A. Aguilar-Aguila-Isaías [1], Isaac E. García-Reyes [1], Ishtiaq Ahmed [2], Roberto Parra-Saldivar [1], Muhammad Bilal [3] and Hafiz M. N. Iqbal [1,*]

1 Tecnologico de Monterrey, School of Engineering and Sciences, Campus Monterrey, Ave. Eugenio Garza Sada 2501, CP 64849, Monterrey, N.L., Mexico; eduardo.sosa@tec.mx (J.E.S.-H.); a00823430@itesm.mx (K.D.R.-C.); a01036078@itesm.mx (L.P.-A.); a00816656@itesm.mx (M.A.A.-A.-I.); a00824289@itesm.mx (I.E.G.-R.); r.parra@tec.mx (R.P.-S.)

2 School of Medical Science, Menzies Health Institute Queensland, Griffith University (Gold Coast campus), Parklands Drive, Southport, QLD 4222, Australia; ishtiaq.ahmed@griffithuni.edu.au

3 School of Life Science and Food Engineering, Huaiyin Institute of Technology, Huaian 223003, China; bilaluaf@hotmail.com

* Correspondence: hafiz.iqbal@my.westminster.ac.uk or hafiz.iqbal@itesm.mx; Tel.: +528183582000 (ext. 5679)

Received: 13 February 2019; Accepted: 9 March 2019; Published: 18 March 2019

Abstract: In recent years, the demand for naturally derived products has hiked with enormous pressure to propose or develop state-of-the-art strategies to meet sustainable circular economy challenges. Microalgae possess the flexibility to produce a variety of high-value products of industrial interests. From pigments such as phycobilins or lutein to phycotoxins and several polyunsaturated fatty acids (PUFAs), microalgae have the potential to become the primary producers for the pharmaceutical, food, and agronomical industries. Also, microalgae require minimal resources to grow due to their autotrophic nature or by consuming waste matter, while allowing for the extraction of several valuable side products such as hydrogen gas and biodiesel in a single process, following a biorefinery agenda. From a Mexican microalgae biodiversity perspective, more than 70 different local species have been characterized and isolated, whereas, only a minimal amount has been explored to produce commercially valuable products, thus ignoring their potential as a locally available resource. In this paper, we discuss the microalgae diversity present in Mexico with their current applications and potential, while expanding on their future applications in bioengineering along with other industrial sectors. In conclusion, the use of available microalgae to produce biochemically revenuable products currently represents an untapped potential that could lead to the solution of several problems through green technologies. As such, if the social, industrial and research communities collaborate to strive towards a greener economy by preserving the existing biodiversity and optimizing the use of the currently available resources, the enrichment of our society and the solution to several environmental problems could be attained.

Keywords: microalgae; biodiversity; bioactive compounds; green extractions; pharmaceutical; secondary metabolites; biofuels

1. Introduction

Current needs demand high-level bio-compounds production coped with cutting-edge biotechnology. Several strategies to produce valuable compounds addressed by pharmaceutical and food industry rely on microorganism production. However, other bioactive products still rely on synthetic production processes. Plants, yeasts, bacteria, fungi, and microalgae are the most used organisms to produce such compounds naturally. Microalgae have a large number of species, and little is known about their potential uses in comparison to the diversity that is reported every day [1]. Microalgae are one of the most used bio-systems to produce different compounds in biotechnology (Figure 1). The utilization of microorganisms' machinery helps to generate high-value bio-products [2]. As this is a bioprocess, it has several advantages over other techniques since it offers new environmental-friendly opportunities. The objective of this work is to compile a list of strains, show the relevance of new extraction techniques, and characterize current applications and potential future biotechnological microalgae opportunities.

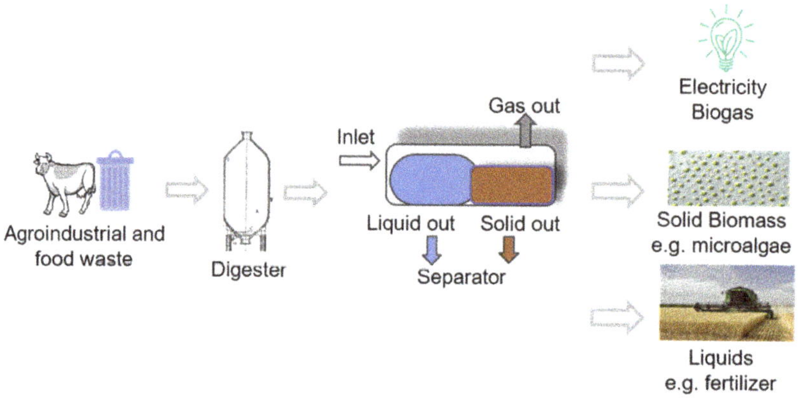

Figure 1. Microalgae biotechnology valorization scheme to produce energy and bio-compounds from agro-industrial and food waste.

Microalgae or cyanobacteria are unicellular, cenobial, pluricellular, or colonial organisms adapted to live in water systems, soils, or as symbionts [1]. Depending on the species, they live in complex systems or as individual cells and interact with light through photosynthesis producing oxygen and consuming carbon dioxide [3]. Microalgae can produce biomass containing high-value bio-compounds and at the same time bio-fixate ions, both important factors to propel microalgae biotechnological applications in the new era of environment remediation [4–6]. Cultivation technologies to produce biomass include open ponds, photo-bioreactors, and fermentation reactors. A lack of attention to microalgae species is evident since only a few hundred have been investigated. It is believed that at least tens of thousands exist in the world [7]. Nonetheless, some countries had already looked for food production through microalgal cultivation. Mexican Aztecs used to cultivate and consume Spirulina from Texcoco salted lake [8]. Japan has been leading since the early 1950s [9] with the first industrial-scale production of *Chlorella* for human consumption to ingest as a nutritional supplement. Leading to use *Chlorella* as the main microalgae source of dietary supplement nowadays. Harvesting and drying of its biomass use expensive centrifuges and cells need to be broken therefor 5000 Mt of *Chlorella* biomass were sold for approximately $20,000/100 kg. Other successful microalgae with great industrial production are *Spirulina*. They have several advantages over *Chlorella* since they require a little inoculum, and is not easy to get contaminated, they grow in temperatures between 15 and 38° Celsius, high pH, and alkalinity. *Spirulina* market value, plant gate, is about $10,000 per ton and its main use is for food supplement [10]. Nowadays, *Chlorella* and *Spirulina* are the principal microalgae used for nutritional supplements, and their producers value them in the global market about $40–50 per kg [11]. The price and volume relations are even higher when pure fine-chemicals are obtained from algal cultivation. β-carotene is a pigment strongly used in the United States. In the market, its price is estimated from $300 to $3,000 USD/kg, the price depends entirely on the production, the fickle market, and the product purity [12]. The animal feeding price is about $10 USD/kg in the nutraceutical sector. On the other hand, for example, the same product for human consumption is sold at $120 US/kg [13].

Microalgal biomass is also used to get biofuels. In comparison with petroleum, biomass is more expensive. Assuming the lipid dry weight content within microalgae, 29.6% (lipid/biomass), the algal biomass must be produced at the cost of US $ 152.00 per ton to be competitive with petroleum [14]. Also, in this area, microalga biomass price along with its valued compound depend on where the product is located and the market status [15]. As discussed previously, it is evident that biotechnology focused on microalgae has a substantial potential application in the industry. This review presents several Mexican microalgae strains along with novel green extraction technologies applied to extract microalgae-based high-value compounds. Then, a comprehensive list of compounds is presented within five fields of applications, to be followed by potential applications and opportunities for improvement. Finally, concluding remarks and future perspectives are summarized.

2. Mexican Microalgae Biodiversity

Mexico is one of the countries with the highest biodiversity in the world thanks to its geography and size that covers several latitudes. The Mesoamerica region provides very different environmental conditions to support life [16]. Algal strains from all around the country were isolated and studied by research groups across México. To our knowledge, this is the first work to gather information from microalgae found in several locations, systems, and types of waterbodies in the country that also addresses its applications and prospect its potential applications in contrast to just freshwater biodiversity [17,18].

The Pacific Ocean is a vast water source with the unique condition of being warm. From this Mexican litoral, in Baja California, 21 species were isolated, but *Aphanocapsa marina*, *Komvophoron* sp., and *Phormidium* sp. were selected thanks to their capacity to produce fatty acids. The remaining strains were also characterized but were not selected for aquaculture farm food [19]. Raw microalgae biomass is used as a nutraceutical product in aquaculture activities directly in the country by increasing its productivity [20]. However, Rodríguez-Palacio et al. focused on a large microalgae diversity that causes algal blooms with toxic consequences for aquatic fauna in twelve locations of the country, where the harmful toxic microalgae affect fishes. In addition, they proposed the culture of those microalgae in order to evaluate changes in water pollution [21]. A list of microalgae found in Mexican water sources and isolated is presented in Table 1. Lately, the discovery of novel microorganisms is increasing, and it is expected to continue thanks to new research groups across the country. The panorama presented by the list of microalgae suggests potential applications since they were found in various environment growth conditions including volcano ponds, salted lakes, freshwaters, and seawaters. Even in extreme physiological conditions, microorganisms are capable of producing compounds with high value. To get an advantage, biotechnological processes like production, extraction, and purification require novel and environmentally friendly methods. The next section focuses on the description of green extraction methodologies.

Table 1. Microalgae biodiversity in Mexico.

State	Municipality/Location	Microalgae	References
Baja California	Ensenada	*Aphanocapsa marina* *Komvophoron* sp. *Phormidium* sp. *Tetraselmis suecica* *Heterococcus* sp. *Amphora* sp. (7) *Cymbella* sp. (2) *Navicula* sp. (4) *Diploneis* sp. *Grammatophora angulosa* *Synedra* sp.	[19]
Veracruz	Catemaco	*Aphanothece comasii* *Cyanotetras aerotopa* *Cylindrospermopsis catemaco* *Cylindrospermopsis taverae* *Planktolyngbya regularis*	[17]
San Luis Potosí		*Cyanobacterium lineatum*	
Puebla	Alchichica	*Cyclotella alchichicana* *Chroococcus deltoids*	
Baja California, Colima, Michoacan, Guerrero, Tamaulipas, Veracruz, Hidalgo, Mexico city	Ensenada, Manzanillo, Lazaro Cardenas, Acapulco and Zihuatanejo, Laguna de Carpintero, Garrapatas and Barberena estuaries, Catemaco and Chalchoapan Lakes, Vicente Aguirre dam, Xochimilco Lake	*Alexandrium tamarense* *Amphidinium* sp. *Cochlodinium polykrikoides* *Heterocapsa pigmea* *Gyrodinium instriatum* *Gymnodinium catenatum* *Karlodinium veneficum* *Prorocentrum gracile* *Prorocentrum micans* *Prorocentrum triestimum* *Prorocentrum mexicanum* *Prorocentrum rathymum* *Protoceratium reticulatum* *Scrippsiella trochoidea* *Bacillaria paxilifera* *Cylindrotheca closterium* *Pseudonitszchia delicatisima* *Chattonella marina*	[21]
Mexico City	Mexico City	*Spirulina maxima*	[22]
Baja California Sur	La Paz	*Rhabdonema* sp. *Schizochytrium* sp. *Nitzchia* sp. *Navicula* sp. *Grammatophora* sp.	[23]
Mexico City	Mexico City	*Spirulina platensis* *Spirulina maxima*	[24]
Queretaro	Not specified	*Oscillatoria* sp.	[25]
Guanajuato	Valle de Santiago	*Actinastrum* sp.	[26]
Baja California Sur	La Paz	*Lyngbya* sp. *Oscillatoria* sp. *Microcoleus* sp. *Anabaena* sp.	[27]
Nuevo León	Apodaca Cadereyta	*Scenedesmus* sp. *Chlorella sorokiniana*	[28]
Campeche	El Carmen	*Anabaena* sp. *Oscillatoria* sp. *Anabaena* sp. *Cylindrospermopsis cuspis*	[29]
Oaxaca	Zipolite	*Dermocarpella* sp.	[30]

Table 1. *Cont.*

State	Municipality/Location	Microalgae	References
Morelos	Tlaquiltenango	*Nostoc* sp.	[31]
Mexico City	Mexico City	*Desmodesmus* sp.	[32]
Coahuila	Cuatrociénegas	*Scenedesmus* sp.	[33]
Mexico City	Mexico City	*Microcystis*	[34]
Michoacan	Michoacan	*Codium giraffa*	[35]
Guerrero	Papanoa	*Codium giraffa*	[36]
Michoacán	Los Azufres	*Trebouxiophyceae* sp.	[37]

3. State-Of-The-Art of Extraction Methods

Currently, most common extraction techniques consist of non-green processes. Millions of liters of organic solvents are used in the extraction process. Consequently, interest in green extraction techniques has recently increased as they are less expensive but cope with the global tendency of green legislation [38]. These processes are named, green extraction, since they do not negatively affect the environment and take advantage of the compound properties such as polarizability, charge, structure, as well as size [38]. Such processes include microwave extraction, supercritical fluid extraction, as well as ultrasound extraction. Using the appropriated method, bioactive compounds are extracted from microalgae, and valuable molecules remain functional after an efficient extraction. A list of compounds extracted from microalgae using ultrasound, microwave, and supercritical fluid extraction methods are presented in Table 2.

Table 2. Compounds from microalgae extracted by novel green techniques.

Compound(s) of Interest	Species	Extraction Technique	References
C-phycocyanin Pigments	*Spirulina maxima*	Ultrasound	[39]
β-carotene	*Chlorella* sp.	Ultrasound	[40]
Polyphenols Flavonoids	*Spirulina platensis*	Microwave and Ultrasound	[41]
Lipids	*Scenedesmus* sp.	Microwave	[42]
Lipids	*Scenedesmus obliquus & Scenedesmus obtusiusculus*	Supercritical-CO_2	[43]
Oil	*Spirulina platensis*	Supercritical-CO_2	[44]
Docosahexaenoic acid	*Schizochytrium limacinum*	Supercritical-CO_2 -vegetable oil	[45]
Lipids, Carotenoids	*Chlorella vulgaris*	Supercritical-CO_2	[46]
Lipids	*Chlorella vulgaris*	Ultrasound & Bligh and Dyer method	[47]
β-carotene	*Spirulina platensis*	Ultrasound	[48]
Vitamins Phycocyanin Fatty Acids	*Spirulina platensis*	Microwave	[49]
Lipids	*Chlorella* sp.	Microwave and Ultrasound	[50]
Long-chain PUFAs	*Schizochytrium* sp.	Supercritical-CO_2	[51]
Carotenoids Fatty Acids	*Spirulina platensis*	Microwave and Supercritical-CO_2 -etOH	[49]
C-phycocyanin	*Spirulina platensis*	Ultrasound	[52]
Neutral Lipids	*Chlorella vulgaris & Nannochloropsis oculata*	Supercritical-CO_2	[53]
Chlorophyll	*Chlorella vulgaris*	Ultrasound	[54]
Lipids	*Scenedesmus obliquus*	Ultrasound + solvent	[55]

3.1. Microwave-Based Extraction

Microwave extraction involves heating of samples in a polar solution such as ionic liquids, ethanol, methanol, chloroform, acetone, and ultra-pure water by placing them in an alternating electric field. The solvent molecules align according to the applied electric field and quickly increase the temperature of the samples as a result of the inter- and intramolecular friction caused by this movement. The algal cell walls break with this sudden increase in temperature and release the compounds of interest (Figure 2). The resulting extract must undergo further purification as this process does not result in the isolated compound of interest [56]. This method differs from conventional heating extraction methods as it does not depend on the diffusion rate of the mixture mass. Therefore, microwaves heat the solvent which interacts with all the sample and prevents the formation of hot-spots and allowing for more homogeneous thermoregulation of the cell mixture. Further, it is quick and has been demonstrated to be at least ten times faster than conventional bath heating extraction methods, as mentioned by Balasubramanian et al. [56]. Additionally, the same study showed that the use of this method is especially beneficial when extracting lipids from microalgae, as it allows for a final product of better quality, with higher unsaturated lipids and antioxidant concentrations in comparison to the conventional Soxhlet extraction. In a second study involving pigment extraction from *Dunaliella tertiolecta* and Cylindrotheca closterium, it was demonstrated that microwave extraction techniques are more efficient than solvent-based techniques in overcoming mechanical resistance factors that limit solvent penetration into the cells [57].

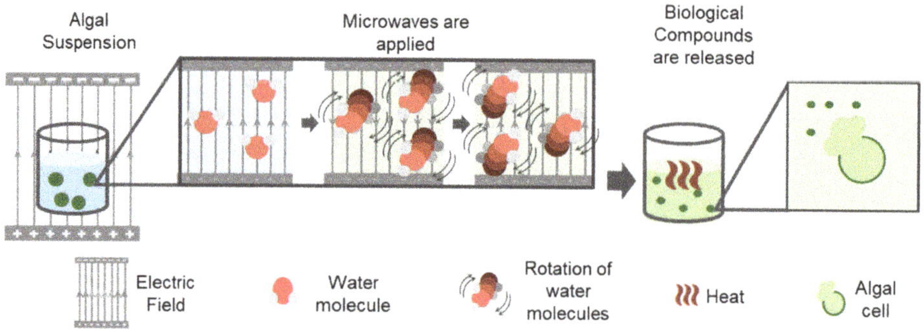

Figure 2. Scheme of microwave algal extraction.

The prospects for industrial implementation of Microwave extraction techniques have been previously discussed by Vinatoru et al. [58], where advantages such as shorter loading and downloading times as well as easier maintenance of the equipment are added to the lower energy consumption and faster extraction times. However, specific advantages depend on the type of material to be extracted (as previously discussed, microwave extraction methods are more efficient for certain mixtures due to their intrinsic properties, e.g., mechanical resistance). Nevertheless, pretreatment methods such as enzymatic digestion or milling could allow for a standardized development of this extraction method by improving its efficiency for a wide range of mixtures [58]. Also, the coupling of this method with other extraction techniques could also improve its efficiency. Still, the feasibility of scaling up microwave extraction techniques into an industrial level is still under research; because its high energy operating costs might present a major drawback of this process. For instance, the use of enzymes is expensive, especially for large scale applications when competing against other methods [59]. Moreover, this method cannot complete the separation process by itself and usually requires a subsequent centrifugation or filtration process [60].

3.2. Supercritical Fluid-Based Extraction

This extraction method depends on the usage of supercritical fluids (e.g., carbon dioxide, water, methane, ethane, methanol, ethanol, acetone, and nitrous oxide), induced either by temperature or pressure excitation, for the recovery of valuable products. Such fluids are capable of crossing the cellular membrane and wall of microalgae and solubilize internal metabolites to extract them from the cell (Figure 3). In most cases, supercritical fluids' induction conditions range between $P_C < P \leq 6P_C$ for pressure and $1.01T_C < T \leq 1.4T_C$ for temperature in order to allow for an energy efficient extraction (where, P_C is the critical pressure constant and T_C is the critical temperature constant for the supercritical fluid) [61]. The most common and preferred solvent used for this method is CO_2 as it has an ambient critical temperature, is non-flammable, is chemically inert, non-toxic, and inexpensive [61]. As such, it is able to meet the ecological and chemical safety standards required for the extraction of high purity biological products (such as pigments for cosmetics and antiviral agent in medicine) as it leaves no harmful solvent residues and prevents thermal degradation of sensitive products. Moreover, with the addition of a polar entrainer (such as water) the solvent is able to dissolve polar compounds as well [61], thus allowing for a robust extraction procedure.

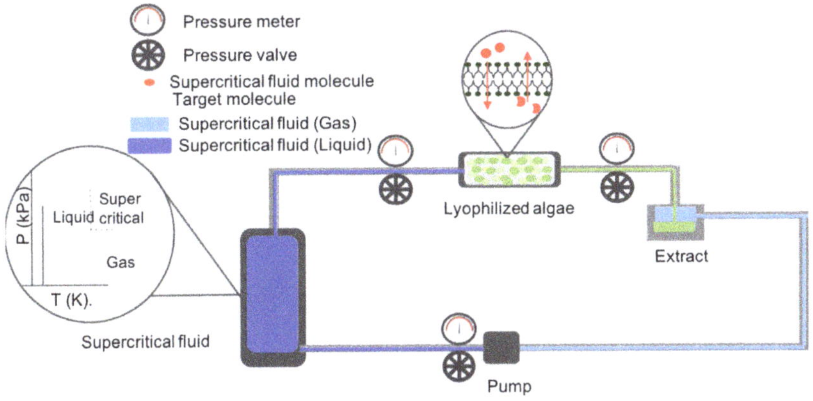

Figure 3. Scheme of the supercritical fluid extraction process in a closed system.

The main advantage this method presents when compared to the conventional Soxhlet extraction method is the fact that it prevents the deposition of residual toxic matter in the extract, while also proving to be quite economical. The mentioned characteristics are because CO_2 can reach a supercritical condition at a temperature of 31 °C (conventionally a temperature of 35 °C is preferred for extraction of biological materials). This critical temperature allows the liquid CO_2 to be used without the consumption of excessive amounts of energy, and with a minimal reduction in temperature, most of the solvent will easily precipitate. Further, it is easily affordable, having a nominal price of 2.65 USD/kg in the year 2017 [62]. Also, as explained before, the non-extreme range of temperatures in which this method can operate prevents the degradation of valuable biological products, thus allowing for a high yield.

A recent study also analyzed the possibility of combining the use of supercritical fluid extraction with cold pressing to improve the extraction of fennel by supercritical fluid extraction alone [63]. The combination of these two extraction methods was originally developed by Johner et al. [64] for the extraction of pequi. This researchers demonstrated some promising results: a faster extraction rate with the consumption of less solvent. These results were validated with the fennel extraction, where the overall yield extraction was improved by 24.5%. Hatami et al. [63] inferred that this might be due to the increased exposure of oil to supercritical CO_2 caused by the release of the substance from the compressed matter. These results also demonstrate that supercritical extraction can reduce operational time and costs while increasing yields if combined with other extraction procedures such as those including solvents like acetone or ethanol. All these factors proved that supercritical fluid extraction might be a promising alternative for a greener future. Nevertheless, supercritical fluid extraction machinery usually represents a high capital cost, regardless of the economic viability in the long run. For example, according to De Aguilar [62], Supercritical Fluid Extraction (SFE) units' nominal prices ranged between 530,000 to 2,600,000 USD in 2017. Further, while temperature extraction conditions are amiable, pressure operating parameters still need to be decreased for general industrial implementation. While previous studies have been able to optimize industrial relevant conditions for supercritical extraction of lipids from *Scenedesmus obliquus, Chlorella protothecoides and Nannochloropsis salina* [65], optimal pressure conditions can range between 30 MPa and 50 MPa in some cases [59], thus representing an area of opportunity for further optimization of the standardized application. Polyunsaturated fatty acids like ω-3 and ω-6 types have been successfully extracted by SFE using CO_2 and n-butane. Feller et al. [66] found a significant relationship between the content of carotenoids and the respective antioxidant activity. They used *Phaeodactylum tricornutum*, *Nannochloropsis oculata*, and *Porphyridium cruentum* strains and attributed the antioxidant activity of the marine microalgae to the carotenoid compounds [66]. In the case of subcritical n-butane, the procedure is the same as for the supercritical system. The difference relays in the control conditions using n-butane at 15 bar, 40 °C and solvent flow rate of 3 mL min^{-1} [66].

3.3. Ultrasound-Based Extraction

The technique of Ultrasound Extraction uses high-frequency sound waves to disrupt algal cell walls leading to the subsequent release of the compound of interest. As shown in Figure 4, the process depends on a physical phenomenon called cavitation where the disruption of the solvent caused by the sound waves, creates small bubbles. The bubbles generate strong jet streams as they implode by the effect of the acoustic cavitation force. When the bubble is close to a cell, allow for the puncturing of the cell wall and membrane [67]. The particular solvent used for this extraction method depends on the physical characteristics of the target compound, and subsequent fractionations are needed to isolate the compound of interest. Ultrasound extraction may occur directly as well as indirectly. Indirect ultrasound consists of placing a transducer touching the outer surface of a water bath. In the case of direct ultrasound extraction, the transducer can be close to the container where the bath occurs or in the form of an ultrasound horn in the sample (Figure 5). The advantages of this method include faster and substantial yields than other conventional techniques and moderate to low costs, in addition to minimal toxicity [68]. According to Kledjus et al. [69], it also allows for a more efficient extraction in freshwater algae species. On the other hand, the technique might negatively affect the quality of the oils as well as the integrity of polyunsaturated fatty acid rich oils. Furthermore, it cannot be scaled up [67].

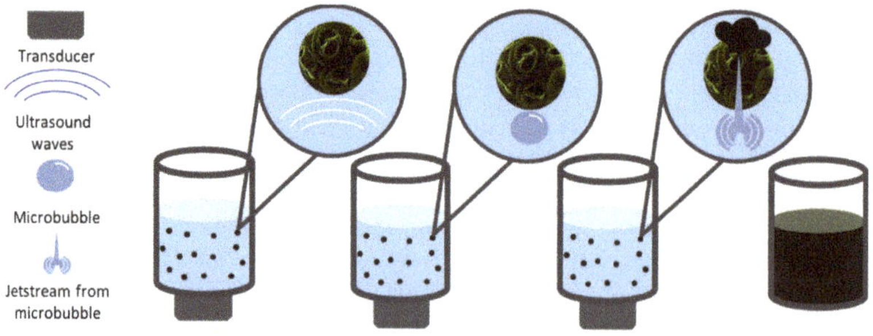

Figure 4. Schematic representation of the steps involved in the ultrasound-assisted extraction method.

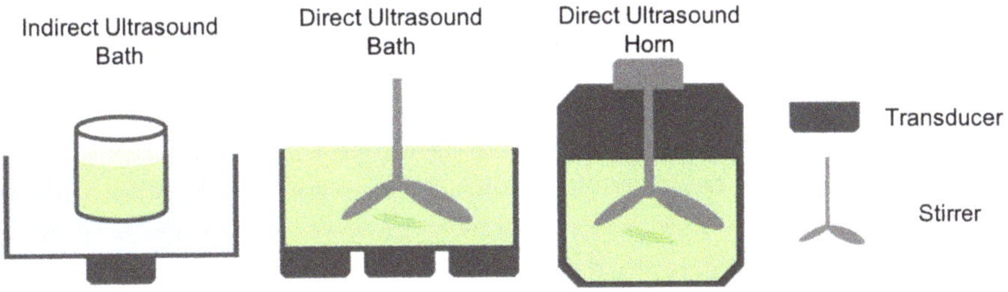

Figure 5. Different methods involved in ultrasound assisted extraction.

4. Current Applications

Cyanobacterial have already shown potential applications in biotechnology, biomedicine, food, biofuel, fertilizers, pigments, waste treatment, among others. The production (general process scheme is presented in Figure 6) of various secondary metabolites includes toxins, antioxidants, vitamins, bio-adsorbents, enzymes, and pharmaceuticals. Considering cyanobacterial pluripotential biotechnological uses, an overview is presented. First, a list of microalgae strains found in Mexico and the bioactive compounds produced are presented in Table 3, followed by the description of the current applications of relevant works with the mentioned microalgae.

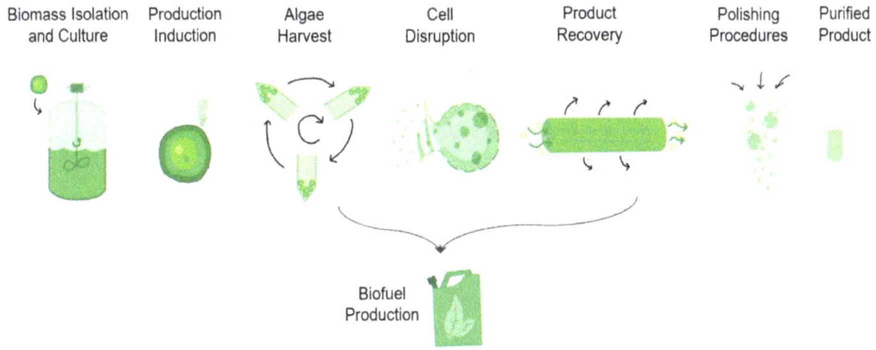

Figure 6. Scheme of the biotechnological process to produce bio-compounds from microalgae biomass.

Table 3. Summary of existing high-value products from Mexican microalgae species.

Microalgae	Bioactive Compounds	Biological Activity	References
Oscillatoriaceae sp.	Malyngolide Lyngbyatoxins Debromoaplysiatoxin	Antibacterial PKC activator Inflammatory	[70]
Lyngbya majuscula	Curacin A Kalkitoxin Cyclic polypeptide	Microtubulin assembly inhibitors Sodium channel blocker Anti-HIV activity	[71]
Oscillatoria raoi	Acetylated sulfoglycolipids	Antiviral	[72]
Spirulina platensis	Spirulan	Antiviral	[73]
Nostocaceae sp.	Nostocyclamide	Antifungal	[74]
Chroococcaceae sp. *Mycrosistis aeuregonosa*	Kawaguchipeptin B	Antibacterial	[75]
Scenedesmus sp.	Lutein	Anti-oxidant	[76–80]
Spirulina (Arthrospira)	γ-Linolenic acid (GLA)	The integrity of tissues, delay of aging	[81]
Spirulina (Arthrospira)	Phycocyanin	Antioxidant, anti-inflammatory	[15,82]
Tetracelmis suecica	α- tocopherol	Antioxidant	[15]
Chlorella sp.	Galactose, rhamnose, mannose, arabinose, N-acetyl glucosamide and N-acetyl galactosamine	Immune stimulatory activity	[83]
Spirulina platensis and Anabaena sp.	Proteins		[84–86]
Anabaena sp.	Superoxide dismutase (SOD)	Antioxidant, anti-inflammatory	[87–90]
Spirulina sp.	Vitamin C; vitamin K; vitamins B_{12}, A and E; α-tocopherol	Antioxidant; blood cell formation; blood clotting mechanism	[15,91]
Chlorella sp.	Lutein, zeaxanthin, canthaxanthin	Antioxidant	[15,92]
Lyngbya majuscula	Microlin- A	Immunosuppressive	[93]
Chlorella sorokiniana and *Scenedesmus* spp.	Mycosporine-like amino acids (MAA)	UV-screening agent; sunscreen	[94–97]
Chlorella sp.	α-carotene Astaxanthin	Lower risk of premature death	[98]
C. sorokiniana	β-carotene	Food colorant; antioxidant property; cancer preventive properties; prevent night blindness; prevent liver fibrosis	[99,100]
Tretraselmis spp.	Zeaxanthin	Protect eye cells; antioxidant activity; neutralizing the free radicals	[101,102]
Nitzschia spp.	Triglycerides and hydrocarbons	Biofuels	[95,103,104]
Tetraselmis spp. and *T. suecica*	Arachidonic acid (AA) Eicosapentaenoic acid (EPA)	Nutritional supplements, aquaculture feeds	[105,106]
T. suecica	Sterols	Antidiabetic; anticancer; anti-inflammatory; anti-photoaging; anti-obesity; anti-inflammatory; antioxidant activities	[107,108]
Chlorella spp. and *C. sorokiniana*	Vitamin B Vitamin C	Decrease fatigue; reducing depression; protect against heart disease; protect the skin; anticancer activity Protect against cardiovascular disease; prenatal health problems; prevent from the eye disease; protect against skin wrinkling	[85,99,109–112]
C. sorokiniana and *T. suecica*	Vitamin E	Protect against toxic pollutants; Premenstrual syndrome protects against eye disorders; anti-Alzheimer's disease; anti-diabetic properties	[85,98,111,113]

4.1. Pigments - Phycobilins, Lutein, and Carotenoids

Phycobilins are produced only by algae such as *Spirulina* [114]. Phycobilins are photosynthetic pigments bonded to water-soluble proteins, building the so-called phycobiliproteins. Phycocyanin, phycoerythrin, and allophycocyanin are water-soluble and have a wide range of applications including food and cosmetic colors, as fluorescent tags for use in flow cytometry and immunology [52]. Other possible applications are as antioxidants in cosmetics, a component of functional foods, and photosensitizers in photodynamic cancer therapy [52,115]. Phycobilins are found in the stroma of chloroplasts of cyanobacteria, rhodophytes (red algae), glaucophytes, and some cryptomonads [116]. They forward the energy of the harvested light to chlorophylls for photosynthesis. Similar to carotenoids, those proteins serve as "secondary light-harvesting pigments" [117]. Besides these highly sophisticated applications as chemical tags, phycobilins are also used as food and cosmetic colorants due to their high yield [118].

Lutein is one of the most important carotenoids. Moreover, it is essential to the macula lutea in the retina and lens of eyes. Lutein industrial applications are as a colorant in food products [119]. Cancer, retinal degeneration, and cardiovascular diseases are some of the health applications [119]. As listed before the applications, the commercial potential of lutein from microalgae is high, but its large-scale production has not yet started to our knowledge [120]. Nonetheless, the basis for lutein production outdoors at a pilot scale for *Scenedesmus* has already been set up [121]. Carotenoids properties, which were discussed by Gille et al., [122], make them outstanding as functional foods. One of the most known is ß-carotene for its nature in sustaining growth and vision. Additionally, other carotenoids have been used as important food colorants [123]. That is the case of astaxanthin, another representative of the xanthophyll group of carotenoid pigments for its properties as a powerful antioxidant. It is important for humans to protect the skin from UV light as UV-induced photo-oxidation, antibody production, and anti-tumor therapy [124].

4.2. Nutraceutical Potentialities

Aztecs in Mexico used *Spirulina* sp. as food [125]. The application of these microalgae as food or dietary supplement has continued and have resulted in the research and finding of new species to be used in food applications. Besides direct consumption, derived products are used in food industry as colorants, antioxidants, and natural preservatives. The following paragraphs describe the most representative used species and respective applications. More recently, microalgae were incorporated into pasta, snack foods, candy bars or gums, and beverages as well [85,126]. Owing to their diverse chemical properties, they can act as a nutritional supplement or represent a source of natural food colorants [126]. The most relevant strains to commercial applications are *Chlorella*, *Spirulina*, *Scenedesmus*, and *Nostoc*. The polysaccharides from type β-1,3-glucan are known for its properties of immune-stimulation, reduction of free radicals and blood lipids, this substance is produced by *Chlorella* [127]. In addition, glucan has also benefited the immune system, reduce depression, protect the skin, and has anticancer properties [83,85,109–112]. Finally, phycobiliproteins and chlorophylls can be found as a food additive produced by *P. cruentum* [128].

As mentioned before, *Spirulina* has been used as a supplement in human nutrition. It is worth mentioning as it produces linolenic acid, which humans cannot synthesize [126], proteins, β-carotene, thiamine, riboflavin, vitamin B12. *Spirulina* also showed to be active against hyperlipidemia, hypertension, oxidative stress, arthritis, and serum glucose levels [129]. One attempt to introduce *Spirulina* into diet was by including it into cookies; in this study, the antioxidant properties were explored [130]. The most common microalgae strains used in the industry are *Chlorella* and *Spirulina* thanks to their high protein content and respective aminoacid profile, nutritive value, and standardized growth protocols with high biomass yield [131]. Although *Scenedesmus* was considered a pioneer as a food source, recently its application has been limited, and some extracts have been used in desserts, fruit puddings, and soups [83]. Besides other nutrients, *Scenedesmus* produces eicosapentaenoic acid (EPA), vitamins, and essential minerals [132].

4.3. Bioactive Compounds

Microalga have become a research target since they are a rich source of bioactive compounds [133–135]. The activities of the secondary metabolites isolated from microalga include antibacterial, antifungal, antialgal, antiprotozoal, and antiviral (Table 3). For example, the cyanobacterium *Phormidium* sp. has been reported to inhibit the growth of different Gram-positive and Gram-negative bacterial strains, yeasts, and fungi [136]. *Lyngbya majuscula* [70] that produces polyketides, lipopeptides, cyclic peptides, and many others compounds that have activities such as anti-HIV, anticancer, antifeedant, antifungal, anti-inflammatory, antimicrobial, antiviral, etc. [71]. Other biological activities of these compounds include protein kinase C activators and tumor promoters, inhibitors of microtubulin assembly, antimicrobial and antifungal, and sodium-channel blockers [71]. Antifungal compounds include fisherellin A, hapalindole, carazostatin, phytoalexin, tolytoxin, scytophycin, toyocamycin, tjipanazole, nostocyclamide and nostodione produced by cyanobacteria belonging to *Nostocales* and *Oscillatoriales* (Table 3) [75].

It is also important to mention the production of long-chain polyunsaturated fatty acids (PUFAs) such as eicosapentaenoic acid (EPA), docosahexaenoic acid (DHA), and arachidonic acid (AA) are important for human diet [15]. Besides, PUFAs have been used to prevent and treat chronic inflammations diseases (e.g., rheumatism, skin diseases, and inflammation of the mucosa of the gastrointestinal tract) [70,71]. In addition, studies show a positive effect on cardio-circulatory diseases, coronary heart diseases, atherosclerosis, hypertension, cholesterol, and cancer treatment [83,137]. Arachidonic acid (ARA), an essential component of membrane phospholipids with a function of vasodilator, shows anti-inflammatory effects [138]. Moreover, ARA is necessary for the repair and growth of skeletal muscle tissue and makes it a powerful dietary component in support of the anabolic muscle formulations [139]. The inclusion of *Spirulina* in malnourished children has shown improvement against anemia by increasing hemoglobin, protein, and vitamin levels [140]. Additionally, phycocyanin, γ-linolenic acid, vitamins, phenolic compounds, and minerals can help with malnourished children [141]. The consumption of *S. platensis* and *S. maxima* showed an increase of lactic acid bacteria increase in the gastrointestinal tract [83].

4.4. Bioremediation Potentialities

The ability to metabolize or bio-transform chemicals is one of the many properties of microalgae. Some of the remarkable studies are shown in the following paragraphs, including treatment against petroleum, herbicides, wastewater, etc. The potential of using the microalgae as a tool and profit from it is huge. Cyanobacteria have shown great potential against surfactants and herbicides as well [142–144]. Radwan et al. [145] showed the degradation of petroleum by using a functionalized mat with microalgae, and fluometuron and lindane degradation were investigated by the group of Mansy and El-Bestway [146], showing promising results when using a wide variety of microalgae.

Wastewater treatment by microalgae for the reduction of different contaminants is another bioremediation potential. The case to reduce calcium and chloride by the use of *Oscillatoria* sp. was studied by Uma and Subramanian [147]. Nitrogen and phosphorous reduction in wastewater by microalgae production is a strategy by combining it with bioremediation of amino acids, enzyme, or food industry effluents. *Chlorella, Spirulina,* and *Scenedesmus* are some of the species most used in these systems to reduce the eutrophication in water bodies [148]. The strategy to use the exopolysaccharides (EPS) produced in high amounts by cyanobacteria and microalgae as emulsifiers are driving the researcher's attention. It can be applied to oil, metal, and dye recovery. Further, Matsunaga et al., [149] used *Anabaena* sp. to remove dyes from textile effluent, and *Phormidium autumnale* was used to degrade indigo dye in 20 days [150].

In addition, exopolysaccharides produced by some cyanobacteria have the capacity of capturing heavy metals suspended in water. The proper function of the EPS needs high purity, which is achieved by ionic resins treatment [151]. Moreover, novel studies suggest green extractions as alternative methods to get high purity EPS using membranes, ultrasound, and microwave. The bio-adsorption process occurs when negative charges present in EPS interact with heavy metal ions producing bonds. Chelation of positively charged ions on the microalgal polysaccharides layer is due to a high crosslink number that promotes fast kinetics. In recent literature, it has been demonstrated that the chelation of zinc, copper, cadmium, lead, arsenic, chromium, and mercury for the potential applications for heavy metals removal currently known as biosorption [152,153].

4.5. Bio-Fuels

The use of microalgae to generate biofuels has huge potential due to its oil content, biomass, and hydrocarbons production. The use of microalgae to produce energy is wide, and the biological conversion method of fermentation to generate hydrogen, ethanol, biodiesel, and biogas are the most important [154]. Hydrogen is the most efficient and cleanest energy carrier and *Chlamydomonas*, *Arthrospira*, and *Chlorella* microalgae species possess all the characteristics to photo produce hydrogen gas (Khetkorn et al.) [155]. The increment of photobiological production of hydrogen is related to the carbon content in biomass [156–158]. Other strains of interest are *Anabaena* able to produce hydrogen [159]. Additionally, *S. platensis* can produce hydrogen in dark conditions with photobiological hydrogen production [157].

4.5.1. Photosynthetically Production of Hydrogen

Cyanobacteria can produce hydrogen in two different ways. First, grown under nitrogen limiting conditions, as a byproduct of nitrogen fixation when the species nitrogenase-containing heterocysts. Second, a reversible activity of hydrogenases enzymes [160]. The two microalgae species studied for hydrogen production were *Anabaena* and *Scenedesmus*. When *Anabaena* was placed into a glass jar it produced hydrogen gas, and after a period of dark anaerobic "adaptation", *Scenedesmus* sp. produces hydrogen at low rates, greatly stimulated by short periods of light [161,162].

4.5.2. Biodiesel/Bioethanol

The substitute for conventional diesel is biodiesel, the result of transesterification of lipids. The production of biodiesel is currently done by processing oily seeds from palm, castor bean, sunflower, corn, and cotton, among others [163–165]. As discussed before, microalgae are a huge producer of fatty acids that can be converted into biodiesel [59]. For instance, around 50% of *Chlorella, Nannochloropsis, Dunaliella, Scenedesmus,* and *Scenedesmus* composition are lipids. Microalgae biofuel has a high calorific value, low viscosity, and low-density properties turning it in a more suitable biofuel than lignocellulosic materials [166].

Among other benefits, the use of ethanol as combustible reduces levels of lead, sulfur, carbon monoxide, and particulates [167]. Normally, ethanol is produced from sugar from byproducts of sugar cane and corn through fermentation of biomass [168]. Microalgae have the fermentable potential substrate since they have high levels of carbon compounds, directly available or after a pre-treatment. Some fermentable microalgae, such as *Chlorella* sp., *Oscillatoria* sp., and *S. platensis,* have already been used to produce ethanol [169]. The ethanol should then be purified and used as efficient fuel and the CO_2 can be recycled in the cultivation of more microalgae or use of residual biomass in the process of anaerobic digestion [170].

4.6. Antioxidants

Microalgae are rich in vitamins [85,112]. They can also accumulate vitamin E and fat-soluble phenols with antioxidant properties. Vitamin E has a wide range of applications. Some of its applications in medicine are to treat cancer, heart, eye, Alzheimer's, Parkinson's disease, and other medical conditions [171]. Harvested microalgae are used in the food industry as added preservatives, health-improving additives, and for photoprotection in skin creams [172].

Phycocyanin purified from cyanobacterium *Synechococcus* sp. R42DM showed antioxidant activity in vitro and in vivo. The cyanobacterium was isolated from a polluted industrial site in India [141].

The conditions showed stability in thermal and oxidative stress with *Caenorhabditis elegans* [141]. *Geitlerinema* sp. H8DM is another microalgae that produced a variation of phycocyanin [173].

4.7. Phycotoxins

One of the groups of microalgae responsible for producing phycotoxins are dinoflagellates that lead to harmful algal blooms and "red tides" [174]. Although, the same microalgae can produce a wide spectrum of secondary metabolites that may be applied to therapy as antitumor, antibiotic, antifungal, immunosuppressant, cytotoxic, and neurotoxic named as phycotoxins [175]. The other group is cyanobacteria. For example, *Nostoc* species are responsible for freshwater toxins with a potential pharmaceutical use such as borophycin used against human carcinoma, borophycin-8 as antibiotic, apratoxin A as a cytotoxin and anticancer, among another more than 30 metabolites [176,177]. Further, *Anabaena* produces bromoana-indolone, an antibiotic compound, along with balticidins and laxaphycins, antifungal metabolites against *Candida albicans*, *Penicillium notatum*, *Saccharomyces cerevisiae*, and *Trichophyton mentagrophytes*. The same species *Anabaena* produces sulfoglycolipids, antivirals that can inhibit the HIV-1 virus. Other antivirus families are lectins, e.g., cyanovirin-N which are produced by *Nostoc* sp. that prevents HI virus infections. It is effective against influenza A and B as well [178].

5. Opportunities for Improvement

Drug discovery through microalgae biotechnology is under-represented in the current pharmaceutical industry. Nevertheless, drug development by natural means like microalgae gives several advantages such as water solubility, membrane permeability, biodegradability, bioavailability, and biocompatibility [7]. Aquaculture feeds require a large volume of biomass for fish, mollusks, and crustaceans. However, accumulation of biomass can be difficult and expensive, but the inclusion of microalgal increases dietary value to feed with essential amino acids, fatty acids, high-quality protein, vitamins, micronutrients, and carotenoids [179]. Products from fisheries and aquaculture combined are supplying the world with 142 million tons of protein every year with a market value of 106 billion dollars calculated in 2008 [179].

Biofuels in the form of gas and liquid products are gaining impact by the world regulations of green economies. The use of microalgae to produce enzymes to be included in specific catalyze processes to generate combustibles. For instance, biodiesel is an opportunity with enzyme-chemistry [180]. More important is to address high-value products, as turbocine with more caloric power for future perspectives and include secondary products generated in the process to stack value and impact the current market. Carbon dioxide capture is another opportunity for microalgae. The utilization of microalgae cultures in industrial processes can capture harmful gas emissions [181]. The accumulation of carbon dioxide can be applied under specific conditions to match with proper algal strains in their mechanisms of photosynthesis, leading to a decrease in pollution and produce biomass [182].

The biopolymer field is a branch of chemistry and material science where the application of novel technologies are required to produce bioplastics. An urgent large-scale production of biodegradable materials for common use, like packaging and containers, is far from current technology. However, the application of biocompatible and biodegradable plastics with zero toxicity to mammal cells offers the initial impulse to study the production of chitosan, cellulose, polyhydroxyalkanoates, and other biopolymers by microalgae. A hot topic is the utilization of scaffolds to support cellular growth in prosthesis and patches to treat skin burns, and missing or destroyed bones [183]. Biosorption is a removal process of potentially toxic elements where adsorption, chelation, ion exchange, and surface precipitation may occur. Through microalgae, heavy metals can be removed from municipal and industrial wastewaters [153]. Its potential increases with the lack of fresh water and recently with the detection of emerging contaminants as pesticides and drug wastes from pharmacological industries [184].

6. Concluding Remarks and Future Perspectives

Discovery, isolation, and preservation of novel microalgae strains are evident as we showed in Table 1, where a large number of species were enumerated in recent years. Still, many more are waiting to be discovered in the vast fresh and marine water resources in Mexico. An opportunity to generate green solutions to local problems through science, innovation, technology development, and transfer becomes one of the most important objectives for the field of microalgae biotechnology applications. Investment in biodiversity has a relevant impact on preserving and studying the natural resources in the country. However, attractive applications for industry investment are imperative to have relevant participation in research. In addition, the involvement of industry, society, and the research community helps to protect Mexico's biodiversity. A green economy means political strategies towards a low-carbon economy, resource efficiency, green investments, technological innovation and more recycling, green jobs, poverty eradication, and social inclusion. The whole idea points to a higher support for novel technologies that help in the mentioned point, especially towards the knowledge development of involving local ecosystems. Local and global problems list include waste management, water treatment and emerging pollutants with potential opportunities to provide innovative solutions. A close collaboration between society, industry, and research institutions will lead to the path for a sustainable development.

Author Contributions: Juan Eduardo Sosa-Hernández and Hafiz M. N. Iqbal conceptualized the overall layout and contents of the review. Kenya D. Romero-Castillo, Lizeth Parra-Arroyo, Mauricio A. Aguilar-Aguila-Isaías, and Isaac E. García-Reyes collected and analyzed the literature and compiled the initial draft. Lizeth Parra-Arroyo, Mauricio A. Aguilar-Aguila-Isaías, and Isaac E. García-Reyes designed the Figures. Juan Eduardo Sosa-Hernández and Kenya D. Romero-Castillo summarized the Tables. Ishtiaq Ahmed, and Roberto Parra-Saldivar pre-checked the collected literature and drafted the manuscript. Muhammad Bilal and Hafiz M. N. Iqbal made revisions and final editing of the final version. Hafiz M. N. Iqbal processed for publication. All the authors read and approved the final manuscript.

Funding: This research received no external funding. The APC (ID: marinedrugs-454602) was funded by MDPI, St. Alban-Anlage 66, 4052 Basel, Switzerland.

Acknowledgments: All authors are grateful to their representative institutes for providing literature facilities. The authors also appreciate the additional support from the Emerging Technologies Research Group of Tecnologico de Monterrey, Mexico. The first author (Juan Eduardo Sosa-Hernández) thankfully acknowledges a postdoctoral fellowship provided by Consejo Nacional de Ciencia y Tecnología (CONACYT), Mexico.

Conflicts of Interest: The authors declare no conflict of interest.

References

1. Centella, M.H.; Arévalo-Gallegos, A.; Parra-Saldivar, R.; Iqbal, H.M. Marine-derived bioactive compounds for value-added applications in bio-and non-bio sectors. *J. Clean. Prod.* **2017**, *168*, 1559–1565. [CrossRef]
2. Posten, C. *Microalgae Biotechnology*; Chen, S.F., Ed.; Springer International Publishing: Berlin/Heidelberg, Germany, 2016.
3. Kasting, J.F.; Siefert, J.L. Life and the evolution of Earth's atmosphere. *Science* **2002**, *296*, 1066–1068. [CrossRef] [PubMed]
4. Arbib, Z.; Ruiz, J.; Álvarez-Díaz, P.; Garrido-Perez, C.; Perales, J.A. Capability of different microalgae species for phytoremediation processes: Wastewater tertiary treatment, CO_2 bio-fixation and low cost biofuels production. *Water Res.* **2014**, *49*, 465–474. [CrossRef] [PubMed]
5. Lei, A.P.; Hu, Z.L.; Wong, Y.S.; Tam, N.F.Y. Removal of fluoranthene and pyrene by different microalgal species. *Bioresour. Technol.* **2007**, *98*, 273–280. [CrossRef] [PubMed]
6. Mennaa, F.Z.; Arbib, Z.; Perales, J.A. Urban wastewater treatment by seven species of microalgae and an algal bloom: Biomass production, N and P removal kinetics and harvestability. *Water Res.* **2015**, *83*, 42–51. [CrossRef]
7. Olaizola, M. Commercial development of microalgal biotechnology: From the test tube to the marketplace. *Biomol. Eng.* **2003**, *20*, 459–466. [CrossRef]
8. Farrar, W.V. Tecuitlatl; a glimpse of Aztec food technology. *Nature* **1966**, *211*, 341–342. [CrossRef]

9. Burlew, J.S. *Algal Culture. From Laboratory to Pilot Plant*; Carnegie Institution of Washington Publication: Washington, DC, USA, 1953; Volume 600.
10. Belay, A.; Gershwin, M.E. Spirulina (Arthrospira). In *Spirulina in Human Nutrition and Health*; CRC Press: Boca Raton, FL, USA, 2007; pp. 11–35.
11. Spolaore, P.; Joannis-Cassan, C.; Duran, E.; Isambert, A. Commercial applications of microalgae. *J. Biosci. Bioeng.* **2006**, *101*, 87–96. [CrossRef]
12. Ben-Amotz, A. Industrial production of microalgal cell-mass and secondary products-major industrial species. In *Handbook of Microalgal Culture: Biotechnology and Applied Phycology*; Blackwell Publishing Ltd.: Hoboken, NJ, USA, 2004; Volume 273.
13. Lamers, P.P.; Janssen, M.; De Vos, R.C.; Bino, R.J.; Wijffels, R.H. Exploring and exploiting carotenoid accumulation in Dunaliella salina for cell-factory applications. *Trends Biotechnol.* **2008**, *26*, 631–638. [CrossRef]
14. Jorquera, O.; Kiperstok, A.; Sales, E.A.; Embirucu, M.; Ghirardi, M.L. Comparative energy life-cycle analyses of microalgal biomass production in open ponds and photobioreactors. *Bioresour. Technol.* **2010**, *101*, 1406–1413. [CrossRef]
15. Pulz, O.; Gross, W. Valuable products from biotechnology of microalgae. *Appl. Microbiol. Biotechnol.* **2004**, *65*, 635–648. [CrossRef]
16. Myers, N.; Mittermeier, R.A.; Mittermeier, C.G.; Da Fonseca, G.A.; Kent, J. Biodiversity hotspots for conservation priorities. *Nature* **2000**, *403*, 853. [CrossRef]
17. Oliva-Martínez, M.G.; Godínez-Ortega, J.L.; Zuñiga-Ramos, C.A. Biodiversidad del fitoplancton de aguas continentales en México. *Rev. Mex. Biodivers.* **2014**, *85*, 54–61. [CrossRef]
18. Muciño-Márquez, R.E.; Figueroa-Torres, M.G.; Aguirre-León, A. Cianofitas de los sistemas fluvio-lagunares Pom-Atasta y Palizada del Este, adyacentes a la Laguna de Términos, Campeche, México. *Polibotánica* **2015**, *39*, 49–78. [CrossRef]
19. Jiménez-Valera, S.; del Pilar Sánchez-Saavedra, M. Growth and fatty acid profiles of microalgae species isolated from the Baja California Peninsula, México. *Lat. Am. J. Aquat. Res.* **2016**, *44*, 689–702. [CrossRef]
20. Dávila-Camacho, C.A.; Galaviz-Villa, I.; Lango-Reynoso, F.; Castañeda-Chávez, M.D.R.; Quiroga-Brahms, C.; Montoya-Mendoza, J. Cultivation of native fish in Mexico: Cases of success. *Rev. Aquac.* **2018**. [CrossRef]
21. Rodríguez-Palacio, M.C.; Crisóstomo-Vázquez, L.; Álvarez-Hernández, S.; Lozano-Ramírez, C. Strains of toxic and harmful microalgae, from waste water, marine, brackish and fresh water. *Food Addit. Contam. Part A* **2012**, *29*, 304–313. [CrossRef]
22. Ciferri, O.; Tiboni, O. The biochemistry and industrial potential of Spirulina. *Annu. Rev. Microbiol.* **1985**, *39*, 503–526. [CrossRef]
23. Pacheco-Vega, J.M.; Cadena-Roa, M.A.; Ascencio, F.; Rangel-Dávalos, C.; Rojas-Contreras, M. Assessment of endemic microalgae as potential food for Artemia franciscana culture. *Lat. Am. J. Aquat. Res.* **2015**, *43*, 23–32. [CrossRef]
24. Ramírez-Moreno, L.; Olvera-Ramírez, R. Uso tradicional y actual de *Spirulina* sp. (*Arthrospira* sp.). *Interciencia* **2006**, *31*, 657–663.
25. Cea-Barcia, G.; Buitrón, G.; Moreno, G.; Kumar, G. A cost-effective strategy for the bio-prospecting of mixed microalgae with high carbohydrate content: Diversity fluctuations in different growth media. *Bioresour. Technol.* **2014**, *163*, 370–373. [CrossRef]
26. Alcocer, J.; Hammer, U.T. Saline lake ecosystems of Mexico. *Aquat. Ecosyst. Health Manag.* **1998**, *1*, 291–315. [CrossRef]
27. Toledo, G.; Bashan, Y.; Soeldner, A. Cyanobacteria and black mangroves in Northwestern Mexico: Colonization, and diurnal and seasonal nitrogen fixation on aerial roots. *Can. J. Microbiol.* **1995**, *41*, 999–1011. [CrossRef]
28. Reyna-Martinez, R.; Gomez-Flores, R.; López-Chuken, U.; Quintanilla-Licea, R.; Caballero-Hernandez, D.; Rodríguez-Padilla, C.; Beltrán-Rocha, J.C.; Tamez-Guerra, P. Antitumor activity of Chlorella sorokiniana and Scenedesmus sp. microalgae native of Nuevo León State, México. *PeerJ* **2018**, *6*, e4358. [CrossRef]
29. Poot-Delgado, C.A.; Okolodkov, Y.B.; Aké-Castillo, J.A. Potentially harmful cyanobacteria in oyster banks of Términos lagoon, southeastern Gulf of Mexico. *Acta Biológica Colomb.* **2018**, *23*, 51–58. [CrossRef]
30. León-Tejera, H.; Montejano, G. Dermocarpella (Cyanoprokaryota/Cyanophyceae/Cyanobacteria) from the pacific coast of Mexico. *Cryptogam. Algol.* **2000**, *21*, 259–272. [CrossRef]

31. Valadez, C.F.; Carmona, J.; Cantoral, U.E. Algas de ambientes lóticos en el estado de Morelos, México. *An. Inst. Biol. Ser. Bot.* **1996**, *67*, 227–282.
32. Komolafe, O.; Orta, S.B.V.; Monje-Ramirez, I.; Noguez, I.Y.; Harvey, A.P.; Ledesma, M.T.O. Biodiesel production from indigenous microalgae grown in wastewater. *Bioresour. Technol.* **2014**, *154*, 297–304. [CrossRef]
33. Toledo-Cervantes, A.; Morales, M.; Novelo, E.; Revah, S. Carbon dioxide fixation and lipid storage by Scenedesmus obtusiusculus. *Bioresour. Technol.* **2013**, *130*, 652–658. [CrossRef]
34. Arzate-Cárdenas, M.A.; Olvera-Ramírez, R.; Martínez-Jerónimo, F. Microcystis toxigenic strains in urban lakes: A case of study in Mexico City. *Ecotoxicology* **2010**, *19*, 1157–1165. [CrossRef]
35. Alvarez-Hernandez, S.; De Lara-Isassi, G.; Arreguin-Espinoza, R.; Arreguin, B.; Hernandez-Santoyo, A.; Rodriguez-Romero, A. Isolation and partial characterization of giraffine, a lectin from the Mexican endemic alga Codium giraffa Silva. *Bot. Mar.* **1999**, *42*, 573–580. [CrossRef]
36. Servín-Garcidueñas, L.E.; Martínez-Romero, E. Complete mitochondrial and plastid genomes of the green microalga Trebouxiophyceae sp. strain MX-AZ01 isolated from a highly acidic geothermal lake. *Eukaryot. Cell* **2012**, *11*, 1417–1418. [CrossRef]
37. Pena-Pereira, F.; Kloskowski, A.; Namieśnik, J. Perspectives on the replacement of harmful organic solvents in analytical methodologies: A framework toward the implementation of a generation of eco-friendly alternatives. *Green Chem.* **2015**, *17*, 3687–3705. [CrossRef]
38. Sosa-Hernández, J.; Escobedo-Avellaneda, Z.; Iqbal, H.; Welti-Chanes, J. State-of-the-Art Extraction Methodologies for Bioactive Compounds from Algal Biome to Meet Bio-Economy Challenges and Opportunities. *Molecules* **2018**, *23*, 2953. [CrossRef] [PubMed]
39. Choi, W.Y.; Lee, H.Y. Effect of Ultrasonic Extraction on Production and Structural Changes of C-Phycocyanin from Marine Spirulina maxima. *Int. J. Mol. Sci.* **2018**, *19*, 220. [CrossRef] [PubMed]
40. Singh, Y.; Mazumder, A.; Giri, A.; Mishra, H.N. Optimization of Ultrasound-Assisted Extraction of β-Carotene from Chlorella Biomass (MCC7) and its Use in Fortification of Apple Jam. *J. Food Process Eng.* **2017**, *40*, e12321. [CrossRef]
41. da Silva, M.F.; Casazza, A.A.; Ferrari, P.F.; Aliakbarian, B.; Converti, A.; Bezerra, R.P.; Porto, A.L.F.; Perego, P. Recovery of phenolic compounds of food concern from Arthrospira platensis by green extraction techniques. *Algal Res.* **2017**, *25*, 391–401. [CrossRef]
42. Guldhe, A.; Singh, B.; Rawat, I.; Bux, F. Synthesis of biodiesel from Scenedesmus sp. by microwave and ultrasound assisted in situ transesterification using tungstated zirconia as a solid acid catalyst. *Chem. Eng. Res. Des.* **2014**, *92*, 1503–1511. [CrossRef]
43. Lorenzen, J.; Igl, N.; Tippelt, M.; Stege, A.; Qoura, F.; Sohling, U.; Brück, T. Extraction of microalgae derived lipids with supercritical carbon dioxide in an industrial relevant pilot plant. *Bioprocess Biosyst. Eng.* **2017**, *40*, 911–918. [CrossRef] [PubMed]
44. Crampon, C.; Nikitine, C.; Zaier, M.; Lépine, O.; Tanzi, C.D.; Vian, M.A.; Chemat, F.; Badens, E. Oil extraction from enriched Spirulina platensis microalgae using supercritical carbon dioxide. *J. Supercrit. Fluids* **2017**, *119*, 289–296. [CrossRef]
45. He, B.; Wang, Y.; Dou, X.; Chen, Y.F. Supercritical CO_2 extraction of docosahexaenoic acid from Schizochytrium limacinum using vegetable oils as entrainer. *Algal Res.* **2017**, *21*, 58–63. [CrossRef]
46. Albarelli, J.Q.; Santos, D.T.; Ensinas, A.V.; Marechal, F.; Cocero, M.J.; Meireles, M.A.A. Comparison of extraction techniques for product diversification in a supercritical water gasification-based sugarcane-wet microalgae biorefinery: Thermoeconomic and environmental analysis. *J. Clean. Prod.* **2018**, *201*, 697–705. [CrossRef]
47. Araujo, G.S.; Matos, L.J.; Fernandes, J.O.; Cartaxo, S.J.; Gonçalves, L.R.; Fernandes, F.A.; Farias, W.R. Extraction of lipids from microalgae by ultrasound application: Prospection of the optimal extraction method. *Ultrason. Sonochem.* **2013**, *20*, 95–98. [CrossRef]
48. Ma, Q.Y.; Fang, M.; Zheng, J.H.; Ren, D.F.; Lu, J. Optimised extraction of β-carotene from Spirulina platensis and hypoglycaemic effect in streptozotocin-induced diabetic mice. *J. Sci. Food Agric.* **2016**, *96*, 1783–1789. [CrossRef]
49. Esquivel-Hernández, D.A.; Ibarra-Garza, I.P.; Rodríguez-Rodríguez, J.; Cuéllar-Bermúdez, S.P.; Rostro-Alanis, M.D.J.; Alemán-Nava, G.S.; García-Pérez, J.S.; Parra-Saldívar, R. Green extraction technologies for high-value metabolites from algae: A review. *Biofuels Bioprod. Biorefining* **2017**, *11*, 215–231. [CrossRef]

50. Ma, Y.A.; Cheng, Y.M.; Huang, J.W.; Jen, J.F.; Huang, Y.S.; Yu, C.C. Effects of ultrasonic and microwave pretreatments on lipid extraction of microalgae. *Bioprocess Biosyst. Eng.* **2014**, *37*, 1543–1549. [CrossRef] [PubMed]
51. Zinnai, A.; Sanmartin, C.; Taglieri, I.; Andrich, G.; Venturi, F. Supercritical fluid extraction from microalgae with high content of LC-PUFAs. A case of study: Sc-CO_2 oil extraction from Schizochytrium sp. *J. Supercrit. Fluids* **2016**, *116*, 126–131. [CrossRef]
52. Tavanandi, H.A.; Mittal, R.; Chandrasekhar, J.; Raghavarao, K.S.M.S. Simple and efficient method for extraction of C-Phycocyanin from dry biomass of Arthospira platensis. *Algal Res.* **2018**, *31*, 239–251. [CrossRef]
53. Obeid, S.; Beaufils, N.; Camy, S.; Takache, H.; Ismail, A.; Pontalier, P.Y. Supercritical carbon dioxide extraction and fractionation of lipids from freeze-dried microalgae Nannochloropsis oculata and Chlorella vulgaris. *Algal Res.* **2018**, *34*, 49–56. [CrossRef]
54. Kong, W.; Liu, N.; Zhang, J.; Yang, Q.; Hua, S.; Song, H.; Xia, C. Optimization of ultrasound-assisted extraction parameters of chlorophyll from Chlorella vulgaris residue after lipid separation using response surface methodology. *J. Food Sci. Technol.* **2014**, *51*, 2006–2013. [CrossRef]
55. Ido, A.L.; de Luna, M.D.G.; Capareda, S.C.; Maglinao, A.L., Jr.; Nam, H. Application of central composite design in the optimization of lipid yield from Scenedesmus obliquus microalgae by ultrasonic-assisted solvent extraction. *Energy* **2018**, *157*, 949–956. [CrossRef]
56. Balasubramanian, S.; Allen, J.D.; Kanitkar, A.; Boldor, D. Oil extraction from Scenedesmus obliquus using a continuous microwave system–design, optimization, and quality characterization. *Bioresour. Technol.* **2011**, *102*, 3396–3403. [CrossRef]
57. Pasquet, V.; Chérouvrier, J.R.; Farhat, F.; Thiéry, V.; Piot, J.M.; Bérard, J.B.; Kaas, R.; Serive, B.; Patrice, T.; Cadoret, J.P.; et al. Study on the microalgal pigments extraction process: Performance of microwave assisted extraction. *Process Biochem.* **2011**, *46*, 59–67. [CrossRef]
58. Vinatoru, M.; Mason, T.J.; Calinescu, I. Ultrasonically assisted extraction (UAE) and microwave assisted extraction (MAE) of functional compounds from plant materials. *TrAC Trends Anal. Chem.* **2017**, *97*, 159–178. [CrossRef]
59. Harris, J.; Viner, K.; Champagne, P.; Jessop, P.G. Advances in microalgal lipid extraction for biofuel production: A review. *Biofuels Bioprod. Biorefining* **2018**, *12*, 1118–1135. [CrossRef]
60. Kumar, S.J.; Kumar, G.V.; Dash, A.; Scholz, P.; Banerjee, R. Sustainable green solvents and techniques for lipid extraction from microalgae: A review. *Algal Res.* **2017**, *21*, 138–147. [CrossRef]
61. Mendes, R.L.; Nobre, B.P.; Cardoso, M.T.; Pereira, A.P.; Palavra, A.F. Supercritical carbon dioxide extraction of compounds with pharmaceutical importance from microalgae. *Inorg. Chim. Acta* **2003**, *356*, 328–334. [CrossRef]
62. de Aguiar, A.C.; Osorio-Tobón, J.F.; Silva, L.P.S.; Barbero, G.F.; Martínez, J. Economic analysis of oleoresin production from malagueta peppers (Capsicum frutescens) by supercritical fluid extraction. *J. Supercrit. Fluids* **2018**, *133*, 86–93. [CrossRef]
63. Hatami, T.; Johner, J.C.F.; Meireles, M.A.A. Extraction and fractionation of fennel using supercritical fluid extraction assisted by cold pressing. *Ind. Crop. Prod.* **2018**, *123*, 661–666. [CrossRef]
64. Johner, J.C.; Hatami, T.; Meireles, M.A.A. Developing a supercritical fluid extraction method assisted by cold pressing for extraction of pequi (Caryocar brasiliense). *J. Supercrit. Fluids* **2018**, *137*, 34–39. [CrossRef]
65. Solana, M.; Rizza, C.S.; Bertucco, A. Exploiting microalgae as a source of essential fatty acids by supercritical fluid extraction of lipids: Comparison between *Scenedesmus obliquus, Chlorella protothecoides* and *Nannochloropsis salina*. *J. Supercrit. Fluids* **2014**, *92*, 311–318. [CrossRef]
66. Feller, R.; Matos, Â.P.; Mazzutti, S.; Moecke, E.H.; Tres, M.V.; Derner, R.B.; Oliveira, J.V.; Junior, A.F. Polyunsaturated ω-3 and ω-6 fatty acids, total carotenoids and antioxidant activity of three marine microalgae extracts obtained by supercritical CO 2 and subcritical n-butane. *J. Supercrit. Fluids* **2018**, *133*, 437–443. [CrossRef]
67. Wei, F.; Gao, G.Z.; Wang, X.F.; Dong, X.Y.; Li, P.P.; Hua, W.; Wang, X.; Wu, X.M.; Chen, H. Quantitative determination of oil content in small quantity of oilseed rape by ultrasound-assisted extraction combined with gas chromatography. *Ultrason. Sonochem.* **2008**, *15*, 938–942. [CrossRef]
68. Mercer, P.; Armenta, R.E. Developments in oil extraction from microalgae. *Eur. J. Lipid Sci. Technol.* **2011**, *113*, 539–547. [CrossRef]

69. Klejdus, B.; Lojková, L.; Plaza, M.; Šnóblová, M.; Štěrbová, D. Hyphenated technique for the extraction and determination of isoflavones in algae: Ultrasound-assisted supercritical fluid extraction followed by fast chromatography with tandem mass spectrometry. *J. Chromatogr. A* **2010**, *1217*, 7956–7965. [CrossRef]
70. Burja, A.M.; Banaigs, B.; Abou-Mansour, E.; Burgess, J.G.; Wright, P.C. Marine cyanobacteria—A prolific source of natural products. *Tetrahedron* **2001**, *57*, 9347–9377. [CrossRef]
71. Shimizu, Y. Microalgal metabolites. *Curr. Opin. Microbiol.* **2003**, *6*, 236–243. [CrossRef]
72. Reshef, V.; Mizrachi, E.; Maretzki, T.; Silberstein, C.; Loya, S.; Hizi, A.; Carmeli, S. New acylated sulfoglycolipids and digalactolipids and related known glycolipids from cyanobacteria with a potential to inhibit the reverse transcriptase of HIV-1. *J. Nat. Prod.* **1997**, *60*, 1251–1260. [CrossRef] [PubMed]
73. Hayashi, K.; Hayashi, T.; Kojima, I. A natural sulfated polysaccharide, calcium spirulan, isolated from Spirulina platensis: In vitro and ex vivo evaluation of anti-herpes simplex virus and anti-human immunodeficiency virus activities. *AIDS Res. Hum. Retrovir.* **1996**, *12*, 1463–1471. [CrossRef]
74. Moore, R.E.; Patterson, G.M.; Carmichael, W.W. New pharmaceuticals from cultured blue-green algae. *Biomed. Importance Mar. Org.* **1988**, *13*, 143–150.
75. Dahms, H.-U.; Xu, Y.; Pfeiffer, C. Antifouling potential of cyanobacteria: A mini-review. *Biofouling* **2006**, *22*, 317–327. [CrossRef] [PubMed]
76. Piccaglia, R.; Marotti, M.; Grandi, S. Lutein and lutein ester content in different types of Tagetes patula and T. erecta. *Ind. Crop. Prod.* **1998**, *8*, 45–51. [CrossRef]
77. Blanco, A.M.; Moreno, J.; Del Campo, J.A.; Rivas, J.; Guerrero, M.G. Outdoor cultivation of lutein-rich cells of Muriellopsis sp. in open ponds. *Appl. Microbiol. Biotechnol.* **2007**, *73*, 1259–1266. [CrossRef] [PubMed]
78. Choudhari, S.M.; Ananthanarayan, L.; Singhal, R.S. Use of metabolic stimulators and inhibitors for enhanced production of β-carotene and lycopene by Blakeslea trispora NRRL 2895 and 2896. *Bioresour. Technol.* **2008**, *99*, 3166–3173. [CrossRef]
79. Sánchez, J.F.; Fernández-Sevilla, J.M.; Acién, F.G.; Cerón, M.C.; Pérez-Parra, J.; Molina-Grima, E. Biomass and lutein productivity of Scenedesmus almeriensis: Influence of irradiance, dilution rate and temperature. *Appl. Microbiol. Biotechnol.* **2008**, *79*, 719–729. [CrossRef]
80. Fernández-Sevilla, J.M.; Fernández, F.A.; Grima, E.M. Biotechnological production of lutein and its applications. *Appl. Microbiol. Biotechnol.* **2010**, *86*, 27–40. [CrossRef]
81. Cohen, Z. Production of polyunsaturated fatty acids (EPA, ARA, and GLA) by the microalgae Porphyridium and Spirulina. *Ind. Appl. Single Cell Oils* **1992**, 243–273.
82. Mao, T.K.; Water, J.V.D.; Gershwin, M.E. Effects of a Spirulina-based dietary supplement on cytokine production from allergic rhinitis patients. *J. Med. Food* **2005**, *8*, 27–30. [CrossRef]
83. Barrow, C.; Shahidi, F. (Eds.) *Marine Nutraceuticals and Functional Foods*; CRC Press: Boca Raton, FL, USA, 2007.
84. Becker, E.W. *Microalgae: Biotechnology and Microbiology*; Cambridge University Press: Cambridge, UK, 1994; Volume 10.
85. Becker, W. Microalgae in Human and Animal Nutrition. In *Handbook of Microalgal Culture: Biotechnology and Applied Phycology*; Blackwell Publishing Ltd.: Hoboken, NJ, USA, 2004; Volume 312.
86. Rasmussen, R.S.; Morrissey, M.T. Marine biotechnology for production of food ingredients. *Adv. Food Nutr. Res.* **2007**, *52*, 237–292.
87. García-González, A.; Ochoa, J.L. Anti-inflammatory activity of Debaryomyces hansenii Cu, Zn-SOD. *Arch. Med. Res.* **1999**, *30*, 69–73. [CrossRef]
88. Guzmán-Murillo, M.A.; López-Bolaños, C.C.; Ledesma-Verdejo, T.; Roldan-Libenson, G.; Cadena-Roa, M.A.; Ascencio, F. Effects of fertilizer-based culture media on the production of exocellular polysaccharides and cellular superoxide dismutase by Phaeodactylum tricornutum (Bohlin). *J. Appl. Phycol.* **2007**, *19*, 33–41. [CrossRef]
89. Priya, B.; Premanandh, J.; Dhanalakshmi, R.T.; Seethalakshmi, T.; Uma, L.; Prabaharan, D.; Subramanian, G. Comparative analysis of cyanobacterial superoxide dismutases to discriminate canonical forms. *BMC Genom.* **2007**, *8*, 435. [CrossRef] [PubMed]
90. Thepenier, C.; Chaumont, D.; Gudin, C. Mass culture of Porphyridium cruentum: A multiproduct stategy for the biomass valorisation. In *Algal Biotechnology*; Stadler, T., Ed.; Elsevier Applied Science Publishers: London, UK, 1988; pp. 413–420.

91. Antia, N.J.; Desai, I.D.; Romilly, M.J. The tocopherol, vitamin K, and related isoprenoid quinone composition of a unicellular red alga (Porphyridium cruentum). *J. Phycol.* **1970**, *6*, 305–312.
92. Shi, X.M.; Chen, F. High yield production of lutein by heterotrophic Chlorella protothecoides in fed-batch systems. In *Algae and Their Biotechnological Potential*; Springer: Dordrecht, The Netherlands, 2001; pp. 107–119.
93. Arya, V.; Gupta, V.K. A review on marine immunomodulators. *Int. J. Pharm. Life Sci.* **2011**, *2*, 751–758.
94. Xiong, F.; Kopecky, J.; Nedbal, L. The occurrence of UV-B absorbing mycosporine-like amino acids in freshwater and terrestrial microalgae (Chlorophyta). *Aquat. Bot.* **1999**, *63*, 37–49. [CrossRef]
95. Chu, W.L. Biotechnological applications of microalgae. *IeJSME* **2012**, *6*, S24–S37.
96. Duval, B.; Shetty, K.; Thomas, W.H. Phenolic compounds and antioxidant properties in the snow alga Chlamydomonas nivalis after exposure to UV light. *J. Appl. Phycol.* **1999**, *11*, 559. [CrossRef]
97. Karsten, U.; Lembcke, S.; Schumann, R. The effects of ultraviolet radiation on photosynthetic performance, growth and sunscreen compounds in aeroterrestrial biofilm algae isolated from building facades. *Planta* **2007**, *225*, 991–1000. [CrossRef]
98. Matsukawa, R.; Hotta, M.; Masuda, Y.; Chihara, M.; Karube, I. Antioxidants from carbon dioxide fixing Chlorella sorokiniana. *J. Appl. Phycol.* **2000**, *12*, 263–267. [CrossRef]
99. Barbosa, M.J.; Zijffers, J.W.; Nisworo, A.; Vaes, W.; van Schoonhoven, J.; Wijffels, R.H. Optimization of biomass, vitamins, and carotenoid yield on light energy in a flat-panel reactor using the A-stat technique. *Biotechnol. Bioeng.* **2005**, *89*, 233–242. [CrossRef]
100. Egeland, E.S.; Guillard, R.R.; Liaaen-Jensen, S. Additional carotenoid prototype representatives and a general chemosystematic evaluation of carotenoids in Prasinophyceae (Chlorophyta). *Phytochemistry* **1997**, *44*, 1087–1097. [CrossRef]
101. Cha, K.H.; Koo, S.Y.; Lee, D.U. Antiproliferative effects of carotenoids extracted from Chlorella ellipsoidea and Chlorella vulgaris on human colon cancer cells. *J. Agric. Food Chem.* **2008**, *56*, 10521–10526. [CrossRef]
102. Leya, T.; Rahn, A.; Lütz, C.; Remias, D. Response of arctic snow and permafrost algae to high light and nitrogen stress by changes in pigment composition and applied aspects for biotechnology. *FEMS Microbiol. Ecol.* **2009**, *67*, 432–443. [CrossRef] [PubMed]
103. Ramaraj, S.; Hemaiswarya, S.; Raja, R.; Ganesan, V.; Anbazhagan, C.; Carvalho, I.S.; Juntawong, N. Microalgae as an attractive source for biofuel production. In *Environmental Sustainability*; Springer: New Delhi, India, 2015; pp. 129–157.
104. Mata, T.M.; Martins, A.A.; Caetano, N.S. Microalgae for biodiesel production and other applications: A review. *Renew. Sustain. Energy Rev.* **2010**, *14*, 217–232. [CrossRef]
105. Reitan, K.I.; Rainuzzo, J.R.; Olsen, Y. Effect of nutrient limitation on fatty acid and lipid content of marine microalgae 1. *J. Phycol.* **1994**, *30*, 972–979. [CrossRef]
106. Cheng-Wu, Z.; Cohen, Z.; Khozin-Goldberg, I.; Richmond, A. Characterization of growth and arachidonic acid production of Parietochloris incisa comb. nov (Trebouxiophyceae, Chlorophyta). *J. Appl. Phycol.* **2002**, *14*, 453–460. [CrossRef]
107. Ponomarenko, L.P.; Stonik, I.V.; Aizdaicher, N.A.; Orlova, T.Y.; Popovskaya, G.I.; Pomazkina, G.V.; Stonik, V.A. Sterols of marine microalgae Pyramimonas cf. cordata (Prasinophyta), Attheya ussurensis sp. nov.(Bacillariophyta) and a spring diatom bloom from Lake Baikal. *Comp. Biochem. Physiol. Part B Biochem. Mol. Biol.* **2004**, *138*, 65–70. [CrossRef]
108. Cardozo, K.H.; Guaratini, T.; Barros, M.P.; Falcão, V.R.; Tonon, A.P.; Lopes, N.P.; Campos, S.; Torres, M.A.; Souza, A.O.; Colepicolo, P.; et al. Metabolites from algae with economical impact. *Comp. Biochem. Physiol. Part C Toxicol. Pharmacol.* **2007**, *146*, 60–78. [CrossRef]
109. Vilchez, C.; Garbayo, I.; Lobato, M.V.; Vega, J. Microalgae-mediated chemicals production and wastes removal. *Enzym. Microb. Technol.* **1997**, *20*, 562–572. [CrossRef]
110. Uhlik, D.J.; Gowans, C.S. Synthesis of nicotinic acid in Chlamydomonas eugametos. *Int. J. Biochem.* **1974**, *5*, 79–84. [CrossRef]
111. Borowitzka, M.A. Commercial production of microalgae: Ponds, tanks, and fermenters. In *Progress in Industrial Microbiology*; Elsevier: Amsterdam, The Netherlands, 1999; Volume 35, pp. 313–321.
112. Running, J.A.; Severson, D.K.; Schneider, K.J. Extracellular production of L-ascorbic acid by *Chlorella protothecoides, Prototheca* species, and mutants of *P. moriformis* during aerobic culturing at low pH. *J. Ind. Microbiol. Biotechnol.* **2002**, *29*, 93–98. [CrossRef] [PubMed]

113. Carballo-Cárdenas, E.C.; Tuan, P.M.; Janssen, M.; Wijffels, R.H. Vitamin E (α-tocopherol) production by the marine microalgae Dunaliella tertiolecta and Tetraselmis suecica in batch cultivation. *Biomol. Eng.* **2003**, *20*, 139–147. [CrossRef]
114. Chandra, R.; Parra, R.; MN Iqbal, H. Phycobiliproteins: A Novel Green Tool from Marine Origin Blue-Green Algae and Red Algae. *Protein Pept. Lett.* **2017**, *24*, 118–125. [CrossRef] [PubMed]
115. Du, S.W.; Zhang, L.K.; Han, K.; Chen, S.; Hu, Z.; Chen, W.; Hu, K.; Yin, L.; Wu, B.; Guan, Y.Q. Combined Phycocyanin and Hematoporphyrin Monomethyl Ether for Breast Cancer Treatment via Photosensitizers Modified Fe3O4 Nanoparticles Inhibiting the Proliferation and Migration of MCF-7 Cells. *Biomacromolecules* **2017**, *19*, 31–41. [CrossRef] [PubMed]
116. Koller, M.; Muhr, A.; Braunegg, G. Microalgae as versatile cellular factories for valued products. *Algal Res.* **2014**, *6*, 52–63. [CrossRef]
117. Parmar, A.; Singh, N.K.; Kaushal, A.; Sonawala, S.; Madamwar, D. Purification, characterization and comparison of phycoerythrins from three different marine cyanobacterial cultures. *Bioresour. Technol.* **2011**, *102*, 1795–1802. [CrossRef] [PubMed]
118. Yu, P.; Wu, Y.; Wang, G.; Jia, T.; Zhang, Y. Purification and bioactivities of phycocyanin. *Crit. Rev. Food Sci. Nutr.* **2017**, *57*, 3840–3849. [CrossRef] [PubMed]
119. Luengo, E.; Martínez, J.M.; Bordetas, A.; Álvarez, I.; Raso, J. Influence of the treatment medium temperature on lutein extraction assisted by pulsed electric fields from Chlorella vulgaris. *Innov. Food Sci. Emerg. Technol.* **2015**, *29*, 15–22. [CrossRef]
120. Lin, J.H.; Lee, D.J.; Chang, J.S. Lutein production from biomass: Marigold flowers versus microalgae. *Bioresour. Technol.* **2015**, *184*, 421–428. [CrossRef]
121. Del Campo, J.A.; García-González, M.; Guerrero, M.G. Outdoor cultivation of microalgae for carotenoid production: Current state and perspectives. *Appl. Microbiol. Biotechnol.* **2007**, *74*, 1163–1174. [CrossRef]
122. Gille, A.; Neumann, U.; Louis, S.; Bischoff, S.C.; Briviba, K. Microalgae as a potential source of carotenoids: Comparative results of an in vitro digestion method and a feeding experiment with C57BL/6J mice. *J. Funct. Foods* **2018**, *49*, 285–294. [CrossRef]
123. Rodriguez-Amaya, D.B. Update on natural food pigments-A mini-review on carotenoids, anthocyanins, and betalains. *Food Res. Int.* **2018**. [CrossRef]
124. Chue, K.T.; Ten, L.N.; Oh, Y.K.; Woo, S.G.; Lee, M.; Yoo, S.A. Carotinoid compositions of five microalga species. *Chem. Nat. Compd.* **2012**, *48*, 141–142. [CrossRef]
125. García, J.L.; de Vicente, M.; Galán, B. Microalgae, old sustainable food and fashion nutraceuticals. *Microb. Biotechnol.* **2017**, *10*, 1017–1024. [CrossRef] [PubMed]
126. Soni, R.A.; Sudhakar, K.; Rana, R.S. Spirulina–From growth to nutritional product: A review. *Trends Food Sci. Technol.* **2017**, *69*, 157–171. [CrossRef]
127. Matos, J.; Cardoso, C.; Bandarra, N.M.; Afonso, C. Microalgae as healthy ingredients for functional food: A review. *Food Funct.* **2017**, *8*, 2672–2685. [CrossRef] [PubMed]
128. Fuentes, M.R.; Fernández, G.A.; Pérez, J.S.; Guerrero, J.G. Biomass nutrient profiles of the microalga Porphyridium cruentum. *Food Chem.* **2000**, *70*, 345–353. [CrossRef]
129. Ovando, C.A.; Carvalho, J.C.D.; Vinícius de Melo Pereira, G.; Jacques, P.; Soccol, V.T.; Soccol, C.R. Functional properties and health benefits of bioactive peptides derived from Spirulina: A review. *Food Rev. Int.* **2018**, *34*, 34–51. [CrossRef]
130. Batista, A.P.; Niccolai, A.; Fradinho, P.; Fragoso, S.; Bursic, I.; Rodolfi, L.; Biondi, N.; Tredici, M.R.; Sousa, I.; Raymundo, A. Microalgae biomass as an alternative ingredient in cookies: Sensory, physical and chemical properties, antioxidant activity and in vitro digestibility. *Algal Res.* **2017**, *26*, 161–171. [CrossRef]
131. Ventura, S.P.M.; Nobre, B.P.; Ertekin, F.; Hayes, M.; Garciá-Vaquero, M.; Vieira, F.; Koc, M.; Gouveia, L.; Aires-Barros, M.R.; Palavra, A.M.F. Extraction of value-added compounds from microalgae. In *Microalgae-Based Biofuels and Bioproducts*; Elsevier: Woodhead Publishing, 2017; pp. 461–483.
132. Markovits, A.; Conejeros, R.; López, L.; Lutz, M. Evaluation of marine microalga *Nannochloropsis* sp. as a potential dietary supplement. Chemical, nutritional and short term toxicological evaluation in rats. *Nutr. Res.* **1992**, *12*, 1273–1284.
133. Rania, M.A.; Hala, M.T. Antibacterial and antifungal activity of Cyanobacteria and green Microalgae evaluation of medium components by Plackett-Burman design for antimicrobial activity of *Spirulina platensis*. *Glob. J. Biotechnol. Biochem.* **2008**, *3*, 22–31.

134. Ruiz-Ruiz, F.; Mancera-Andrade, E.I.; Iqbal, H.M. Marine-derived bioactive peptides for biomedical sectors: A review. *Protein Pept. Lett.* **2017**, *24*, 109–117. [CrossRef] [PubMed]
135. de Vera, C.; Díaz Crespín, G.; Hernández Daranas, A.; Montalvão Looga, S.; Lillsunde, K.E.; Tammela, P.; Perälä, M.; Hongisto, V.; Virtanen, J.; Rischer, H.; et al. Marine Microalgae: Promising Source for New Bioactive Compounds. *Mar. Drugs* **2018**, *16*, 317. [CrossRef]
136. Bloor, S.; England, R.R. Elucidation and optimization of the medium constituents controlling antibiotic production by the cyanobacterium Nostoc muscorum. *Enzym. Microb. Technol.* **1991**, *13*, 76–81. [CrossRef]
137. Galano, J.M.; Roy, J.; Durand, T.; Lee, J.C.Y.; Le Guennec, J.Y.; Oger, C.; Demion, M. Biological activities of non-enzymatic oxygenated metabolites of polyunsaturated fatty acids (NEO-PUFAs) derived from EPA and DHA: New anti-arrhythmic compounds? *Mol. Asp. Med.* **2018**, *64*, 161–168. [CrossRef]
138. Abdulrazaq, M.; Innes, J.K.; Calder, P.C. Effect of ω-3 polyunsaturated fatty acids on arthritic pain: A systematic review. *Nutrition* **2017**, *39*, 57–66. [CrossRef] [PubMed]
139. Markworth, J.F.; Mitchell, C.J.; D'Souza, R.F.; Aasen, K.M.; Durainayagam, B.R.; Mitchell, S.M.; Chan, A.H.; Sinclair, A.J.; Garg, M.; Cameron-Smith, D. Arachidonic acid supplementation modulates blood and skeletal muscle lipid profile with no effect on basal inflammation in resistance exercise trained men. *Prostaglandins Leukot. Essent. Fat. Acids* **2018**, *128*, 74–86. [CrossRef]
140. Habib, M.A.B. *Review on Culture, Production and Use of Spirulina as Food for Humans and Feeds for Domestic Animals and Fish*; Food and Agriculture Organization of the United Nations: Quebec, QC, Canada, 2008.
141. Sonani, R.R.; Patel, S.; Bhastana, B.; Jakharia, K.; Chaubey, M.G.; Singh, N.K.; Madamwar, D. Purification and antioxidant activity of phycocyanin from Synechococcus sp. R42DM isolated from industrially polluted site. *Bioresour. Technol.* **2017**, *245*, 325–331. [CrossRef]
142. Yan, G.A.; Jiang, J.W.; Wu, G.; Yan, X. Disappearance of linear alkylbenzene sulfonate from different cultures with Anabaena sp. HB 1017. *Bull. Environ. Contam. Toxicol.* **1998**, *60*, 329–334. [CrossRef]
143. Radwan, S.S.; Al-Hasan, R.H. Oil pollution and cyanobacteria. In *The Ecology of Cyanobacteria*; Springer: The Netherlands, 2000; pp. 307–319.
144. Raghukumar, C.; Vipparty, V.; David, J.; Chandramohan, D. Degradation of crude oil by marine cyanobacteria. *Appl. Microbiol. Biotechnol.* **2001**, *57*, 433–436.
145. Radwan, S.S.; Al-Hasan, R.H.; Salamah, S.; Al-Dabbous, S. Bioremediation of oily sea water by bacteria immobilized in biofilms coating macroalgae. *Int. Biodeterior. Biodegrad.* **2002**, *50*, 55–59. [CrossRef]
146. Mansy, A.E.R.; El-Bestawy, E. Toxicity and biodegradation of fluometuron by selected cyanobacterial species. *World J. Microbiol. Biotechnol.* **2002**, *18*, 125–131. [CrossRef]
147. Uma, L.; Subramanian, G. Effective use of cyanobacteria in effluent treatment. In Proceedings of the National Symposium Cyanobacerial Nitrogen Fixation, IARI, New Delhi, India; 1990; pp. 437–444.
148. Scherer, M.D.; de Oliveira, A.C.; Magalhães Filho, F.J.C.; Ugaya, C.M.L.; Mariano, A.B.; Vargas, J.V.C. Environmental study of producing microalgal biomass and bioremediation of cattle manure effluents by microalgae cultivation. *Clean Technol. Environ. Policy* **2017**, *19*, 1745–1759. [CrossRef]
149. Matsunaga, T.; Sudo, H.; Takemasa, H.; Wachi, Y.; Nakamura, N. Sulfated extracellular polysaccharide production by the halophilic cyanobacterium *Aphanocapsa halophytia* immobilized on light-diffusing optical fibers. *Appl. Microbiol. Biotechnol.* **1996**, *45*, 24–27. [CrossRef]
150. Dellamatrice, P.M.; Silva-Stenico, M.E.; de Moraes, L.A.B.; Fiore, M.F.; Monteiro, R.T.R. Degradation of textile dyes by cyanobacteria. *Braz. J. Microbiol.* **2017**, *48*, 25–31. [CrossRef]
151. Pierre, G.; Zhao, J.M.; Orvain, F.; Dupuy, C.; Klein, G.L.; Graber, M.; Maugard, T. Seasonal dynamics of extracellular polymeric substances (EPS) in surface sediments of a diatom-dominated intertidal mudflat (Marennes–Oléron, France). *J. Sea Res.* **2014**, *92*, 26–35. [CrossRef]
152. Bhunia, B.; Uday, U.S.P.; Oinam, G.; Mondal, A.; Bandyopadhyay, T.K.; Tiwari, O.N. Characterization, genetic regulation and production of cyanobacterial exopolysaccharides and its applicability for heavy metal removal. *Carbohydr. Polym.* **2018**, *179*, 228–243. [CrossRef]
153. Bilal, M.; Rasheed, T.; Sosa-Hernández, J.; Raza, A.; Nabeel, F.; Iqbal, H. Biosorption: An Interplay between Marine Algae and Potentially Toxic Elements—A Review. *Mar. Drugs* **2018**, *16*, 65. [CrossRef]
154. Shuba, E.S.; Kifle, D. Microalgae to biofuels:'Promising'alternative and renewable energy, review. *Renew. Sustain. Energy Rev.* **2018**, *81*, 743–755. [CrossRef]
155. Khetkorn, W.; Rastogi, R.P.; Incharoensakdi, A.; Lindblad, P.; Madamwar, D.; Pandey, A.; Larroche, C. Microalgal hydrogen production–A review. *Bioresour. Technol.* **2017**, *243*, 1194–1206. [CrossRef]

156. Batyrova, K.; Hallenbeck, P.C. Hydrogen production by a Chlamydomonas reinhardtii strain with inducible expression of photosystem II. *Int. J. Mol. Sci.* **2017**, *18*, 647. [CrossRef]
157. Ainas, M.; Hasnaoui, S.; Bouarab, R.; Abdi, N.; Drouiche, N.; Mameri, N. Hydrogen production with the cyanobacterium Spirulina platensis. *Int. J. Hydrog. Energy* **2017**, *42*, 4902–4907. [CrossRef]
158. Sengmee, D.; Cheirsilp, B.; Suksaroge, T.T.; Prasertsan, P. Biophotolysis-based hydrogen and lipid production by oleaginous microalgae using crude glycerol as exogenous carbon source. *Int. J. Hydrog. Energy* **2017**, *42*, 1970–1976. [CrossRef]
159. Vargas, S.R.; dos Santos, P.V.; Zaiat, M.; do Carmo Calijuri, M. Optimization of biomass and hydrogen production by Anabaena sp. (UTEX 1448) in nitrogen-deprived cultures. *Biomass Bioenergy* **2018**, *111*, 70–76. [CrossRef]
160. Nagarajan, D.; Lee, D.J.; Kondo, A.; Chang, J.S. Recent insights into biohydrogen production by microalgae–From biophotolysis to dark fermentation. *Bioresour. Technol.* **2017**, *227*, 373–387. [CrossRef] [PubMed]
161. Wünschiers, R.; Lindblad, P. Hydrogen in education—A biological approach. *Int. J. Hydrog. Energy* **2002**, *27*, 1131–1140. [CrossRef]
162. Benemann, J.R. Hydrogen production by microalgae. *J. Appl. Phycol.* **2000**, *12*, 291–300. [CrossRef]
163. Milano, J.; Ong, H.C.; Masjuki, H.H.; Chong, W.T.; Lam, M.K.; Loh, P.K.; Vellayan, V. Microalgae biofuels as an alternative to fossil fuel for power generation. *Renew. Sustain. Energy Rev.* **2016**, *58*, 180–197. [CrossRef]
164. Park, J.Y.; Park, M.S.; Lee, Y.C.; Yang, J.W. Advances in direct transesterification of algal oils from wet biomass. *Bioresour. Technol.* **2015**, *184*, 267–275. [CrossRef] [PubMed]
165. Lee, S.Y.; Cho, J.M.; Chang, Y.K.; Oh, Y.K. Cell disruption and lipid extraction for microalgal biorefineries: A review. *Bioresour. Technol.* **2017**, *244*, 1317–1328. [CrossRef]
166. Miao, X.; Wu, Q.; Yang, C. Fast pyrolysis of microalgae to produce renewable fuels. *J. Anal. Appl. Pyrolysis* **2004**, *71*, 855–863. [CrossRef]
167. Willke, T.H.; Vorlop, K.D. Industrial bioconversion of renewable resources as an alternative to conventional chemistry. *Appl. Microbiol. Biotechnol.* **2004**, *66*, 131–142. [CrossRef]
168. Gaurav, N.; Sivasankari, S.; Kiran, G.S.; Ninawe, A.; Selvin, J. Utilization of bioresources for sustainable biofuels: A Review. *Renew. Sustain. Energy Rev.* **2017**, *73*, 205–214. [CrossRef]
169. Rizza, L.S.; Smachetti, M.E.S.; Do Nascimento, M.; Salerno, G.L.; Curatti, L. Bioprospecting for native microalgae as an alternative source of sugars for the production of bioethanol. *Algal Res.* **2017**, *22*, 140–147. [CrossRef]
170. Harun, R.; Danquah, M.K.; Forde, G.M. Microalgal biomass as a fermentation feedstock for bioethanol production. *J. Chem. Technol. Biotechnol.* **2010**, *85*, 199–203. [CrossRef]
171. Pham-Huy, L.A.; He, H.; Pham-Huy, C. Free radicals, antioxidants in disease and health. *Int. J. Biomed. Sci.* **2008**, *4*, 89–96.
172. Alberts, D.S.; Goldman, R.; Xu, M.J.; Dorr, R.T.; Quinn, J.; Welch, K.; Guillen-Rodriguez, J.; Aickin, M.; Peng, Y.M.; Loescher, L.; et al. Disposition and metabolism of topically administered α-tocopherol acetate: A common ingredient of commercially available sunscreens and cosmetics. *Nutr. Cancer* **1996**, *26*, 193–201. [CrossRef]
173. Patel, H.M.; Rastogi, R.P.; Trivedi, U.; Madamwar, D. Structural characterization and antioxidant potential of phycocyanin from the cyanobacterium Geitlerinema sp. H8DM. *Algal Res.* **2018**, *32*, 372–383. [CrossRef]
174. Camacho, F.G.; Rodríguez, J.G.; Mirón, A.S.; García, M.C.; Belarbi, E.H.; Chisti, Y.; Grima, E.M. Biotechnological significance of toxic marine dinoflagellates. *Biotechnol. Adv.* **2007**, *25*, 176–194. [CrossRef]
175. Sathasivam, R.; Radhakrishnan, R.; Hashem, A.; Abd_Allah, E.F. Microalgae metabolites: A rich source for food and medicine. *Saudi J. Biol. Sci.* **2017**. [CrossRef]
176. Vijayakumar, S.; Menakha, M. Pharmaceutical applications of cyanobacteria—A review. *J. Acute Med.* **2015**, *5*, 15–23. [CrossRef]
177. Nowruzi, B.; Haghighat, S.; Fahimi, H.; Mohammadi, E. Nostoc cyanobacteria species: A new and rich source of novel bioactive compounds with pharmaceutical potential. *J. Pharm. Health Serv. Res.* **2018**, *9*, 5–12. [CrossRef]
178. Niedermeyer, T.H.J. Anti-infective natural products from Cyanobacteria. *Planta Med.* **2015**, *81*, 1309–1325. [CrossRef]

179. Yaakob, Z.; Ali, E.; Zainal, A.; Mohamad, M.; Takriff, M.S. An overview: Biomolecules from microalgae for animal feed and aquaculture. *J. Biol. Res.-Thessalon.* **2014**, *21*, 6. [CrossRef]
180. Sandoval, G.; Casas-Godoy, L.; Bonet-Ragel, K.; Rodrigues, J.; Ferreira-Dias, S.; Valero, F. Enzyme-Catalyzed Production of Biodiesel as Alternative to Chemical-Catalyzed Processes: Advantages and Constraints. *Curr. Biochem. Eng.* **2017**, *4*, 109–141. [CrossRef]
181. Hosseini, N.S.; Shang, H.; Scott, J.A. Biosequestration of industrial off-gas CO_2 for enhanced lipid productivity in open microalgae cultivation systems. *Renew. Sustain. Energy Rev.* **2018**, *92*, 458–469. [CrossRef]
182. Packer, M. Algal capture of carbon dioxide; biomass generation as a tool for greenhouse gas mitigation with reference to New Zealand energy strategy and policy. *Energy Policy* **2009**, *37*, 3428–3437. [CrossRef]
183. Kavitha, G.; Rengasamy, R.; Inbakandan, D. Polyhydroxybutyrate production from marine source and its application. *Int. J. Biol. Macromol.* **2018**, *111*, 102–108. [CrossRef]
184. Archer, E.; Petrie, B.; Kasprzyk-Hordern, B.; Wolfaardt, G.M. The fate of pharmaceuticals and personal care products (PPCPs), endocrine disrupting contaminants (EDCs), metabolites and illicit drugs in a WWTW and environmental waters. *Chemosphere* **2017**, *174*, 437–446. [CrossRef]

© 2019 by the authors. Licensee MDPI, Basel, Switzerland. This article is an open access article distributed under the terms and conditions of the Creative Commons Attribution (CC BY) license (http://creativecommons.org/licenses/by/4.0/).

marine drugs

Article

New Source of 3D Chitin Scaffolds: The Red Sea Demosponge *Pseudoceratina arabica* (Pseudoceratinidae, Verongiida)

Lamiaa A. Shaala [1,2,*], Hani Z. Asfour [3], Diaa T. A. Youssef [4,5], Sonia Żółtowska-Aksamitowska [6,7], Marcin Wysokowski [6,7], Mikhail Tsurkan [8], Roberta Galli [9], Heike Meissner [10], Iaroslav Petrenko [7], Konstantin Tabachnick [11], Viatcheslav N. Ivanenko [12], Nicole Bechmann [13], Lyubov V. Muzychka [14], Oleg B. Smolii [14], Rajko Martinović [15], Yvonne Joseph [7], Teofil Jesionowski [6] and Hermann Ehrlich [7,*]

1 Natural Products Unit, King Fahd Medical Research Centre, King Abdulaziz University, Jeddah 21589, Saudi Arabia
2 Suez Canal University Hospital, Suez Canal University, Ismailia 41522, Egypt
3 Department of Medical Parasitology, Faculty of Medicine, Princess Al-Jawhara Center of Excellence in Research of Hereditary Disorders, King Abdulaziz University, Jeddah 21589, Saudi Arabia; hasfour@kau.edu.sa
4 Department of Natural Products, Faculty of Pharmacy, King Abdulaziz University, Jeddah 21589, Saudi Arabia; dyoussef@kau.edu.sa
5 Department of Pharmacognosy, Faculty of Pharmacy, Suez Canal University, Ismailia 41522, Egypt
6 Institute of Chemical Technology and Engineering, Faculty of Chemical Technology, Poznan University of Technology, Poznan 60965, Poland; soniazolaks@gmail.com (S.Ż.-A.); marcin.wysokowski@put.poznan.pl (M.W.); teofil.jesionowski@put.poznan.pl (T.J.)
7 Institute of Electronics and Sensor Materials, Technische Universität Bergakademie-Freiberg, Freiberg 09599, Germany; iaroslavpetrenko@gmail.com (I.P.); yvonne.joseph@esm.tu-freiberg.de (Y.J.)
8 Leibniz Institute of Polymer Research Dresden, Dresden 01069, Germany; tsurkanmv@gmail.com
9 Clinical Sensoring and Monitoring, Department of Anesthesiology and Intensive Care Medicine, Faculty of Medicine, Technische Universität Dresden, Dresden 01307, Germany; roberta.galli@tu-dresden.de
10 Department of Prosthetic Dentistry, Faculty of Medicine, Technische Universität Dresden, Dresden 01307, Germany; heike.meissner@uniklinikum-dresden.de
11 P.P. Shirshov Institute of Oceanology, Russian Academy of Sciences, Moscow 117997, Russia; tabachnick@mail.ru
12 Department of Invertebrate Zoology, Biological Faculty, Lomonosov Moscow State University, Moscow 119992, Russia; ivanenko.slava@gmail.com
13 Institute of Clinical Chemistry and Laboratory Medicine, University Hospital Carl Gustav Carus at the Technische Universität Dresden, Dresden 01307, Germany; nicole.bechmann@uniklinikum-dresden.de
14 V.P. Kukhar Institute of Bioorganic Chemistry and Petrochemistry, National Academy of Science of Ukraine, Kiev 02094, Ukraine; lmuzychka@rambler.ru (L.V.M.); smolii@bpci.kiev.ua (O.B.S.)
15 Institute of Marine Biology, University of Montenegro, Kotor 85330, Montenegro; rajko.mar@ucg.ac.me
* Correspondence: lshalla@kau.edu.sa (L.A.S.); hermann.ehrlich@esm.tu-freiberg.de (H.E.)

Received: 7 January 2019; Accepted: 30 January 2019; Published: 1 February 2019

Abstract: The bioactive bromotyrosine-derived alkaloids and unique morphologically-defined fibrous skeleton of chitin origin have been found recently in marine demosponges of the order Verongiida. The sophisticated three-dimensional (3D) structure of skeletal chitinous scaffolds supported their use in biomedicine, tissue engineering as well as in diverse modern technologies. The goal of this study was the screening of new species of the order Verongiida to find another renewable source of naturally prefabricated 3D chitinous scaffolds. Special attention was paid to demosponge species, which could be farmed on large scale using marine aquaculture methods. In this study, the demosponge *Pseudoceratina arabica* collected in the coastal waters of the Egyptian Red Sea was examined as a potential source of chitin for the first time. Various bioanalytical tools including scanning electron microscopy (SEM), fluorescence microscopy, FTIR analysis, Calcofluor white staining, electrospray ionization mass spectrometry (ESI-MS), as well as a chitinase digestion assay were successfully used to confirm the discovery of α-chitin within the skeleton of *P. arabica*. The current finding should make an important contribution to the field of application of this verongiid sponge as a novel renewable source of biologically-active metabolites and chitin, which are important for development of the blue biotechnology especially in marine oriented biomedicine.

Keywords: chitin; scaffolds; biological materials; demosponges; *Pseudoceratina arabica*

1. Introduction

Structural aminopolysaccharide chitin is one of the oldest biopolymers due to its presence in fungi which appeared on our planet around 2.4 billion years ago [1]. In 1811, Henri Braconnot discovered chitin in the form of an alkali-resistant fraction during his studies on higher fungi and, consequently, termed it as *fungine* (for review see [2]). The currently used term *chitin*, however, has been proposed in 1823 by Auguste Odier who used beetle cuticles to isolate similar biomaterial during alkali treatment with hot KOH solutions [3]. Chitin has been found in skeletal structures of diverse unicellular organisms (yeasts, protists) and invertebrate organisms (corals, annelids, molluscs, arthropods) with exception of crustose coralline algae; cell walls of diatoms and skeletons of sponges (see for review [4,5]). The existence of chitin within the marine demosponges and glass sponges' skeletons was reported for the first time only in 2007 [6,7]. The first report on chitin identification in siliceous cell walls (frustules) of diatoms was carried out in 2009 [8]. Intriguingly, the presence of chitin in crustose coralline algae has been described in 2014 [9]. Nowadays, chitin has been reported in 17 species of marine [10] and in two species of freshwater sponges [11,12]. One of the special characteristics of poriferan chitin is the 3D fibrous nature, which has been recognized as a naturally prefabricated tubular scaffold that follows the morphology especially of keratosan demosponges [13–15]. These unique 3D architectures of such scaffolds are typical for representatives of the Verongiida order (subclass Verongimorpha, class Demospongiae) and open perspectives for their applications in waste treatment [16], tissue engineering [14,17,18], electrochemistry [19] as well as extreme biomimetics [2,20–23]. Due to the fact that manufacturing of fungi, as well as crustaceans chitin into 3D sponge-like scaffolds, is difficult and expensive, the extensive research of species-specific morphology and structure of the chitin-scaffolds of sponge origin as "ready to use" materials still remain important for practical applications.

Representatives of Verongiida demosponges contain aplystane-type and bromotyrosine-derived secondary metabolites, which is a unique feature within Demospongiae. This is a very distinct chemotaxonomic marker for all members of the order Verongiida [24–26]. It has been proved that bromotyrosine-derived alkaloids possess antimicrobial, antifungal, cytotoxic, and antimalarial activity (for review see [27–34]). Interestingly, only nudibranchs represent the natural predator of the verongiid sponges [35]. As reported previously [36], some of bromotyrosines also showed anti-chitinase activity. Consequently, it was suggested that bromotyrosine related compounds localized within chitinous skeletons of verongiid sponges can inhibit the chitinases of bacterial and fungal origins and in this way protect the integrity of sponge skeleton [13].

So far, only two representative species of the Verongiida order exist in the Red Sea, namely *Pseudoceratina arabica* and *Suberea mollis*. Both sponges have been extensively investigated by our group to identify their bioactive compounds. Recently, several bromotyrosine alkaloids and halogenated compounds with different biological activities have been reported from these two sponges [27–31,37,38]. Due to the ability of diverse chitin-producing sponges to grow under marine ranching conditions (see for overview [39]), poriferan chitin constitutes a renewable source of such unique naturally occurring scaffolds. This encouraged studies on monitoring of novel demosponge species with chitinous skeletons. Therefore, this study focused on the bromotyrosines producing Red Sea demosponge *Pseudoceratina arabica* (Figure 1) where the presence of chitin has never been reported before.

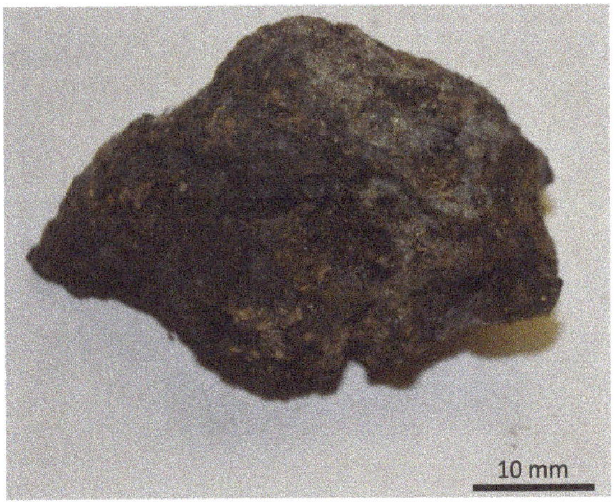

Figure 1. The fragment of the dried specimens of *P. arabica* demosponge used in this study.

2. Results

Figure 2 clearly shows that the alkali treatment resulted in depigmented, protein-free, fibrous scaffolds with residual siliceous spicules and foreign, sandy microparticles within the fibers (Figure 3). Observations of these contaminants into the NaOH-treated fragments of *P. arabica* support our previous suggestion about the allochronic origin of sponges from Pseudoceratinidae family [33].

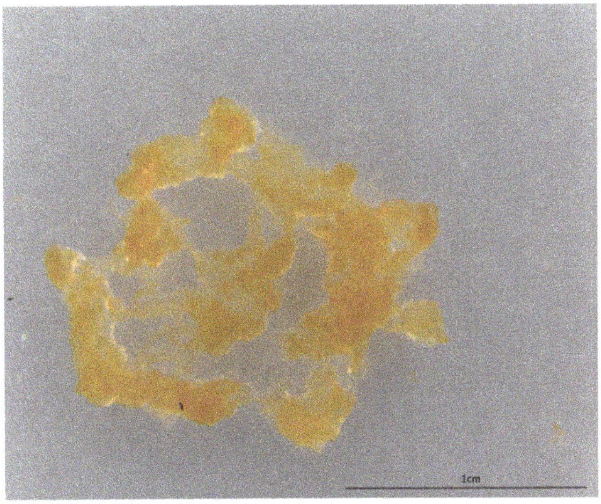

Figure 2. Completely demineralized and pigment-free scaffolds isolated from the sponge *P. arabica*.

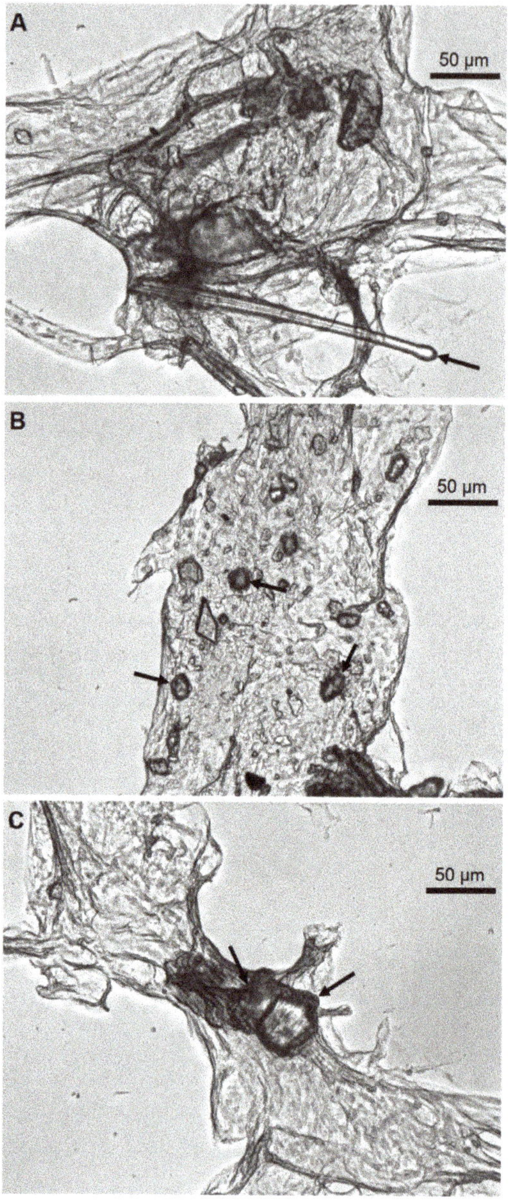

Figure 3. Alkali-treated fibers of *P. arabica* under the optical microscope showing foreign spicules (**A**) and microparticles of sand (**B**, **C**) (arrows).

SEM microphotographs of the scaffolds isolated from *P. arabica* before (Figure 4) and after (Figure 5) HF-treatment show that only treatment using diluted HF water solution leads to dissolution and removal of sand microparticles as well as spicules and result in silica-free, pure, microfibers with high structural integrity, as observed before in other verongiid sponges [6,13,15,40] (Figure 5). These results were also confirmed using light as well as fluorescent microscopy (Figure 6).

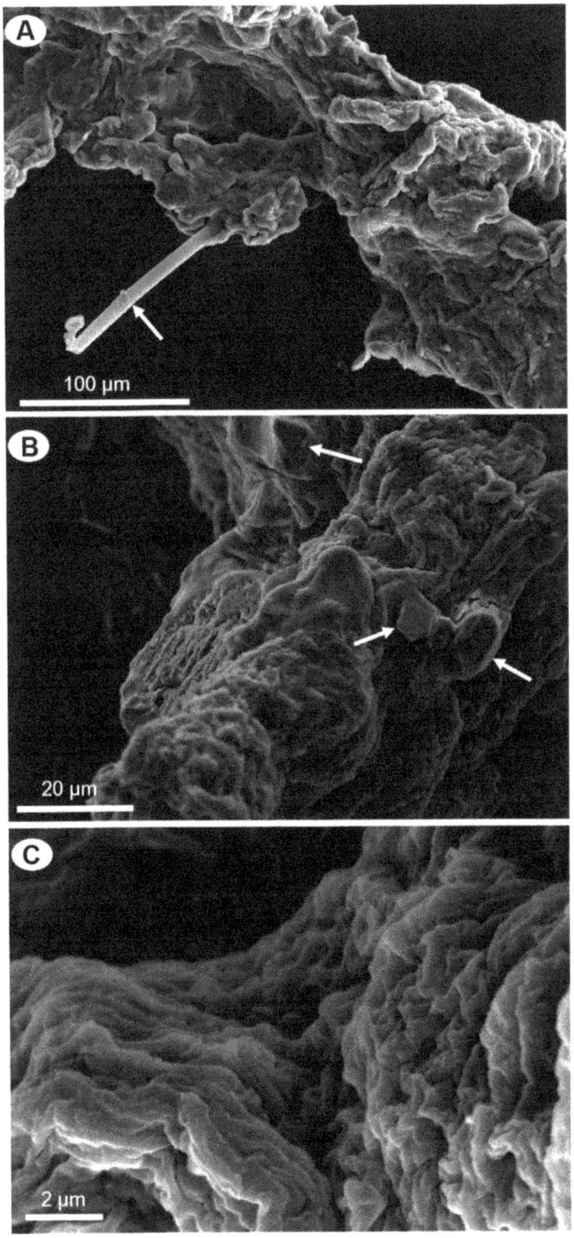

Figure 4. SEM images of alkali-treated skeletal fibers of *P. arabica*. Microparticles of siliceous foreign sponge spicules (**A**) and sand particles (**B**) are marked with arrows. Some parts of partially demineralized fibers remain to be free from foreign particles (**C**).

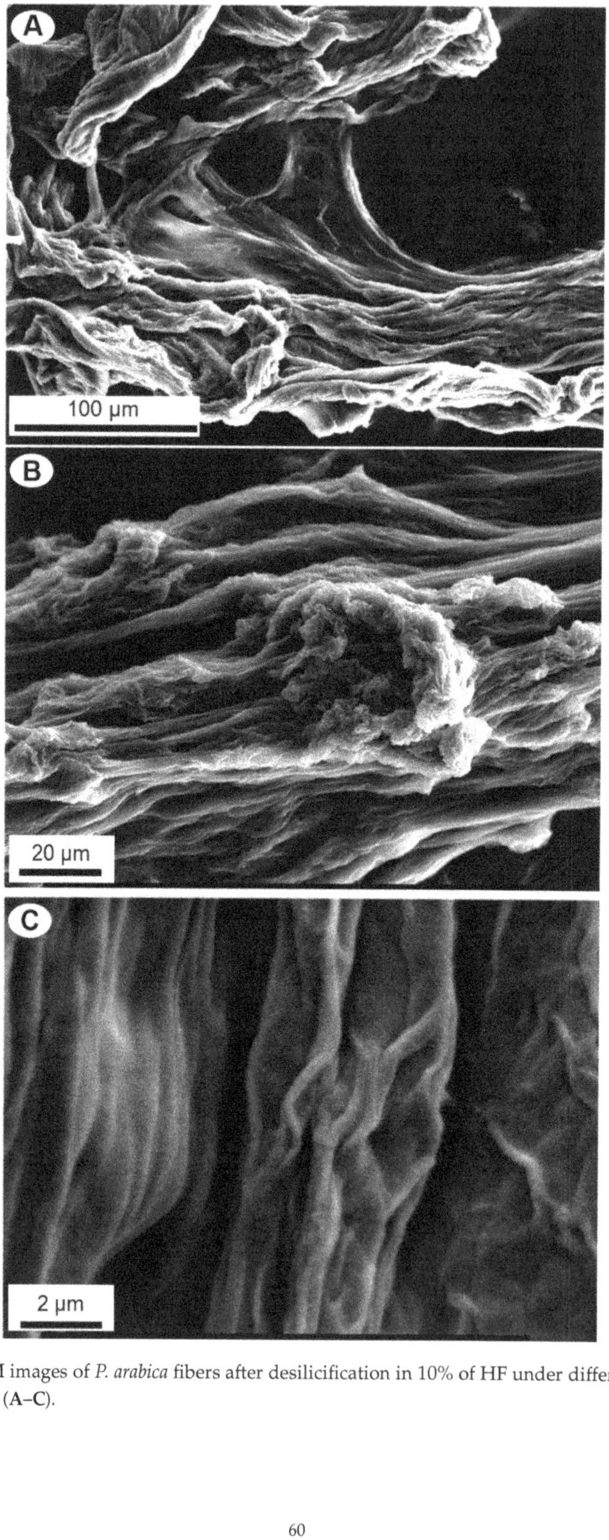

Figure 5. SEM images of *P. arabica* fibers after desilicification in 10% of HF under different levels of magnification (**A–C**).

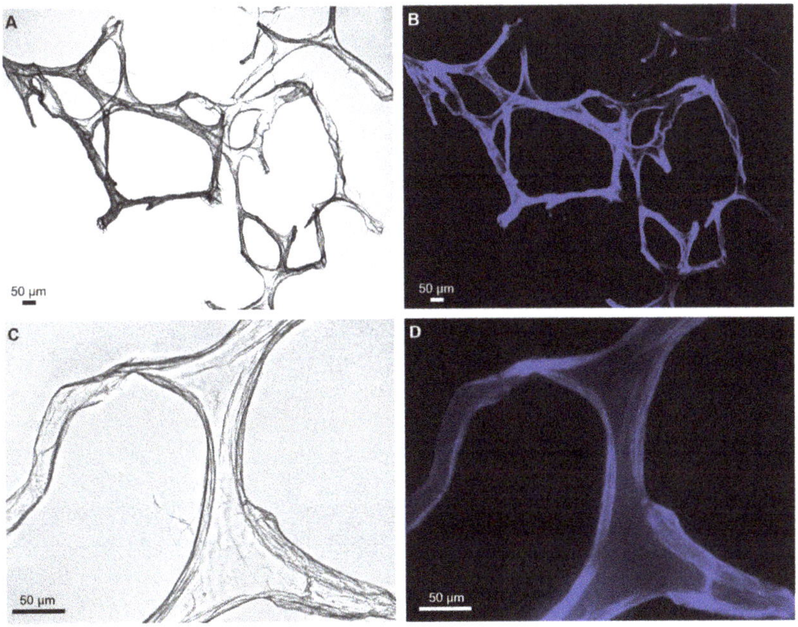

Figure 6. Light microscopy (**A**,**B**) and fluorescence (**C**,**D**) microscopy images of *P. arabica* fibers after desilicification in 10% HF lacking of spicules and other foreign contaminants in investigated fibers.

Typically, Calcofluor white staining (CFW) was used as the first stage of chitin identification in completely demineralized (including HF-based treatment) sponge skeletons. This fluorescent dye is commonly used for staining β-(1→3) and β-(1→4) linked polysaccharides including chitin. Consequently, after binding to polysaccharides, CFW dye exhibits bright blue light under UV excitations [41].

Examination of the scaffolds isolated from *P. arabica* after CFW staining using fluorescent microscopy demonstrate strong fluorescence under light exposure time as short as 1/4800 s (Figure 7B). Similar conclusions were reported previously for chitin isolated from sponges of marine [6,10,15,32,33,40] as well as freshwater [12] origin and fossilized chitin-containing remains [11,41].

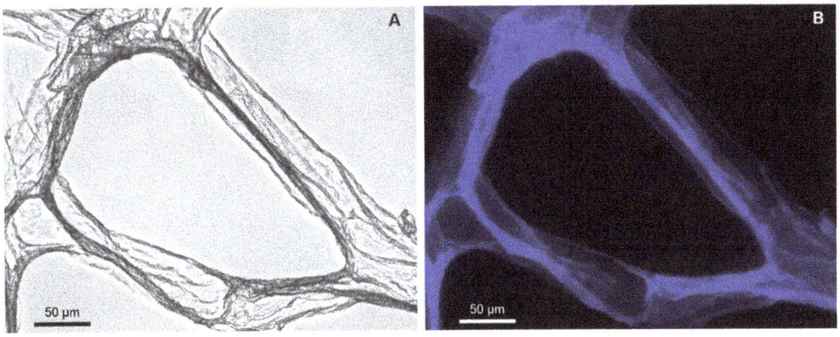

Figure 7. Completely purified fibers of *P. arabica* after CFW staining: (**A**) light microscopy image and (**B**) fluorescence microscopy image of the same location (light exposure time 1/4800) confirm the chitinous nature of the fibers.

More precise methods were applied to study in details the presence and identification of chitin in isolated scaffolds. FTIR spectroscopy is considered as an effective technique for structural analysis of different polysaccharides including chitin. Recently, FTIR analysis was successfully used to obtain information about of type of polymorph form of chitin [42].

The acquired FTIR spectra of demineralized scaffolds of *P. arabica* and standard α-chitin are presented in Figure 8. Between 1700 and 1500 cm^{-1}, the different signatures characteristic for chitin polymorphs were observed. In this amidic moiety region, the investigated sample showed strong band related to the stretching vibrations of C=O group characteristic for band I of the amidic moiety. This band, registered for studied sample, possessed twin peaks at 1651 and 1633 cm^{-1}, which is related with the presence of two types of carbonyl groups within the chitin chain, and it is also typical for α-chitin. The first peak derives from the specific intermolecular hydrogen bond of carbonyl group and hydroxymethyl group on the next chitin residue in the same chain. The second peak is a result of the intramolecular hydrogen bonds of carbonyl with the amide groups. Additionally, in the purified sponge chitin sample, as well as in the α-chitin standard, the characteristic intense band at v_{max} 948 cm^{-1} which is referred to γCH_x bond was observed. Moreover, the α-chitin characteristic band assigned to β-glycosidic bond at 895 cm^{-1} is well visible in the studied samples. However, it should be noted that the characteristic bands for $CaCO_3$ (855–876 cm^{-1}) and SiO_2 (720 cm^{-1}) were not observed in the spectrum of *P. arabica*, suggesting that procedure of chitin isolation resulted in chitin of high purity. Additionally, the comprehensive analysis of acquired spectra shows that recorded bands correspond with those referred in the α-chitin reference sample.

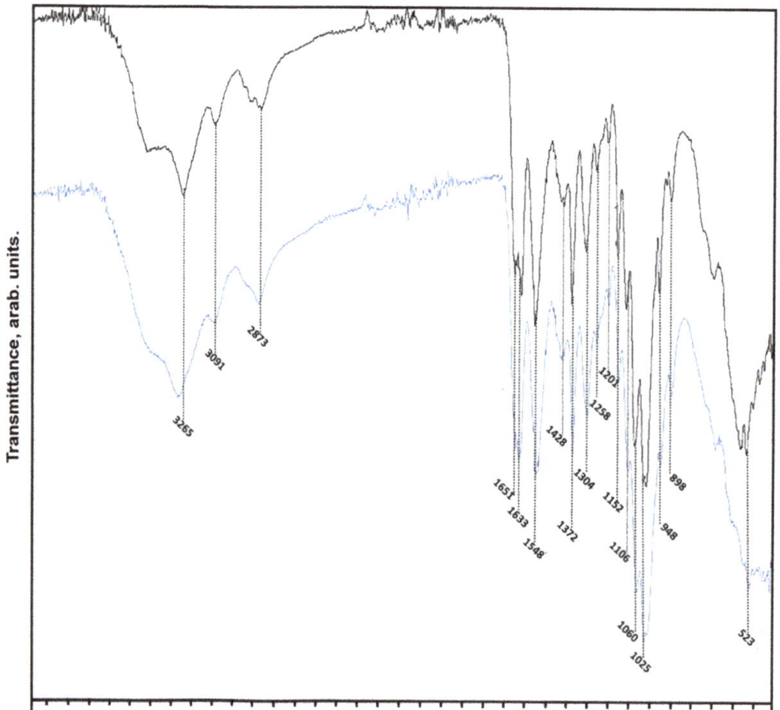

Figure 8. FTIR spectra of the chitin isolated from *P. arabica* compared to standard *a*-chitin.

Figure 9 shows the Raman spectrum of chitin isolated from *P. arabica* compared with the spectrum of the α-chitin reference. Characteristic bands for α-chitin can be found in the spectrum of the isolated chitin within the spectral resolution of the measurement. The existence of two bands characteristic to amine band I at v_{max} 1657 and 1624 cm^{-1} as well as intense band related to the β-glycosidic bond at v_{max} 895 cm^{-1} clearly indicate that chitin isolated from *P. arabica* is of α isomorph. Moreover, the bands in the spectrum are in good agreement with previously published data [5,10,43,44].

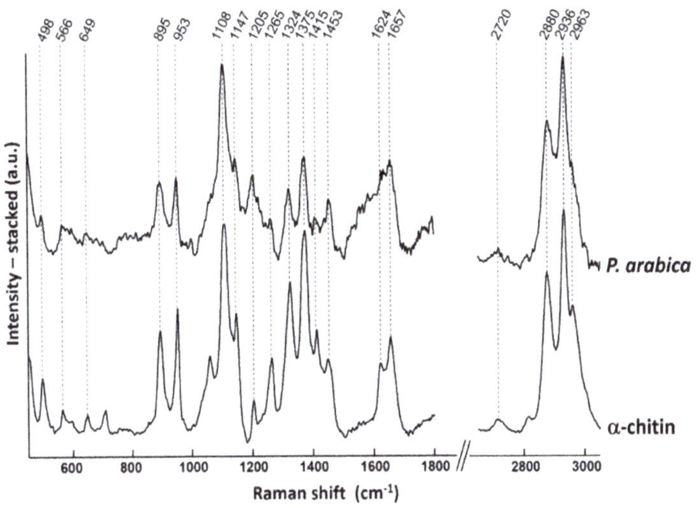

Figure 9. A Raman spectrum of chitin isolated from *P. arabica* compared with the spectrum of reference α-chitin. The bands of *P. arabica* are in good agreement with those of α-chitin standard within the spectral resolution of the measurements.

Previously, in order to confirm the presence of chitin in diverse sponges, the chitinase digestion test has been successfully applied [6,10,15,32,33,40]. This enzyme has unique ability to decompose chitin into low-molecular oligomers such as *N*-acetyl-*D*-glucosamine (GlcNAc). Therefore, the action of chitinase leads to the loss of chitin integrity and the release of residual chitin microfibers of steadily decreasing size. The changes in the structure of treated fibers can be observed using light microscopy (Figure 10). This test is unequivocal and provides additional confirmation of the successful chitin isolation from the sponge under study here.

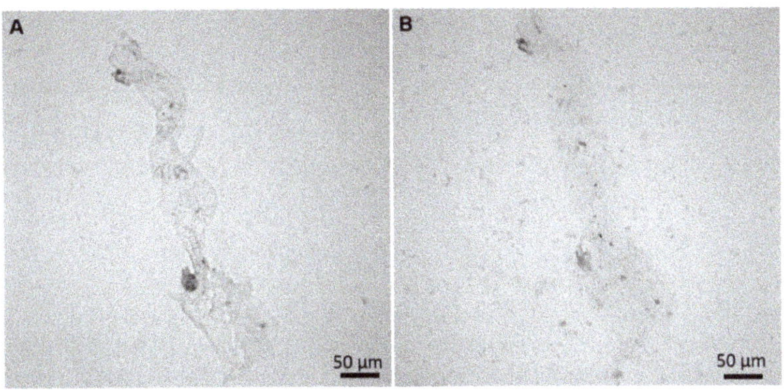

Figure 10. Results of chitinase digestion test on the purified skeletal fibers of *P. arabica*. Fibers before the digestion (**A**) and after 2 h of treatment with chitinase solution (**B**) are well visible.

D-glucosamine (dGlcN) is the product of chitin's acidic hydrolysis which can be readily identified by electrospray-ionization mass spectroscopy (ESI-MS) measurements. Thus, ESI-MS spectroscopy becomes a standard method for chitin identification which usability was shown in complex organisms [40,45,46] and even in 505-million-year-old chitin-containing fossil remnants [47].

In the positive ESI-MS spectra, D-glucosamine (dGlcN) standard revealed several main ion peaks with m/z = 162.08, 180.09, 202.07, 359.17, and 381.15 (Figure 11). The ion peak at m/z = 180.09 and 202.07 correspond to a $[M + H]^+$ and $[M + Na]^+$ species with molecular weight of 179.09 which is dGlcN molecule (calculated: 179.1). The ion peak at m/z = 161.85 corresponds to a $[M + H]^+$ specie with molecular weight of 160.85 that is dGlcN ion $[M-H_2O + H]^+$ without one water molecule (calculated: 161.1). There are also week ion peaks at m/z = 359.17 and 381.15 corresponding to $[2M + H]^+$ and $[2M + Na]^+$ species which are proton- or sodium-bound dGlcN noncovalent dimmer. The ESI-MS spectra of the *P. arabica* hydrolysate has revealed nearly identical ion peaks to those of the *D*-glucosamine standard signal composition (Figure 12). This result clearly demonstrates the presence of dGlcN in the hydrolysate and correspondingly chitin in the sample.

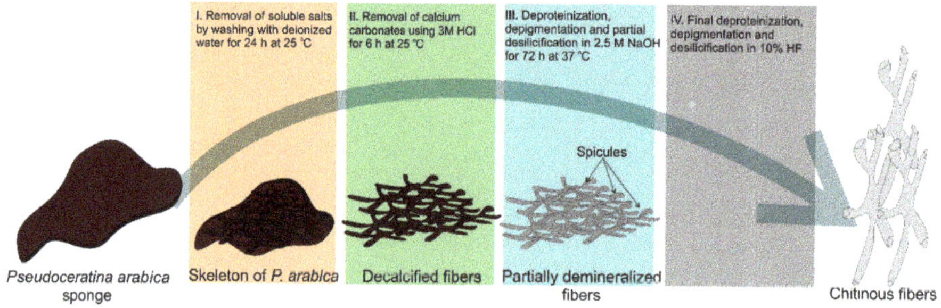

Figure 11. Schematic diagram showing the step-by-step procedure of chitin isolation from the skeleton of *P. arabica*.

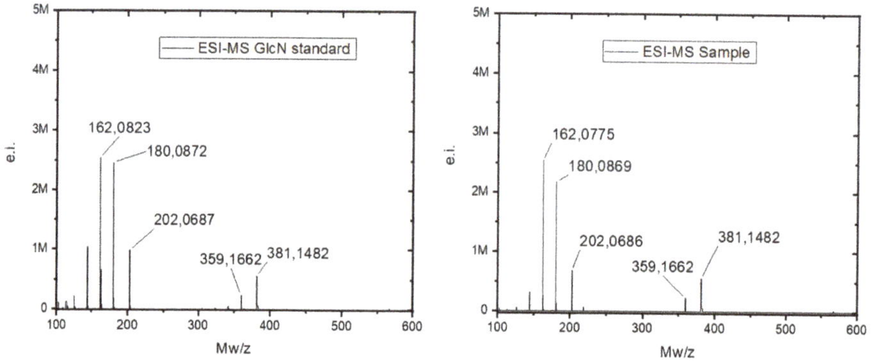

Figure 12. The positive ESI-MS spectra of *D*-glucosamine (dGlcN) standard (**left**) and of acid-hydrolyzed chitin (**right**) from *P. arabica*.

3. Discussion

Seas and oceans are a huge source of various invertebrate animals with potential to be used in biomedicine. For this reason, these organisms are frequently being tested for the presence of various useful products (unique secondary metabolites, biopolymers and biological materials), and many of them have been found in marine sponges. The order Verongiida has been recognized to be divided into four families, which differ in the structure and composition of skeletal fibers [48,49]. The largest verongiid family is Aplysinidae (52 species from three genera: *Aiolochroia*, *Aplysina*, and *Verongula*).

This family is characterized by an anastomosing fiber skeleton with both pith and bark elements. The second largest verongiid family is Ianthellidae (21 species in four genera: *Anomoianthella*, *Hexadella*, *Ianthella*, and *Vansoestia*). The presence of eurypylous choanocyte chambers is a feature distinguishing this family from the others verongiids. Aplysinellidae includes 17 species in three genera (*Aplysinella*, *Porphyra*, and *Suberea*) with dendritic fiber skeleton possessing both pith and bark elements, which are typical morphological features characteristic for representatives of this family. The verongiid *P. arabica* (Keller, 1889) that has been investigated in this study belongs to the family Pseudoceratinidae, which is currently including four species representing the only genus *Pseudoceratina*. Representatives of this family are characterized by a dendritic fiber skeleton with only pith elements. Interestingly, sponges of the genus *Pseudoceratina* are assumedly the richest sources of pharmacologically active alkaloids with diverse chemical skeletons within the order Verongiida [33]. Among various secondary metabolites isolated from *Pseudoceratina* species are: moloka'iamine derivatives, phenolic halogenated compounds, psammaplysins, pseudoceratinamide A and B, ceratinines, moloka'iakitamide, aplysterol, and aplysamine [33]. To date, a variety of secondary metabolites obtained from *P. arabica* have been purified using the solvent extraction method. Surprisingly, there are no literature reports on the extraction of these metabolites using the alkaline-based solution as well as about structural stability of such biomolecules at pH above 7. Alkaline stepwise extraction procedures were recently reported as effective methods for isolation of chitin-based scaffolds with bromotyrosines from other representatives of the order Verongiida and to "squeeze the full potential" of marine sponges [39]. However, it is necessary to prove, the pharmacological and biotechnological potential of the Red Sea verongiid sponges especially because of the recently published intriguing results concerning anti-tumorigenic and anti-metastatic activity of Aeroplysinin-1 which is one of the main bromotyrosine derivatives extracted from Verongiida [34]. All Verongiida sponge samples analyzed until now were found to exhibit a chitin-based scaffold, and here it was proved that *P. arabica* is the new example of chitin-containing sponge from this order. Apart from the bioactive metabolites of *P. arabica*, which are excellently described in the literature, here it was strongly demonstrated that this marine sponge can be effectively used also as a source of naturally prefabricated 3D chitinous scaffold with open-pore structure. Unfortunately, there is still lack of information concerning the interrelationships between the secondary metabolites and chitinous skeleton of *P. arabica*, especially with respect to their localization within so called spherulous cells. However, it known that spherulous cells are rich on bromotyrosines and have been found within skeletal fibres of verongiids [50]. The questions about the role of bromotyrosines in regeneration of chitinous skeleton as well as the growth rate of this species are still open. However, these data are crucial for the future estimation of the biotechnological, biomedical and pharmaceutical potential of *P. arabica* in the region.

It is worth to mention that, the 3D macroporous biomaterials of sponge origin gain a particular interest in tissue engineering, water purification, catalysis, and electrochemistry [51]. Preliminary research done with the use of corresponding 3D chitinous-scaffolds isolated from *A. aerophoba* [17] and *Ianthella basta* [18] confirm their biocompatibility with human mesenchymal stromal cells; supporting their adhesion, viability, growth, and proliferation. Additional, useful features of chitinous scaffolds of poriferan origin are their simplicity and ease of isolation. Calculated swelling capacity for chitinous matrices isolated from *P. arabica* is equal to 255 $\pm$ 8%. There are no doubts that comparative studies on interconnected porosity and swelling ability between chitinous matrices of *P. arabica* and that from other verongiid species [17,18] should be carried out. Consequently, the discovery of chitin in other members of the genus *Pseudoceratina* would be the next stage in the evaluation of the possibility to accept these organisms as a new source of 3D chitin scaffolds with macroporosity which range between 150–350 µm for biomedical applications. We suggest that the opportunity for ex situ cultivation of *P. arabica* can be an important advantage, which enables the use of this sponge for large scale applications in diverse advanced technologies.

4. Materials and Methods

4.1. Collection of Samples

Specimens of marine sponge *Pseudoceratina arabica* (Keller, 1889) (Porifera: Demospongiae: Verongiida: Pseudoceratinidae) described initially as *Psammaplysilla arabica* Keller, 1889 were collected by hands using SCUBA from the southern part of the Egyptian Hurghada (N 27°02′46.8″ E 33°54′21.4″) in July 2017 at depths up to 25 m. The yellowish green encrusting sponge with its conulose surface measuring about 1–2 cm thick. The preserved sponge in ethanol is completely black in color with dark-discolored ethanol. The conules on the sponge surface are bluntly rounded in shape, compressible and rubbery. The individual conules measure about 2–5 mm. The sponge skeleton consists of irregular and scattered fibers composed of pith. The outline and branching were irregular with thickness measuring between 80 and 300 μm. The sponge is similar to the sample collected in Red Sea from Eritrea. The sponge voucher (10.0 × 4.0 × 1.0 cm) was kept in the Zoological Museum of the University of Amsterdam with reference no. 17951. A similar specimen of the sponge was kept at Suez Canal University with collection reference DY-61. Collected specimens were kept on ice after collection. After returning to our laboratory, the specimens were freeze-dried (Figure 1) and transferred to the bioanalytical laboratories at TU Bergakademie Freiberg (Freiberg, Germany).

4.2. Isolation of Chitin from P. Arabica

The isolation of chitin scaffolds from *P. arabica* (Figure 1) was carried out according to our previous reports [12,40,52]. The methodology consists of four steps (Figure 11): first, the skeleton of *P. arabica* was incubated in deionized water at room temperature for one hour to remove possible water-soluble sediment particles and salts. In the second step, the samples were treated with 3 M HCl at room temperature for 6 h in order to eliminate possible residual calcium carbonate-based debris (micro fragments of crustacean carapaces and mollusc shells) from the skeleton of *P. arabica*. Afterwards, the samples were washed several times with deionized water until achieving a pH of 6.5 followed by treatment with 2.5 M NaOH at 37 °C for 72 h to remove pigments and proteins. Due to the observation of the foreign spicules and their fragments in the samples after 72 h of alkali treatment, additional desilicification was needed. Consequently, alkali-treated samples were accurately rinsed with deionized water and stored in a plastic vessel containing appropriate amount of 10% hydrofluoric acid (HF) solution (step four). The vessel was covered in order to prevent the evaporation of HF. The desilicification process was conducted at room temperature for 12 h. The influence of alkaline and strong acidic treatments on the structure of skeleton of the studied sponge was investigated using stereo, white light and fluorescence microscopy. Finally, the isolated material was washed several times with deionized water up to a pH level of 6.5. The fibrous translucent scaffolds (Figure 2) were placed into 250 mL large GLS 80 Duran glass bottles containing deionized water and stored at 4 °C for further analyses.

4.3. Light and Fluorescent Microscopy Analyses and Imaging

Collected sponge samples and isolated chitinous scaffolds were observed using BZ-9000 microscope (Keyence, Osaka, Japan) in the light as well as in the fluorescent microscopy modus.

4.4. Scanning Electron Microscopy Analysis

The morphology and microstructure of isolated and purified chitinous scaffolds, as well as untreated samples of *P. arabica*, were studied on the basis of SEM images using a Philips ESEM XL 30 scanning electron microscope (FEI Company, Peabody, MA, USA). Before analysis, samples were covered with a carbon layer for one minute using an Edwards S150B sputter coater (BOC Edwards, Wilmington, MA, USA).

4.5. Calcofluor White Staining Test

Due to the fact that Calcofluor White (Fluorescent Brightener M2R, Sigma-Aldrich, Taufkirchen, Germany) exhibits enhanced fluorescence after binding to chitin [53,54], this staining method was applied to investigate the location of chitin in the completely purified fibers of *P. arabica*. The selected chitinous fibers were soaked in 0.1 M KOH-glycerine-water solution and few drops of the 0.1% CFW solution were added. This mixture was incubated for 3 h in darkness, washed several times with demineralized water, dried at room temperature and examined using BZ-9000 microscope (Keyence, Osaka, Japan).

4.6. FTIR and Raman Spectroscopy

FTIR spectra of chitinous scaffolds were acquired using a Nicolet 210c FTIR spectrometer. The samples were analysed using the ATR system with resolution equals 4 cm^{-1}. A micro-Raman system composed by a spectrometer (RamanRxn1™, Kaiser Optical Systems Inc., Ann Arbor, MI, USA), a 785 nm excitation laser diode (Invictus 785, Kaiser Optical Systems Inc., Ann Arbor, MI, USA) and an upright microscope (DM2500 P, Leica Microsystems GmbH, Wetzlar, Germany) was used to acquire the Raman spectra from the sample surface. Each spectrum was registered in the range 150–3250 cm^{-1} with resolution of 4 cm^{-1}, using a total acquisition time of 80 s. The fluorescence background was subtracted in MATLAB (MathWorks Inc., Natick, MA, USA) with a baseline procedure.

4.7. Chitinase Digestion Test

Yatalase®from culture supernatants of *Corynebacterium* sp. OZ-21 (Cosmo Bio, Tokyo, Japan) was used for the digestion test. Yatalase is a complex enzyme, consisting mainly of chitinase, chitobiase and β-1,3-glucanase. One unit of this enzyme released one μmol of *N*-acetylglucosamine from 0.5% chitin solution and 1 μmol of p-nitrophenol from p-nitrophenyl-*N*-acetyl-β-*D*-glucosaminide solution in 1 min at 37 °C and pH 6.0. The selected, completely demineralized chitinous scaffolds of *P. arabica* (Figure 3) were incubated in an enzyme solution containing 10 mg/mL Yatalase dissolved in phosphate buffer at pH 6.0 for 2 h. The progress of digestion was monitored under light microscopy using BZ-9000 microscope (Keyence, Osaka, Japan).

4.8. Estimation of N-Acetyl-D-Glucosamine (NAG) Content and Electrospray Ionization Mass Spectrometry (ESI-MS)

The Morgan–Elson assay was used in order to evaluate the *N*-acetyl-*D*-glucosamine released after chitinase treatment, as described previously. For more details see [6,11,12].

Sample preparation for the ESI-MS analysis was performed by the hydrolysis of organic matrixes obtained after HF-treatment of the biological samples in 6M HCl (24 h at 90 °C). The samples, after HCl hydrolysis were filtrated with a 0.4 micron filter and freeze-dried in order to remove any excess HCl. The standard D-glucosamine as a control was purchased from Sigma (Sigma-Aldrich, Taufkirchen, Germany Both the commercial standard and the prepared sample were dissolved in water before ESI-MS analysis. ESI-MS measurements were performed on an Agilent Technologies 6230 TOF LC/MS spectrometer (Applied Biosystems, Foster City, CA, USA) in line as a detector in the analytical HPLC instrument. Nitrogen was used as the nebulizing and desolation gas.

5. Conclusions

The results of this investigation showed the need to develop new, simultaneous, more effective methods of extraction of both biologically active compounds and chitinous scaffolds from *P. arabica* and other species. The possibility of farming of *Pseudoceratina* species from primmorph-based cultures and under marine ranching conditions possesses high potential for advanced blue biotechnology. Due to the fact that, the *P. arabica* species live at low depths (around 10 m) development of a new method for their aquaculture in tropical areas become very attractive from the industrial and economical point of view. It is already confirmed that chitinous scaffolds isolated from representatives of the order Verongiida are lucrative for the development of regenerative medicine. Further research could also be conducted to determine the possibility of technological application of chitinous scaffolds of *P. arabica* origin as advanced 3D composite materials under conditions of extreme biomimetics or adsorbents. We suggest that this study will trigger the future research dedicated to both (i) discovery of chitin within other representatives of the family Pseudoceratinidae (ii) and their utilization in modern technologies improving the quality of human life and health.

Author Contributions: H.E., T.J., Y.J., L.A.S., and S.Ż.-A. designed the study protocol and wrote the manuscript; D.T.A.Y. collected the sponge materials; L.A.S., H.Z.A., D.T.A.Y., M.T., L.V.M., O.B.S., R.G., K.T., V.N.I., and I.P. prepared samples and performed chemical characterization of chitin from *P. arabica*; R.M., N.B., H.M., and M.W. conducted SEM and other microscopy investigations and analyzed the data. All the authors critically reviewed and approved the final version of the manuscript.

Funding: This work was partially supported by DFG Project HE 394/3-2 (Germany) and PUT Research Grant no. 03/32/DSMK/0810 (Poland). Marcin Wysokowski was supported by Foundation for Polish Science—START 097.2017 and Sonia Żółtowska-Aksamitowska was supported by DAAD as well as Erasmus Plus programs. A special thanks for technical assistance and discussions goes to BromMarin GmbH and INTIB GmbH (Germany). There was no additional external funding received for this study.

Conflicts of Interest: The authors declare no conflict of interest.

References

1. Bengtson, S.; Rasmussen, B.; Ivarsson, M.; Muhling, J.; Broman, C.; Marone, F.; Stampanoni, M.; Bekker, A. Fungus-like mycelial fossils in 2.4-billion-year-old vesicular basalt. *Nat. Ecol. Evol.* **2017**, *1*, 0141. [CrossRef]
2. Wysokowski, M.; Petrenko, I.; Stelling, A.L.; Stawski, D.; Jesionowski, T.; Ehrlich, H. Poriferan chitin as a versatile template for extreme biomimetics. *Polymers* **2015**, *7*, 235–265. [CrossRef]
3. Roberts, G.A.F. *Chitin Chemistry*; MacMillian: London, UK, 1992.
4. Ehrlich, H. Chitin and collagen as universal and alternative templates in biomineralization. *Int. Geol. Rev.* **2010**, *52*, 661–669. [CrossRef]
5. Kaya, M.; Mujtaba, M.; Ehrlich, H.; Salaberria, A.M.; Baran, T.; Amemiya, C.T.; Galli, R.; Akyuz, L.; Sargin, I.; Labidi, J. On chemistry of γ-chitin. *Carbohydr. Polym.* **2017**, *176*, 177–186. [CrossRef] [PubMed]
6. Ehrlich, H.; Malando, M.; Spindler, K.D.; Eckert, C.; Hanke, T.; Born, R.; Goebel, C.; Simon, P.; Heinemann, S.; Worch, H. First evidence of chitin as a component of the skeletal fibers of marine sponges. Part I. Verongidae (Demospongia: Porifera). *J. Exp. Zool. B Mol. Dev. Evol.* **2007**, *308*, 347–356. [CrossRef]
7. Ehrlich, H.; Krautter, M.; Hanke, T.; Simon, P.; Knieb, C.; Heinemann, S.; Worch, H. First Evidence of the presence of chitin in skeletons of marine sponges. Part II. Glass sponges (Hexactinellida: Porifera). *J. Exp. Zool. B Mol. Dev. Evol.* **2007**, *306*, 473–483. [CrossRef]
8. Brunner, E.; Richthammer, P.; Ehrlich, H.; Paasch, S.; Simon, P.; Ueberlein, S.; van Pée, K.H. Chitin-based organic networks: An integral part of cell wall biosilica in the diatom *Thalassiosira pseudonana*. *Angew. Chem. Int. Ed.* **2009**, *48*, 9724–9727. [CrossRef] [PubMed]
9. Rahman, M.A.; Halfar, J. First evidence of chitin in calcified coralline algae: New insights into the calcification process of *Clathromorphum compactum*. *Sci. Rep.* **2014**, *4*, 6162. [CrossRef]
10. Ehrlich, H.; Shaala, L.A.; Youssef, D.T.A.; Żoltowska-Aksamitowska, S.; Tsurkan, M.; Galli, R.; Meissner, H.; Wysokowski, M.; Petrenko, I.; Tabachnick, K.R.; et al. Discovery of chitin in skeletons of non-verongiid Red Sea demosponges. *PLoS ONE* **2018**, *13*, e0195803. [CrossRef] [PubMed]
11. Ehrlich, H.; Kaluzhnaya, O.V.; Tsurkan, M.V.; Ereskovsky, A.; Tabachnick, K.R.; Ilan, M.; Stelling, A.; Galli, R.; Petrova, O.V.; Nekipelov, S.V.; et al. First report on chitinous holdfast in sponges (Porifera). *Proc. Biol. Sci.* **2013**, *280*, 20130339. [CrossRef]
12. Ehrlich, H.; Kaluzhnaya, O.V.; Brunner, E.; Tsurkan, M.V.; Ereskovsky, A.; Ilan, M.; Tabachnick, K.R.; Bazhenov, V.V.; Paasch, S.; Kammer, M.; et al. Identification and first insights into the structure and biosynthesis of chitin from the freshwater sponge *Spongilla lacustris*. *J. Struct. Biol.* **2013**, *183*, 474–483. [CrossRef] [PubMed]

13. Brunner, E.; Ehrlich, H.; Schupp, P.; Hedrich, R.; Hunoldt, S.; Kammer, M.; Machill, S.; Paasch, S.; Bazhenov, V.V.; Kurek, D.V.; et al. Chitin-based scaffolds are an integral part of the skeleton of the marine demosponge *Ianthella basta*. *J. Struct. Biol.* **2009**, *168*, 539–547. [CrossRef] [PubMed]
14. Ehrlich, H.; Steck, E.; Ilan, M.; Maldonado, M.; Muricy, G.; Bavestrello, G.; Kljajic, Z.; Carballo, J.L.; Schiaparelli, S.; Ereskovsky, A.; et al. Three-dimensional chitin-based scaffolds from Verongida sponges (Demospongiae: Porifera). Part II. Biomimetic potential and applications. *Int. J. Biol. Macromol.* **2010**, *47*, 141–145. [CrossRef] [PubMed]
15. Ehrlich, H.; Ilan, M.; Maldonado, M.; Muricy, G.; Bacestrello, G.; Kljajic, Z.; Carballo, J.L.; Schiaparelli, R.; Ereskovsky, A.; Schupp, P.; et al. Three-dimensional chitin-based scaffolds from Verongida sponges (Demospongiae: Porifera). Part I. Isolation and identification of chitin. *Int. J. Biol. Macromol.* **2010**, *47*, 132–140. [CrossRef] [PubMed]
16. Schleuter, D.; Günther, A.; Paasch, S.; Ehrlich, H.; Kljajić, Z.; Hanke, T.; Bernhard, G.; Brunner, E. Chitin-based renewable materials from marine sponges for uranium adsorption. *Carbohydr. Polym.* **2013**, *92*, 712–718. [CrossRef] [PubMed]
17. Mutsenko, V.V.; Bazhenov, V.V.; Rogulska, O.; Tarusin, D.N.; Schütz, K.; Brüggemeier, S.; Gossla, E.; Akkineni, A.R.; Meissner, H.; Lode, A.; et al. 3D chitinous scaffolds derived from cultivated marine demosponge *Aplysina aerophoba* for tissue engineering approaches based on human mesenchymal stromal cells. *Int. J. Biol. Macromol.* **2017**, *104*, 1966–1974. [CrossRef] [PubMed]
18. Mutsenko, V.V.; Gryshkov, O.; Lauterboeck, L.; Rogulska, O.; Tarusin, D.N.; Bazhenov, V.V.; Schütz, K.; Brüggemeier, S.; Gossla, E.; Akkineni, A.R.; et al. Novel chitin scaffolds derived from marine sponge *Ianthella basta* for tissue engineering approaches based on human mesenchymal stromal cells: Biocompatibility and cryopreservation. *Int. J. Biol. Macromol.* **2017**, *104*, 1955–1965. [CrossRef]
19. Stepniak, I.; Galinski, M.; Nowacki, K.; Wysokowski, M.; Jakubowska, P.; Bazhenov, V.V.; Leisegang, T.; Ehrlich, H.; Jesionowski, T. A novel chitosan/sponge chitin origin material as a membrane for supercapacitors—Preparation and characterization. *RSC Adv.* **2016**, *6*, 4007–4013. [CrossRef]
20. Ehrlich, H.; Simon, P.; Motylenko, M.; Wysokowski, M.; Bazhenov, V.V.; Galli, R.; Stelling, A.L.; Stawski, D.; Ilan, M.; Stöcker, H.; et al. Extreme Biomimetics: Formation of zirconium dioxide nanophase using chitinous scaffolds under hydrothermal conditions. *J. Mater. Chem. B* **2013**, *1*, 5092–5099. [CrossRef]
21. Wysokowski, M.; Motylenko, M.; Bazhenov, V.V.; Stawski, D.; Petrenko, I.; Ehrlich, A.; Behm, T.; Kljajic, Z.; Stelling, A.L.; Jesionowski, T.; et al. chitin as a template for hydrothermal zirconia deposition. *Front. Mater. Sci.* **2013**, *7*, 248–260. [CrossRef]
22. Wysokowski, M.; Motylenko, M.; Beyer, J.; Makarova, A.; Stöcker, H.; Walter, J.; Galli, R.; Kaiser, S.; Vyalikh, D.; Bazhenov, V.V.; et al. Extreme biomimetic approach for developing novel chitin-GeO_2 nanocomposites with photoluminescent properties. *Nano Res.* **2015**, *8*, 2288–2301. [CrossRef]
23. Petrenko, I.; Bazhenov, V.V.; Galli, R.; Wysokowski, M.; Fromont, J.; Schupp, P.J.; Stelling, A.L.; Niederschlag, E.; Stöker, H.; Kutsova, V.Z.; et al. Chitin of poriferan origin and the bioelectrometallurgy of copper/copper oxide. *Int. J. Biol. Macromol.* **2017**, *104*, 1626–1632. [CrossRef]
24. Harper, M.K.; Bugni, T.S.; Copp, B.R.; James, R.D.; Lindsay, B.S.; Richardson, A.D.; Schnabel, P.C.; Tasdemir, D.; van Wagoner, R.M.; Verbitski, S.M. Introduction to the chemical ecology of marine natural products. In *Marine Chemical Ecology*; McClintock, J.B., Baker, B.J., Eds.; CRC Press LLC: Boca Raton, FL, USA, 2011; pp. 3–70.
25. Bergquist, P.R.; Wells, R.J. Chemotaxonomy of the Porifera: The development and current status of the field. In *Marine Natural Products. Chemical and Biological Perspectives*; Scheue, P.J., Ed.; Academic Press: New York, NY, USA, 1983; Volume V, pp. 1–50.
26. Bergquist, P.R.; Hofheinz, W.; Oesterhelt, G. Sterol composition and the classification of the demospongiae. *Biochem. Syst. Ecol.* **1991**, *19*, 17–24. [CrossRef]
27. Shaala, L.A.; Bamane, F.H.; Badr, J.M.; Youssef, D.T.A. Brominated arginine-derived alkaloids from the red sea sponge *Suberea mollis*. *J. Nat. Prod.* **2011**, *74*, 1517–1520. [CrossRef] [PubMed]
28. Shaala, L.A.; Youssef, D.T.A.; Badr, J.M.; Sulaiman, M.; Khedr, A. Bioactive secondary metabolites from the Red Sea marine Verongid sponge *Suberea* species. *Mar. Drugs* **2015**, *13*, 1621–1631. [CrossRef] [PubMed]
29. Shaala, L.A.; Youssef, D.T.A.; Sulaiman, M.; Behery, F.A.; Foudah, A.I.; El Sayed, K.A. Subereamolline A as a potent breast cancer migration, invasion and proliferation inhibitor and bioactive dibrominated alkaloids from the red sea sponge *Pseudoceratina arabica*. *Mar. Drugs* **2012**, *10*, 2492–2508. [CrossRef] [PubMed]

30. Shaala, L.A.; Youssef, D.T.A.; Badr, J.M.; Sulaiman, M.; Khedr, A.; El Sayed, K.A. Bioactive alkaloids from the Red Sea marine Verongid sponge *Pseudoceratina arabica*. *Tetrahedron* **2015**, *71*, 7837–7841. [CrossRef]
31. Shaala, L.A.; Khalifa, S.I.; Mesbah, M.K.; van Soest, R.W.M.; Youssef, D.T.A. Subereaphenol A, a new cytotoxic and antimicrobial dibrominated phenol from the red sea sponge *Suberea mollis*. *Nat. Prod. Commun.* **2008**, *3*, 219–222.
32. Żółtowska-Aksamitowska, S.; Shaala, L.A.; Youssef, D.T.A.; Elhady, S.S.; Tsurkan, M.V.; Petrenko, I.; Wysokowski, M.; Tabachnick, K.; Meissner, H.; Ivanenko, V.N.; et al. First report on chitin in a non-verongiid marine demosponge: The *Mycale euplectellioides* case. *Mar. Drugs* **2018**, *16*, 68. [CrossRef]
33. Żółtowska-Aksamitowska, S.; Tsurkan, M.V.; Lim, S.C.; Meissner, H.; Tabachnick, K.; Shaala, L.A.; Youssef, D.T.A.; Ivanenko, V.N.; Petrenko, I.; Wysokowski, M.; et al. The demosponge *Pseudoceratina purpurea* as a new source of fibrous chitin. *Int. J. Biol. Macromol.* **2018**, *112*, 1021–1028. [CrossRef] [PubMed]
34. Bechmann, N.; Ehrlich, H.; Eisenhofer, G.; Ehrlich, A.; Meschke, S.; Ziegler, C.G.; Bornstein, S.R. Anti-tumorigenic and anti-metastatic activity of the sponge-derived marine drugs aeroplysinin-1 and isofistularin-3 against pheochromocytoma in vitro. *Mar. Drugs* **2018**, *16*, 172. [CrossRef] [PubMed]
35. Karuso, P. Chemical ecology of the nudibranchs. *Bioorg. Med. Chem.* **1987**, *1*, 31–60.
36. Tabudravu, J.N.; Eijsink, V.G.H.; Gooday, G.W.; Jaspars, M.; Komander, D.; Legg, M.; Synstad, B.; Van Aalten, D.M.F. Psammaplin A, a chitinase inhibitor isolated from the Fijian marine sponge *Aplysinella rhax*. *Bioorg. Med. Chem.* **2002**, *10*, 1123–1128. [CrossRef]
37. Abbas, A.T.; Shaala, L.A.; Ali, S.S.; Azhar, E.I.; Abdel-Dayem, U.A.; El-Shitany, N.A.; Youssef, D.T.A. Assessment of protective effects of the Red Sea Sponge *Suberea mollis* against CCl_4 -induced acute liver injury in rats. *Evid.-Based Complement. Altern. Med.* **2014**, *3*, 745606. [CrossRef]
38. Abu-Shoer, M.I.; Shaala, L.A.; Youssef, D.T.A.; Badr, J.M.; Habib, A.M. Bioactive brominated metabolites from the Red Sea sponge *Suberea mollis*. *J. Nat. Prod.* **2008**, *71*, 1464–1467. [CrossRef] [PubMed]
39. Ehrlich, H.; Bazhenov, V.V.; Meschke, S.; Burger, M.M.; Ehrlich, A.; Petovic, S.; Durovic, M. Marine invertebrates of Boka Kotorska Bay unique sources for bioinspired materials science. In *The Boka Kotorska Bay Environment, Series: The Handbook of Environmental Chemistry*; Djurović, M., Semenov, A., Zonn, I., Kostianoy, A., Eds.; Springer: Berlin/Heidelberg, Germany, 2016; pp. 313–334.
40. Ehrlich, H.; Bazhenov, V.V.; Debitus, C.; de Voogd, N.; Galli, R.; Tsurkan, M.V.; Wysokowski, M.; Meissner, H.; Bulut, E.; Kaya, M.; et al. Isolation and identification of chitin from heavy mineralized skeleton of *Suberea clavata* (Verongida: Demospongiae: Porifera) marine demosponge. *Int. J. Biol. Macromol.* **2017**, *104*, 1706–1712. [CrossRef] [PubMed]
41. Wysokowski, M.; Zatoń, M.; Bazhenov, V.V.; Behm, T.; Ehrlich, A.; Stelling, A.L.; Hog, M.; Ehrlich, H. Identification of chitin in 200-million-year-old gastropod egg capsules. *Paleobiology* **2014**, *40*, 529–540. [CrossRef]
42. Kumirska, J.; Czerwicka, M.; Kaczyński, Z.; Bychowska, A.; Brzozowski, K.; Thoming, J.; Stepnowski, P. Application of spectroscopic methods for structural analysis of chitin and chitosan. *Mar. Drugs* **2010**, *8*, 1567–1636. [CrossRef] [PubMed]
43. Galat, A.; Popowicz, J. Study of the Raman scattering spectra of chitins. *Bull. Acad. Pol. Sci. Ser. Sci. Biol.* **1987**, *26*, 519–524.
44. De Gussem, K.; Vandenabeele, P.; Verbeken, A.; Moens, L. Raman spectroscopic study of *Lactarius* spores (Russulales, Fungi). *Spectrochim. Acta Part A Mol. Biomol. Spectrosc.* **2005**, *61*, 2896–2908. [CrossRef]
45. Ehrlich, H.; Maldonado, M.; Parker, A.R.; Kulchin, Y.N.; Schilling, J.; Köhler, B.; Skrzypczak, U.; Simon, P.; Reiswig, H.M.; Tsurkan, M.V.; et al. Supercontinuum generation in naturally occurring glass sponges spicules. *Adv. Opt. Mater.* **2016**, *4*, 1608–1613. [CrossRef]
46. Nickerl, J.; Tsurkan, M.; Neinhuis, C.; Werner, C. The multilayered protective cuticle of *Collembola*: A chemical analysis. *J. R. Soc. Interface* **2014**, *11*, 20140619. [CrossRef] [PubMed]
47. Ehrlich, H.; Rigby, J.K.; Botting, J.P.; Tsurkan, M.V.; Werner, C.; Schwille, P.; Petrášek, Z.; Pisera, A.; Simon, P.; Sivkov, V.N.; et al. Discovery of 505-million-year old chitin in the basal demosponge *Vauxia gracilenta*. *Sci. Rep.* **2013**, *3*, 17–20. [CrossRef] [PubMed]
48. Bergquist, P.R.; Kelly-Borges, M. Systematics and biogeography of the genus *Ianthella* (Demospongiae: Verongida: Ianthellidae) in the South-West Pacific. The Beagle. *Rec. Museums Art Gall. North. Territ.* **1995**, *12*, 151–176.

49. Erwin, P.M.; Thacker, R.W. Phylogenetic analyses of marine sponges within the order Verongida: A comparison of morphological and molecular data. *Invertebr. Biol.* **2007**, *126*, 220–234. [CrossRef]
50. Thompson, J.E.; Barrow, K.D.; Faulkner, D.J. Localization of two brominated metabolites, aerothionin and homoaerothionin, in spherulous cells of the marine sponge *Aplysina fistularis* (=*Verongia thiona*). *Acta Zool.* **1983**, *64*, 199–210. [CrossRef]
51. Jesionowski, T.; Norman, M.; Żółtowska-Aksamitowska, S.; Petrenko, I.; Joseph, Y.; Ehrlich, H. Marine spongin: Naturally prefabricated 3D scaffold-based biomaterial. *Mar. Drugs* **2018**, *16*, 88. [CrossRef]
52. Wysokowski, M.; Bazhenov, V.V.; Tsurkan, M.V.; Galli, R.; Stelling, A.L.; Stöcker, H.; Kaiser, S.; Niederschlag, E.; Gärtner, G.; Behm, T.; et al. Isolation and identification of chitin in three-dimensional skeleton of *Aplysina fistularis* marine sponge. *Int. J. Biol. Macromol.* **2013**, *62*, 94–100. [CrossRef]
53. Monheit, J.E.; Cowan, D.F.; Moore, D.G. Rapid detection of fungi in tissues using Calcofluor White and fluorescence microscopy. *Arch. Pathol. Lab. Med.* **1984**, *108*, 616–618.
54. Hickey, P.C.; Swift, S.R.; Roca, M.G.; Read, N.D. Live-cell imaging of filamentous fungi using vital fluorescent dyes and confocal microscopy. *Methods Microbiol.* **2004**, *34*, 63–87.

© 2019 by the authors. Licensee MDPI, Basel, Switzerland. This article is an open access article distributed under the terms and conditions of the Creative Commons Attribution (CC BY) license (http://creativecommons.org/licenses/by/4.0/).

marine drugs

MDPI

Article

From Aggregates to Porous Three-Dimensional Scaffolds through a Mechanochemical Approach to Design Photosensitive Chitosan Derivatives

Kseniia N. Bardakova [1,2,*], Tatiana A. Akopova [3], Alexander V. Kurkov [1], Galina P. Goncharuk [3], Denis V. Butnaru [1], Vitaliy F. Burdukovskii [4], Artem A. Antoshin [1], Ivan A. Farion [4], Tatiana M. Zharikova [1,5], Anatoliy B. Shekhter [1], Vladimir I. Yusupov [2], Peter S. Timashev [1,2,6] and Yury A. Rochev [1,7]

1 Institute for Regenerative Medicine, Sechenov University, 8-2 Trubetskaya st., Moscow 119991, Russia; a-kurkov@yandex.ru (A.V.K.); butnaru.dw@gmail.com (D.V.B.); antoshin.art@gmail.com (A.A.A.); zharikova.tm@gmail.com (T.M.Z.); a.shehter@yandex.ru (A.B.S.); timashev.peter@gmail.com (P.S.T.); yury.rochev@nuigalway.ie (Y.A.R.)

2 Institute of Photonic Technologies, Research center "Crystallography and Photonics", Russian Academy of Sciences, 2 Pionerskaya st., Troitsk, Moscow 108840, Russia; iouss@yandex.ru

3 Enikolopov Institute of Synthetic Polymer Materials, Russian Academy of Sciences, 70 Profsoyuznaya st., Moscow 117393, Russia; akopova@ispm.ru (T.A.A.); duna2011@yandex.ru (G.P.G.)

4 Baikal Institute of Nature Management, Siberian Branch of the Russian Academy of Sciences, 6 Sakhyanovoy st., Ulan-Ude 670047, Russia; burdvit@mail.ru (V.F.B.); fariv@mail.ru (I.A.F.)

5 Institute for Urology and Reproductive Health, Sechenov University, 2-1 Bolshaya Pirogovskaya st., Moscow 119435, Russia

6 Semenov Institute of Chemical Physics, Russian Academy of Sciences, 4 Kosygina st., Moscow 119991, Russia

7 National Centre for Biomedical Engineering Science, National University of Ireland, Galway (NUI Galway), University Road, Galway H91 TK33, Ireland

* Correspondence: arie5@yandex.ru; Tel.: +7-495-609-1400

Received: 11 December 2018; Accepted: 8 January 2019; Published: 10 January 2019

Abstract: The crustacean processing industry produces large quantities of waste by-products (up to 70%). Such wastes could be used as raw materials for producing chitosan, a polysaccharide with a unique set of biochemical properties. However, the preparation methods and the long-term stability of chitosan-based products limit their application in biomedicine. In this study, different scale structures, such as aggregates, photo-crosslinked films, and 3D scaffolds based on mechanochemically-modified chitosan derivatives, were successfully formed. Dynamic light scattering revealed that aggregation of chitosan derivatives becomes more pronounced with an increase in the number of hydrophobic substituents. Although the results of the mechanical testing revealed that the plasticity of photo-crosslinked films was 5–8% higher than that for the initial chitosan films, their tensile strength remained unchanged. Different types of polymer scaffolds, such as flexible and porous ones, were developed by laser stereolithography. In vivo studies of the formed structures showed no dystrophic and necrobiotic changes, which proves their biocompatibility. Moreover, the wavelet analysis was used to show that the areas of chitosan film degradation were periodic. Comparing the results of the wavelet analysis and X-ray diffraction data, we have concluded that degradation occurs within less ordered amorphous regions in the polymer bulk.

Keywords: mechanochemical synthesis; chitosan; laser stereolithography; long-term stability; scaffold; tissue reaction

1. Introduction

Formation of waste by-products from commercial fish and seafood production is a topical problem nowadays. For example, in the case of the crustacean processing industry, the amount of waste by-products reaches 50–70% of the raw material [1]. Such wastes require additional economic costs for their disposal and, therefore, the industry should pay close attention to the waste recycling process.

Sea crustaceans are known to contain a large amount of chitin, a polysaccharide which is the second most abundant biopolymer after cellulose. It is also found in the exoskeleton of insects, cell walls of fungi, and in green algae [2]. Partial deacetylation of chitin results in the formation of chitosan [3], a biopolymer with a unique set of biological and physicochemical properties. In addition to biodegradability and biocompatibility, chitosan is a non-immunogenic material, which also demonstrates antifungal and antimicrobial activities [4], with an almost absent reaction to a foreign body, no formation of a fibrous capsule [5], and the ability to penetrate through the intestinal barrier [6]. Free amino groups give chitosan many specific properties, distinguishing it from chitin. The amino groups of the D-glucosamine residues can be protonated, and the resulting polycation can subsequently form ionic complexes with various proteins, lipids, DNA and negatively-charged synthetic polymers [2]. Moreover, such polycations have the ability to interact with the negative charges of the cell surface [7]. Materials based on chitosan and its derivatives may be presented in different physical forms. Their mucoadhesive properties allow them to be used as excipients for the preparation of buccal, vaginal and nasal dosage forms [8,9].

Despite extensive renewable sources of chitosan and its universal properties, there are practically no available pharmaceutical products based on this biopolymer. This fact has several explanations. First, chitosan is sensitive to storage and processing conditions. Significant heating or cooling can cause stress to its structure and cause polymer degradation or oxidative transformation of its functional groups [8]. It limits the number of reagents suitable for chemical modification of chitosan. In the numerous studies devoted to the application of chitosan-based materials in the pharmaceutical and biomedical fields, chitosan and its derivatives were obtained mainly through a classical chemical synthesis [10–13]. Application of toxic solvents as well as a low final product yield do not allow the extrapolation of the synthesis schemes developed in the scientific studies onto an industrial scale.

There is another reason limiting the application of chitosan and its derivatives in the pharmaceutical industry and biomedicine. Being a natural polymer, chitosan has highly variable properties. Its mean molecular weight, molecular weight distribution, degree of deacetylation, and purity are highly dependent on the production methods, as well as on the choice of the raw material source [14]. These characteristics affect the physicochemical (e.g., viscosity, solubility) and biological (e.g., biodegradability, stability) properties of chitosan and its derivatives.

Long-term stability is one of the problems associated with the introduction of drug delivery systems into a wider clinical application. Chitosan-based delivery systems must be thermally, chemically, and mechanically stable thereby maintaining the effectiveness of the dosage form for a long time [15]. Several strategies to increase the long-term stability of chitosan-based products are known: polymer-analogous transformations of functional groups, application of stabilizing agents, and physical and chemical cross-linking [8,16,17].

In our study, we used the technique of processing solid mixtures which combines chemical reagents, pressure and shear stress. This method is known as mechanochemical synthesis [18–20]. Compared to the conventional solvent-based chemical synthesis, mechanochemical synthesis is a convenient and effective approach to targeted chemical modification of non-melting or poorly soluble polysaccharides, since it does not require melting the reaction mixtures [21,22]. Mechanochemical synthesis can be adopted to different production conditions as well as scaled and, therefore, this method has been employed across a number of industries including food, polymer, and pharmaceutical manufacturing [23]. Currently, there is a global trend towards using environmentally friendly and safe processes to modify medical polymers. Mechanochemical synthesis has attracted the attention of researchers in the field of biomedical materials science, since it does not require solvents, catalysts, and initiators of chemical processes, thus reducing the negative impact on the environment. As a result, the economic costs of solvent disposal and purification of synthesized medical polymers are excluded.

In our study, we used the same extruder either for alkaline deacetylation of chitin or for its modification with allyl groups on a pilot-industrial scale. Introduction of hydrophobic unsaturated substituents allows us not only to increase the long-term stability of chitosan-based materials, but also to obtain a photosensitive biopolymer. When exposed to ultraviolet and laser radiation, it can crosslink and form stable three-dimensional networks.

Thus, the presented work is aimed at determining the physicochemical properties and long-term stability of chitosan materials modified by mechanochemical synthesis at various levels of their structural organization including aggregates, films and three-dimensional structures. In other words, from submicron structures to macrostructures of high resolution.

To achieve this goal, our work was divided into the following stages, according to Figure 1.

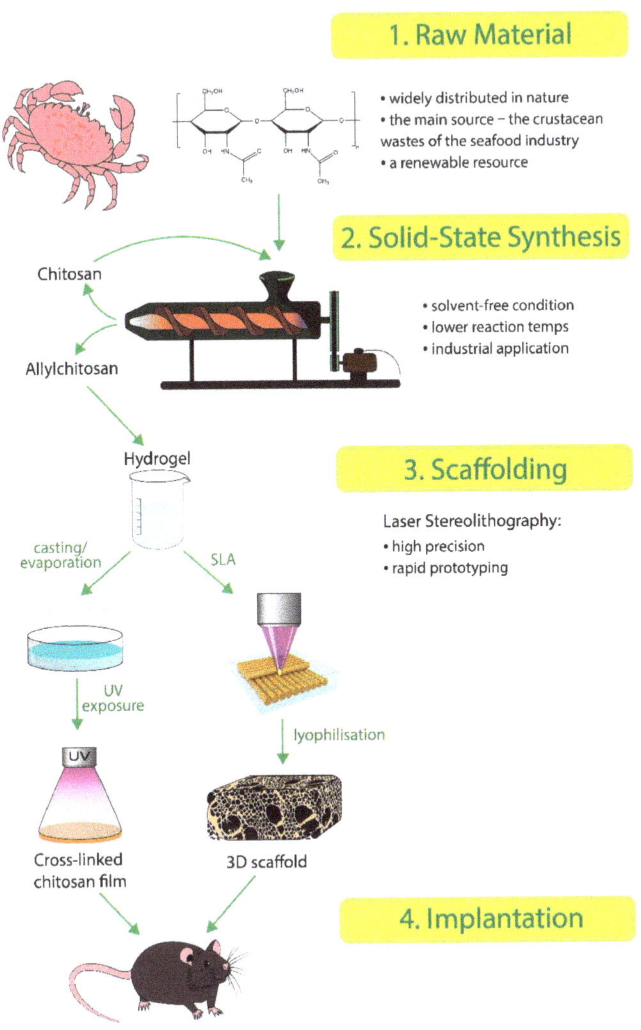

Figure 1. Scheme of the experimental work.

Chitosan was synthesized by deacetylation of crab chitin in a pilot-industrial extruder. Later, in the same extruder, hydrophobic fragments were introduced into the structure of chitosan. The obtained derivatives were used to prepare polymer solutions, in which forming aggregates were studied by dynamic light scattering. At the next step, photocrosslinked polymer films and three-dimensional structures (3D scaffolds) were formed. Previously, we had applied the two-photon polymerization technique to produce three-dimensional microstructures from synthesized photosensitive polysaccharides [24,25]. In this study, we used laser stereolithography, a simple and fast technique of three-dimensional prototyping requiring no expensive equipment [26,27]. The technique implies a layer-by-layer formation of a three-dimensional scaffold from a photosensitive material according to a computer-aided design (CAD) blueprint. The photosensitive material usually consists of monomers or oligomers with a photoinitiator. It is of note that, in the case of laser stereolithography, it is possible to regulate the mechanical properties of a scaffold and subsequently obtain a construct with the properties close to those of the tissues to be substituted. This is achieved by varying the parameters of laser structuring (e.g., the number of laser passes for one layer, distance both between passes and layers, laser fluence, and the scanning speed of galvanometric mirrors); regulating the number of chromophore groups in the raw material; varying the physico-mechanical characteristics of the polymer component in the composition. In addition, the long-term stability of the formed photocrosslinked films and 3D scaffolds was studied in vivo.

2. Results and Discussion

2.1. *Synthesis of Allylchitosans (AC) and Their Properties*

According to the NMR spectra-based calculations, the degree of substitution (per 100 polymer units) of the sample AC2 was 5% and it grew on increasing the allyl bromide (AB) in the initial mixtures: 17–20% for samples AC3, AC4 and up to 50% for the sample AC5. In the alkaline medium, O-substituted products were formed predominantly, but not selectively. The observed structure of the obtained derivatives was in total agreement with the difference in the nucleophilicity of the polymer hydroxy and amino groups under the catalytic reaction conditions. When compared to the initial polymer, the solubility of chitosan samples modified with hydrophobic allyl fragments in acetic acid (2%), a conventional solvent of chitosan, decreased insignificantly (1–2%), which allowed us to use solution methods for the preparation of such materials. Generally, our studies have shown that, for the synthesis of chitosan derivatives, mechanical activation of solid reaction mixtures is preferable since it substantially reduces the consumption of reagents, the process duration (up to several minutes), and the process temperature in contrast to a similar process in an organic solvent (isopropyl alcohol, 70 °C, 1–4 h) [28].

2.1.1. Hydrodynamic Diameter of Aggregates in the Samples in Aqueous Solutions

Since the use of chitosan and its derivatives is mainly associated with their aqueous solutions, it is necessary to investigate the materials' behavior in such media. Spontaneously-formed chitosan aggregates, which can be used as drug and gene carriers [29,30], are of special interest. Figure 2 shows the relation between the hydrodynamic diameter and the degree of substitution (DS) of chitosan amino groups.

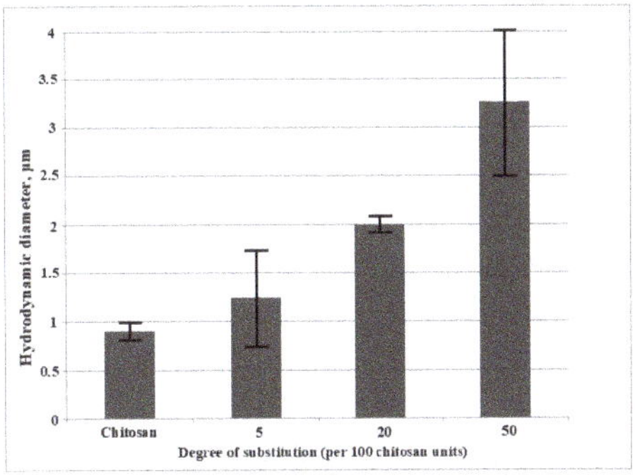

Figure 2. The relation between the hydrodynamic diameter and the degree of substitution of chitosan amino groups with allyl fragments. Solutions were prepared with acetic acid (2%) at a final concentration of 0.02 g/dL.

The same results for the average size of chitosan aggregates were obtained in the study by Popa-Nita et al. [31]: for 0.01 wt% chitosan solutions, aggregate sizes (diameters) ranged from 200 nm to 2000 nm. Moreover, the authors showed an increase in the aggregate sizes with an increase in the degree of acetylation, i.e., with an increase in the number of hydrophobic substituents in the chitosan structure [31]. Other studies [32,33] also showed more pronounced aggregation caused by acetamide groups left as a result of incomplete chitin deacetylation. In these articles, the aggregation was caused by either a change in the degree of protonation of dissolved macromolecules or by enhancement of hydrophobic intermolecular interactions.

However, the available data on the chitosan intermolecular aggregation are highly contradictory. The complex behavior of chitosan macromolecules in solutions is determined by the ability of their functional groups to form hydrogen bonds, both intermolecular and intramolecular, that stabilize the conformational structure. For example, some studies [34,35] showed a suppression of aggregation with an increase in the degree of acetylation, which was explained by the decrease in the chitosan crystallinity. Apparently, chitosan is prone to aggregate due to several factors, with each of them contributing to the association energy. In our experiments with dilute solutions of allylchitosan samples, dynamic light scattering revealed the formation of intermolecular lipophilic interactions. When the degree of substitution reached a significant value (sample AC5), these interactions led to the formation of aggregates, whose sizes were greater than those of the initial chitosan. Thus, the mechanical activation of solid reaction mixtures allows for the preparation of chitosan aggregates—of the required sizes by selecting the conditions for mechanochemical synthesis and varying the number of hydrophobic fragments introduced into the chitosan structure.

2.1.2. Mechanical Properties of the Film Samples

Table 1 shows the effect of mechanochemical modification with allyl fragments, as well as of ultraviolet (UV) irradiation, on the mechanical properties of chitosan films.

Table 1. Deformation-strength characteristics of allylchitosans.

Sample	DS (mol%)	Before UV Exposure			After UV Exposure		
		σ (MPa)	E (MPa)	ε (%)	σ (MPa)	E (MPa)	ε (%)
Chitosan	0	37 ± 2	1800 ± 200	18 ± 3	39 ± 3	1900 ± 200	18 ± 3
AC2	5	37 ± 2	1800 ± 200	26 ± 3	41 ± 3	1900 ± 100	21 ± 3
AC4	20	38 ± 2	2100 ± 200	25 ± 3	38 ± 2	1800 ± 200	19 ± 3
AC5	50	33 ± 2	1900 ± 200	23 ± 3	33 ± 2	1400 ± 200	17 ± 3

For the initial chitosan, the obtained values of tensile strength and elongation at break are higher than those in the study by Souza et al. [36] (σ = 13 MPa and ε = 16%) and they also exceed values for chitosan films treated with various monomers and UV irradiation by Khan et al. [37] (σ up to 29.1 MPa and ε up to 16.2%). This difference can be explained by the following factors: the origin and characteristics of chitosan source, the degree of acetylation and the molecular weight of chitosan, the solvent type, the polymer concentration in molding solutions, and the conditions for film preparation and storage [38,39].

Additional lipophilic interactions provided by allyl fragments in the structure of AC samples did not significantly contribute to their tensile strength. Moreover, UV irradiation also had no effect on the tensile strength of the films. For allylchitosan-based films, elongation at break (or plasticity) prior to UV exposure was 5–8% higher than that of the initial chitosan films. Obviously, the introduction of hydrophobic substituents into a chitosan macromolecule results in a change in the films' crystalline morphology [40]. The UV treatment led to some decrease in the elongation at break for the AC films, especially for samples with a high degree of substitution. Such a result is expectable. UV irradiation has the ability to induce formation of cross-links in a polymer film containing unsaturated fragments. This leads to a decrease in the mobility of polymer chains, which is reflected in a lower material plasticity. The increased film hydrophobicity also causes a reduction of the water content in the film, while water acts as a plasticizer [41].

2.1.3. X-Ray Diffraction (XRD) Analysis of Film Samples

The results of the XRD analysis for mechanochemically modified chitosan before and after UV irradiation are demonstrated in Figure 3.

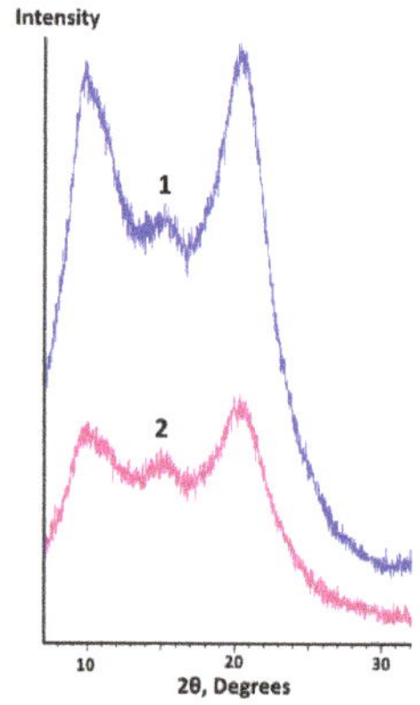

Figure 3. XRD analysis of allylchitosan film (sample AC2) before (spectrum 1) and after (spectrum 2) UV cross-linking.

When comparing the XRD data of the two samples, one can notice that cross-linking did not change the positions of the peaks. The presence of a broad intense maximum corresponding to $2\theta \approx 20$ deg (d_1 = 4.434 Å) for the mechanochemically modified chitosan is similar to other published results [36,42–44]. This maximum is explained by the presence of amorphous as well as "pseudocrystalline" regions (crystallites) in the polymer. These crystallites represent ordered regions where polymer chains are oriented parallel to each other. Another broad intense maximum at $2\theta \approx 10$ deg (d_2 = 8.835 Å) is assigned to the hydrated crystalline structure of chitosan, which was also observed in other studies [36,45]. The values of the interplanar distance, d_2 and d_1, had an approximate ratio of 2:1, which could correspond to two reflection periods between two planes of crystallites. In other words, the minimum distance between these planes was 4.434 Å. The maximum of low intensity at 2θ ≈ 15 deg (d_3 = 5.899 Å) can also relate to the presence of crystalline regions in the structure of the initial chitosan, as was shown in several studies [43,46].

2.2. Three-Dimensional Scaffolds

Three-dimensional scaffolds based on mechanochemically modified chitosan were successfully formed by laser stereolithography. The scaffold thicknesses of 1 mm or 2 mm were obtained, i.e., approximately six or 11 layers respectively were cross-linked layer-by-layer. The advantage of this approach to structuring chitosan derivatives is the production of three-dimensional scaffolds which have sufficient dimensions for regenerating tissue defects. After stereolithography, the scaffolds were slightly yellowish and transparent. The transparency of the allylchitosan materials allows us not only to sterilize them with UV radiation [47], but also to develop 3D structures for easy microscopy imaging [48]. In addition, the selected structuring parameters resulted in the preparation of a flexible and mechanically strong scaffold (Figure 4a).

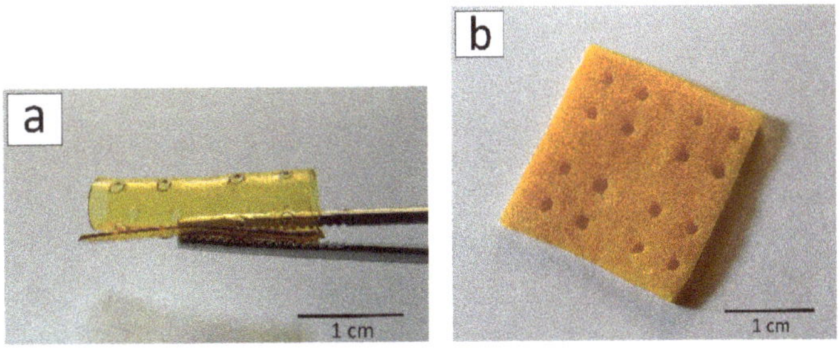

Figure 4. Three-dimensional scaffold after laser stereolithography (**a**) and freeze drying (**b**).

However, there is no internal pore architecture in such 3D scaffolds, which is a disadvantage of this structuring method since the scaffold porosity plays an important role in the diffusion of oxygen, nutrients and cellular waste [49], and supports cells' attachment and proliferation following seeding [50]. To form allylchitosan porous structures, we used the freeze-drying method. Freeze-drying is not associated with any chemical reaction and, therefore, there are no complications with the scaffold purification from by-products. As can be seen in Figure 4b, the three-dimensional scaffold does not lose its integrity and architectonics after the process of freeze drying, and it may be rehydrated. At the same time, the scaffold loses its transparency, which is caused by phase separation during the freezing of the solvent. Freezing, in turn, forms macropores and tightly crosslinked pore walls [51,52]. The 3D scaffold becomes slightly brittle, although in general its mechanical properties are still suitable for suturing.

Evaluation of a typical pore in the scanning electron microscopy (SEM) image (Figure 5a) revealed that the pore surface occupied 30% of the total surface area.

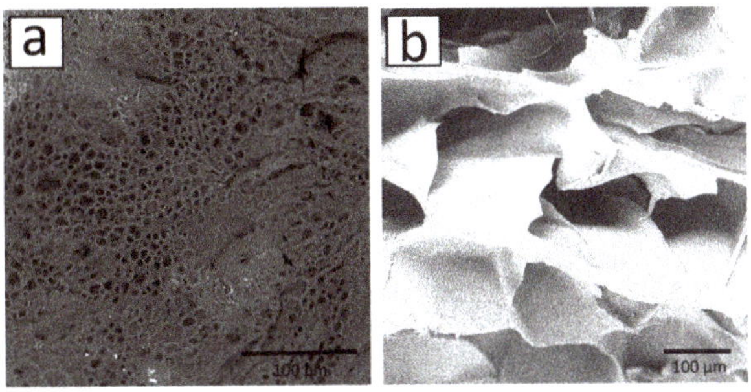

Figure 5. Surface SEM images of the 3D scaffold (**a**) and freeze-dried matrix (**b**), bar = 100 µm.

About 66% of pores had a size of 3–6 μm. It should be noted that the pore surface area was determined by the method of treating scaffolds after stereolithography, UV photocuring. The photocuring process was expected to additionally photo-crosslink chitosan derivatives and, as a consequence, to form more durable polymeric networks on the scaffold surface. The obtained pore sizes, as well as the presence of hydrophobic allyl fragments in the structure of chitosan, will provide a long-time efficiency of the subsequently prepared drug forms.

Based on the evaluation of a two-dimensional section in Figure 5b, the typical pore size was 20–60 μm. Thicker parallel pore walls of the 3D scaffold are also visible in a two-dimensional section. Most likely, the walls were formed by the freeze drying of more tightly crosslinked contact regions of the previous laser-crosslinked layer with the subsequent layer.

2.3. Implantation of Films and Porous 3D Scaffolds based on Allylchitosans

On day 30 after the implantation, there were no signs of biodegradation of any of the film types or 3D scaffolds. There were no significant differences in the tissue reaction to them. Tinctorial and optical properties of these scaffolds were close (Figure 6a,b; Supplementary Figures S1–S3; Figure S4a,b; Table S1).

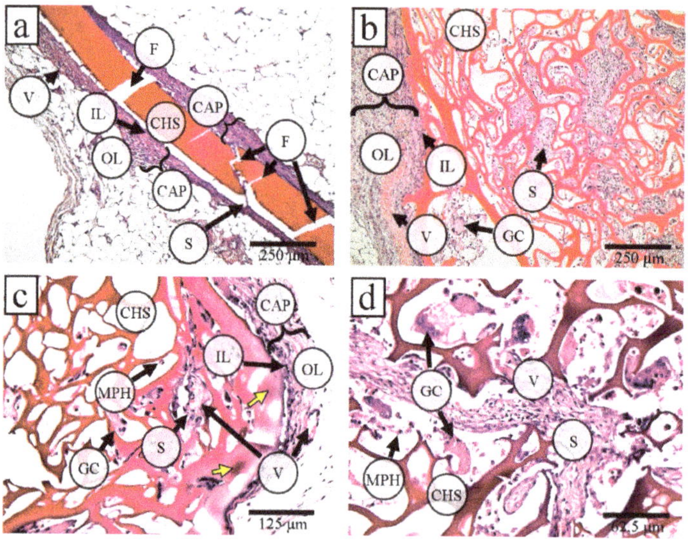

Figure 6. Tissue reaction to the films and the porous 3D scaffolds based on allylchitosans: the connective tissue formed the capsule (CAP) with blood vessels (V) around the implanted chitosan films (CHF) and the chitosan sponges (CHS); CAP consisted of two layers: the inner layer (IL) was an immature connective tissue (granulation tissue) with macrophages (MPH) and giant cells (GC), while the outer layer (OL) consisted of a more mature connective tissue; IL grew into the film fractures (F) and CHS pores forming connective tissue septa (S); some MPH and GC adhered to the surface of scaffolds, hematoxylin and eosin staining, simple microscopy (**a**) CHF (AC2) implantation (30 days): the CHF material was oxyphilic, 100×; (b–d)—3D scaffold implantation: (**b**) 30 days: the CHS material was oxyphilic, 100×; (**c**) a basophilic foci (yellow arrows) in the surface septa of the CHS material, 60 days, 200×; and (**d**) deep CHS sections: most of the scaffold septa were moderately basophilic, 90 days, 400×.

Connective tissue capsules surrounded all implanted scaffolds. Additionally, connective tissue carried of varying thickness and maturity. It grew into the pores of 3D scaffolds and the chitosan films fracture sites together with blood vessels. There were moderate macrophage and foreign-body giant cell reactions without any necrosis or dystrophy in surrounding tissues.

Since the film material was brittle (see Figure 6a; Supplementary Figure S1; Figure S2a,b,d,f), for the subsequent studies of the long-term stability of samples from solid-phase modified chitosan we only used porous 3D scaffolds.

On days 60 and 90 after the implantation, there were no macroscopic signs of scaffold biodegradation. On day 60 after implantation, focal changes in the tinctorial properties of the scaffolds became noticeable (Figure 6c; Supplementary Figure S5; Table S1). We clearly observed these changes in the scaffold septa (mainly near macrophages and giant cells), which had small foci of lysis of scaffold material. These changes slightly increased on day 90 (Figure 6d; Supplementary Figure S6; Tables S1 and S2). The tissue reaction to scaffolds did not significantly differ during all the post-implantation periods, except for a decrease in the maximum capsule thickness (Supplementary Figure S4c). Additionally, we observed the intensification of connective tissue ingrowth and vascularization and a giant cell reaction, the connective tissue around and inside the 3D scaffolds became more mature, grew deeper, but it did not fill the scaffold pores completely (Supplementary Tables S1 and S2).

In summary, the implanted films and 3D scaffolds caused the foreign body reaction with the development of fibrosis without any necrosis or dystrophy in surrounding tissues, which was generally similar to the morphological results in other experiments [53–59].

The resorption of chitosan-based materials was also confirmed by basophilicity in other studies [54,56]. Kim et al. [56] used hematoxylin and eosin staining combined with Luxol fast blue. They suggested that, when chitosan degrades with lysozyme, the hydrolyzed β1–4 glycosidic bond results in the formation of a free anomeric hydroxyl group on the cleaved residue. Together with the C2-amino group, it is capable of forming a complex with aluminum-containing hematoxylin dye. Apparently, introduction of allyl groups does not block the access of enzymes (lysozyme, chitinase, chitosanase, glucosaminidase) capable of breaking glycosidic bonds in chitosan [60]. There is no detailed study of the relationship between the tinctorial and physicochemical characteristics of chitosan with respect to other dyes.

It should be added that in our study, there were no necrotic tissue changes or acute inflammatory reactions, reported in a number of other studies on chitosan implantation [53,55,57,58]. Most likely, we suppressed the neutrophil infiltration by introducing allyl groups in the chitosan structure, which led to an increase in the basic properties of a chitosan molecule's fragments. This result, in turn, was similar to the proposals [57,59,61–63] to increase the amino group concentration (or decrease N-acetylation of chitosan) to reduce the chemotactic effect of chitosan on neutrophils.

Internal Structure of Film Samples

We used the wavelet analysis to characterize the microstructure of a chitosan film stained with picrosirius red. In principle, the wavelet analysis has already been suggested for applying in the clinical interpretation of histological images. For example, in the study by Haar and Daubechies [64], transform wavelets were tested as a diagnostic tool for the detection and classification of breast tumors. However, there are no studies in the field of materials science which use a wavelet transform to reveal the internal structure of scaffolds which biodegrade in vivo.

In Figure 7, we present an example of the wavelet analysis applied in our study.

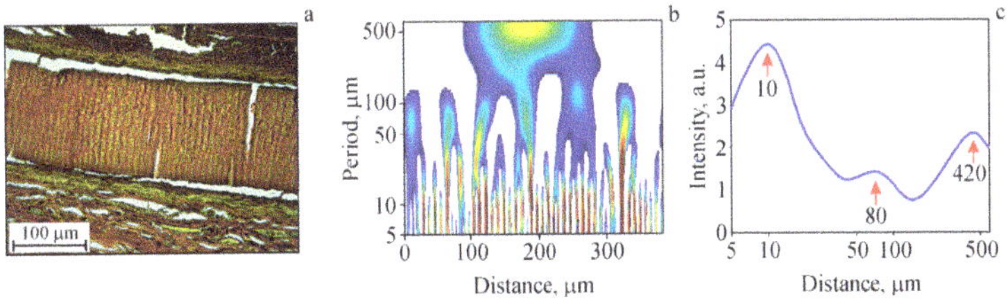

Figure 7. A histological section of chitosan film (**a**), a waveletgram (**b**), and the integral spatial spectrum of the structural optical inhomogeneities along the film section in the direction of its surface (**c**).

In Figure 7a, a chitosan film histological section is shown. Its structural optical inhomogeneities, yellow (picrinophilic) fragments and brown-red strips, were investigated with a constructed waveletgram. Figure 7b shows the corresponding waveletgram with vertical strips in the period range of 5 μm to 100 μm. Some of these strips join together forming a "tree structure", while the other strips are separated from the others forming a "grass structure". There is also a large "tree structure" in the range from 5 μm to 500 μm in the center of the waveletgram. The "tree structures" indicate that the periodicities of different scales are interrelated [65] (so-called cascade process where multiscale structures are genetically related). Using waveletgrams, an integral spatial spectrum may be plotted (Figure 7c), which characterizes the strongest periodicities for the entire processed image. For this procedure, we averaged the waveletgram along the abscissa (the distance). In the integral spatial spectrum three pronounced maxima are seen with a spatial periodicity of 10 μm, 80 μm and 420 μm. Thus, the transverse striation visualized by picrosirius red staining, depicting the areas of allylchitosan degradation, demonstrates that such areas are located periodically rather than chaotically.

When stained with picrosirius red, chitosan was colored dark-red [53–55], while in the study by Park et al. [66] it was picrinophilic. Most likely, the different chitosan coloration can be explained by its varying degree of degradation as well as by the diversity of chitosan crystalline forms. It is known that chitosan can exist in two distinct crystal forms, and its XR diffractogram depends on the ratio of these forms [36]. Comparing the integral spatial spectrum of the structural optical inhomogeneities along the film section (Figure 7c) and the XR diffractogram of modified chitosan films in the range of $7 < 2\theta < 30$ deg (see Section 2.1.3, Figure 3), one can note the "reverse" similarity of the obtained spectra. This effect indicates that crystallites are distributed throughout the entire film volume (long-range order) that apparently causes the observed structural optical inhomogeneities (the brown-red strips in picrosirius red staining). In other words, at the first stage, the degradation of film samples occurs within less ordered amorphous regions, following the increase in the chitosan degree of deacetylation due to β-1,4-glycosidic bond cleavage (depolymerization) with the subsequent N-acetyl linkage [8]. The newly released basic groups react with sulfide groups of picrosirius red. This leads to the formation of brown-red strips on day 30 after the film implantation and to the expansion of red-stained areas on day 60 after the 3D scaffold implantation.

3. Materials and Methods

3.1. Synthesis of Allylchitosans

The synthesis of unsaturated chitosan derivatives (Figure 8) was carried out by treating chitosan powders with AB in the absence of solvents under shear strain in a pilot-industrial twin-screw extruder ("Berstorff ZE 40", Munich, Germany).

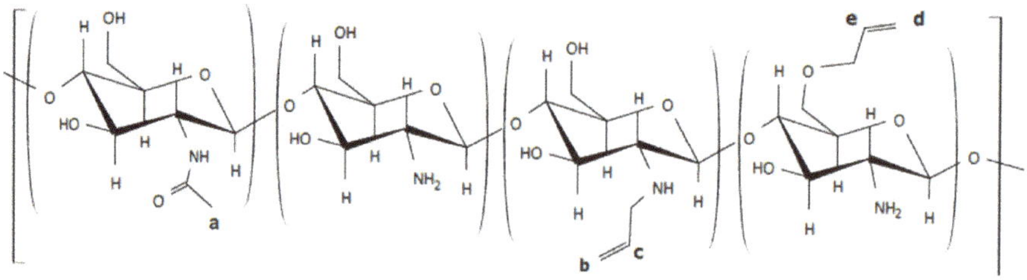

Figure 8. The structure of the synthesized allylchitosans.

Chitosan was prepared by mechanochemical alkaline deacetylation of crab chitin (Xiamen Fine Chemical Import and Export Co., Ltd., Xiamen, China) with a three-fold molar excess of sodium hydroxide, according to the published procedure [67], and had the following characteristics: degree of acylation (DA) = 15 mol% (evaluated by potentiometric titration of a hydrochloric solution of a sample and by NMR spectroscopy (Bruker, Billerica, MA, USA), and molecular weight (MW) = 80 kDa (evaluated by viscosimetry). The working chambers of extruder were cooled to −5 °C before adding AB to the reactive mixture. The relative number of AB molecules per elementary unit of chitosan in the mixtures was 0.5 (sample AC2), 1.0 (sample AC3), 1.5 (sample AC4), and 2.0 (sample AC5). In the case of AC3–AC5 samples, the reactive mixture contained also sodium hydroxide (2 molecules per elementary unit of chitosan), while AC2 sample was prepared using neat chitosan powder. The reaction products were purified by extraction of unreacted allyl bromide with isopropanol. The removal of alkaline impurities was performed by dialysis against distilled water until the rinsing water became neutral. The purified products were freeze-dried.

The ^{1}H NMR spectra were recorded with a Bruker-Avance II-300 instrument operating at 300 MHz in D_2O solutions at a temperature of 90 °C. A deuterated DMSO signal (δ = 2.5 ppm) was used to calibrate the chemical shift scale (Supplementary Figure S7).

The content of allyl groups in the modified chitosan was determined by measuring and comparing the integrated intensities of proton signals in the following structural fragments: >C**H**-NH_2 (at 3.0–3.2 ppm); **H_3**C-CONH- (Figure 8a; 1.9 ppm); **H_2**C=CH-CH_2-NH- (Figure 8b,c; 5.3–5.5 ppm); **H_2**C=CH-CH_2-O- (Figure 8d,e; 5.1–5.2 ppm).

3.2. Preparation of Films and 3D Scaffolds

The films were prepared by casting solutions of polymers (2%) in acetic acid (2%) onto a plastic substrate with subsequent drying at the temperature of 20 °C for 48 h in a laminar flow cabinet. The solutions were preliminarily filtered through a membrane with a pore size of 0.45 μm, the volume was calculated based on the amount of the polymer necessary to form homogeneous films with a thickness of 100 μm. Before carrying out the mechanical tests, the films were stored in a vacuum desiccator above KOH for a week to remove the excess acid. For the biological studies, the films were immersed for 2 h in an aqueous ammonia solution (25%) for the polymer transfer from the salt to the basic form and washed with distilled water to neutral pH.

For each type of allylchitosan, photocrosslinked films were prepared as follows: 0.5 wt% of a photoinitiator (Irgacure 2959; Ciba Specialty Chemicals, Switzerland) was added into the molding solutions of allylchitosan, and the films were illuminated for 30 min by a DRSH-500 mercury lamp. The radiation intensity at the surface of the films was 3.1 mW/cm^2. The detailed studies of the crosslinking process of the films are given in [68].A photosensitive composition (PSC) for the preparation of 3D scaffolds by single-photon laser stereolithography was prepared as follows: an acetic acid solution (4.7 wt%) of sample AC5 was mixed with polyethylene glycol diacrylate (8 wt%; Sigma-Aldrich, MO, USA), and the mixture was stirred for 24 h at 35 °C until a homogeneous solution was achieved. Subsequently, 1 wt% of the Irgacure 2959 photoinitiator was added, and the mixture was again stirred at 35 °C for 24 h. The shelf life of PSC is three days.

The three-dimensional scaffolds were structured by laser stereolithography (LS 120, IPT RAS, Russia) according to the previous study [26]. HeCd laser (with the wavelength of 325 nm, laser power of 15 mW) was used to initiate the three-dimensional cross-linking process in the PSC. The laser beam movement along the surface of the PSC and its focusing were performed with a scanner. Then, a single scaffold layer was formed, the stage was lowered with a Z-axis motor stage to a predetermined layer thickness (200 μm), and the next scaffold layer was formed.

A 20 mm × 20 mm plate with a thickness of 1 mm or 2 mm with reach-through oval holes measuring 1 mm by 2 mm was used as a computer-aided design (CAD) blueprint. The distance between the centers of the holes was 4 mm or 6 mm (changed alternately). After the laser structuring, the samples were washed from unreacted PSC with distilled water and additionally photocured for 20 s under UV-LED light (λ = 365 nm, Epileds, Taiwan) at an intensity of 3.9 mW/cm^2. The scaffolds were stored at +5 °C at constant humidity.

At the next stage, the obtained allylchitosan 3D scaffolds were freeze-dried using a FreeZone freeze-dryer by Labconco. When the temperature of the 3D scaffolds reached −83 °C, the pressure in the chamber was reduced to 6 μBar, and the scaffolds were left inside for one more day.

3.3. *Characterization of Film Samples and 3D Scaffolds*

3.3.1. Hydrodynamic Diameter of Samples in Aqueous Solutions

The dynamic light scattering method was applied to determine the sizes of aggregates formed by dissolving the synthesized derivatives (0.02 wt%) in acetic acid (2%). The measurements were performed with a Zetatrac (Microtrac, Inc., Montgomeryville, PA, USA) instrument using Microtrac V 10.5.3 software.

3.3.2. Mechanical Properties of Film Samples

Mechanical studies were carried out using an AG-E universal testing machine (Shimadzu, Japan) at a speed of 1 mm/min. Before testing, the films were kept in a desiccator at a constant humidity of 81% above a $(NH_4)_2SO_4$ saturated solution for a week.

3.3.3. XRD Analysis

X-ray diffraction analysis was carried out with a D8 Advance diffractometer (Bruker AXS GmbH, Karlsruhe, Germany) using CuKα radiation and a "Vantec-1" detector. An allylchitosan film was fixed to a silicon single crystal substrate with liquid paraffin. The scanning step was 0.021 deg.

3.3.4. SEM and the Pore Surface Area Estimation

The surface and internal structure of 3D scaffolds were characterized using a Phenom ProX scanning electron microscope (15 nm resolution; Phenom-World, Eindhoven, the Netherlands). The pore surface area was quantified with ImageJ software (National Institutes of Health, Bethesda, MD, USA [69]).

3.4. *Implantation*

All animal experiments were performed according to the national regulations of the usage and welfare of laboratory animals and approved by the Institutional Animal Care and Use Committee in Sechenov University (Moscow, Russia) (protocol SU2018-052, approval date 12.03.2018). The laboratory rats (Wistar, average weight 450 $\pm$ 20 g) were divided into two groups. Each animal in group 1 ($n = 5$) received four film samples of different types (AC2–AC5). Animals in group 2 ($n = 15$) received 3D scaffolds (2 mm thick) and were subdivided into 3 subgroups: day 30 ($n = 5$), day 60 ($n = 5$), and day 90 ($n = 5$). The film samples and 3D scaffolds were implanted subcutaneously in the interscapular region of white rats. All manipulations were performed under anesthesia. For the premedication, a combination of 0.03 mL of Atropine solution (0.1%), 0.02 mL of diphenhydramine (10 mg/mL), and 0.05 mL of droperidol (2.5 mg/mL) was injected intramuscularly into the right thigh. General anesthesia was induced with an intramuscular injection of 0.06 mL of Zoletil (100 mg/mL) combined with 0.04 mL of Xyla (20 mg/mL) into the left thigh. The samples (0.8 cm $\times$ 0.8 cm) were implanted subcutaneously and fixed with non-absorbable sutures at the four corners of the sample to the muscles in the interscapular area. After the experiment completion, the animals were sacrificed via an intracardiac injection of 10 mL of novocaine solution (2.5%) on day 30 in group 1; on days 30, 60 and 90 in group 2. For the histological analysis, excision of a 2.0 cm $\times$ 2.0 cm interscapular area was performed.

3.5. *Histological Analysis*

Tissue fragments with implanted scaffolds ($n = 35$) were fixed in a 10% neutral phosphate-buffered formalin solution then paraffin blocks were prepared by a standard procedure. For all the samples, transverse serial sections with a thickness of 4–5 μm were stained with hematoxylin and eosin and picrosirius red for collagen fibers. We investigated the samples by light, phase-contrast, and polarization microscopies using a LEICA DM4000 B LED microscope equipped with a LEICA DFC7000 T digital video camera and LAS V4.8 software (Leica Microsystems, Wetzlar, Germany).

The connective tissue capsule thickness was measured by morphometric studies (see below). We assessed the change in tinctorial properties and material resorption, maturity of the connective tissue capsule, intensity of macrophage and giant foreign-body cell infiltration by a morphological semi-quantitative evaluation. This method was used in other similar studies [70,71]. For porous 3D scaffolds, the connective tissue ingrowth into pores and their vascularization were also assessed by a semi-quantitative evaluation.

The connective tissue capsule thickness was measured by examination of 10 selected fields of view located at an equal distance from each other at a 100× magnification. In each field the sections with the maximum, mean and minimum capsule thickness in the sample were taken into account.

In a semi-quantitative evaluation, a four-point system was used: 0 points corresponded to the absence of changes, 1 to minimal changes, 2 to moderate changes, and 3 to the maximum changes. A histological semi-quantitative scoring system for the evaluation of macrophage and foreign-body giant cell reaction to the scaffolds was based on an algorithm for semi-quantitative evaluation of inflammatory infiltration around the implantation of nanocomposites (Supplementary Table S3) [70]. Other original histological semi-quantitative scoring systems for the evaluation of chitosan scaffold's changes and tissue reaction were original (Supplementary Tables S4–S6).

The statistical data were analyzed in GraphPad Prism 7.00 software. For each parameter, the data were tested for a normal distribution using Shapiro-Wilk test or D'Agostino and Pearson normality test. If the data fitted a normal distribution, the statistical comparison in groups was performed by the two-way ANOVA followed by Tukey's or Sidak's test for the comparison between groups. The correlation between different parameters was estimated with Pearson's correlation coefficient. A difference was considered statistically significant when p-value < 0.05.

Identification of the Internal Film Structure (Wavelet Analysis)

Sections of allylchitosan films were analyzed for periodic structures by the wavelet method [65]. In contrast to Fourier transform, wavelets allow an optimal analysis of spatial fields with a complex multiscale structure [65]. To isolate the patterns of the spatial structure at different scales, the MHAT-wavelet (Mexican HAT) was set as the basic one [72]. Moreover, such an approach could explain the mechanisms for the destruction of implanted samples. Initially, from the obtained image fragment, two one-dimensional rows were formed representing the spatial distributions of the averaged (along and across the visible surface of the chitosan film) pixel intensities. Subsequently, for each such row, a waveletgram and a spatial spectrum of structural non-uniformities were calculated [65,72].

4. Conclusions

Chitin and chitosan, its deacetylated product, have unique properties for use in the pharmaceutical industry and biomedicine. In the present study, we used the method of mechanochemical synthesis in a pilot setup to obtain chitosan and its derivatives with a different content of hydrophobic allyl substituents. Mechanochemical synthesis provides a high yield of products in a shorter time and at a lower temperature than a similar synthesis carried out in an organic solvent. We have shown that aggregation of chitosan derivatives becomes more pronounced with an increase in the number of hydrophobic substituents. The introduction of hydrophobic unsaturated fragments into the structure of chitosan also allows for the obtaining a photosensitive polymer, which crosslinks and forms stable three-dimensional networks under UV photocuring and laser exposure. Although photocured film samples from the obtained derivatives demonstrated no increase in the tensile strength compared to the initial chitosan, their plasticity increased.

We have demonstrated a principal possibility of structuring the synthesized derivatives by laser stereolithography to obtain three-dimensional porous structures. Of note, the selected structuring technique allows obtaining biopolymer matrices at a centimeter scale with a high productivity, which is important for restoring large tissue defects (from 1 cm).

The long-term stability of the films and 3D scaffolds based on allylchitosan has been investigated. The histological study has shown that additional allyl fragments cause no significant changes in the tissue response for the chitosan derivatives with different degrees of substitution. No dystrophic and necrobiotic changes were detected in the surrounding tissues, which proves the biocompatibility of allylchitosan materials. We have also shown the ability of 3D scaffolds to biodegrade, with their biodegradation starting on day 60 after implantation, with its rate increased by day 90. This should be taken into consideration when producing tissue engineered scaffolds. Moreover, for the first time, we used the wavelet analysis to show that the areas of allylchitosan film degradation were periodic rather than chaotic. Comparing the results of the wavelet analysis and the XRD data, we have concluded that the degradation of the film samples occurs within less ordered amorphous regions in the polymer bulk.

Supplementary Materials: The following are available online at http://www.mdpi.com/1660-3397/17/1/48/s1, Figure S1–S2: Tissue reaction to the films based on allylchitosan (day 30); Figure S3: Tissue reaction to the 3D scaffolds based on allylchitosan (day 30); Figure S4: The data of connective tissue capsule thickness around the implanted films and 3D scaffolds based on allylchitosan; Figure S5: Tissue reaction to the 3D scaffolds based on allylchitosan (day 60); Figure S6: Tissue reaction to the 3D scaffolds based on allylchitosan (day 90); Figure S7: ^{1}H NMR spectra of chitosan (1), AC2 (2) and AC5 (3); Table S1: Summary table of histological semi-quantitative analysis results; Table S2: Correlation analysis: correlations between the time after implantation and the histological findings in samples of 3D-scaffold implantations; Table S3: A histological semi-quantitative scoring system for the evaluation of macrophage and foreign-body giant cell reactions to the scaffolds; Table S4: A histological semi-quantitative scoring system for the evaluation of changes in tinctorial properties of scaffolds and scaffolds' lysis; Table S5: A histological semi-quantitative scoring system for the evaluation of a maturity of connective tissue capsules around scaffolds; Table S6: A histological semi-quantitative scoring system for the evaluation of a connective tissue ingrowth and vascularization in pores of 3D scaffolds.

Author Contributions: Y.A.R. and P.S.T. conceived and designed the experiments and analyzed the data; K.N.B., T.A.A., and A.V.K. wrote the manuscript; G.P.G. prepared film samples, conducted mechanical investigations, and analyzed the data; T.A.A. designed and performed the synthesis of unsaturated chitosan derivatives and performed chemical characterization of the allylchitosans; K.N.B. prepared a photosensitive composition and structured the scaffolds by laser stereolithography; A.V.K. and A.B.S. conducted a histological analysis and analyzed the data; A.A.A. conducted SEM and DLS analysis; D.V.B. and T.M.Z. designed the study protocol and performed an implantation; V.I.Y. analyzed the internal film structure by the wavelet method; and V.F.B. and I.A.F. conducted XRD analysis and analyzed the data. All the authors critically reviewed and approved the final version of the manuscript.

Funding: This work was supported by the Russian academic excellence project '5-100' (in vivo and morphological studies, the development of a photosensitive composition), the Russian Science Foundation grant 15-15-00132 (formation of film and three-dimensional samples, their characterization), by RFBR according to the research projects no. 18-32-00222 (laser stereolithography of hydrogel matrices), no. 18-29-17050 (mechanochemical synthesis of AC), and by the Ministry of Science and Higher Education within the State assignment FSRC "Crystallography and Photonics" RAS (wavelet analysis of samples).

Acknowledgments: We thank Alexandra V. Butenko (Sechenov University, Russia) for her help in the histological analysis and Georgii V. Cherkaev (ISPM RAS, Russia) for his help in recording and interpretation of the ^{1}H NMR spectra.

Conflicts of Interest: The authors declare no conflict of interest.

References

1. Sayari, N.; Sila, A.; Abdelmalek, B.E.; Abdallah, R.B.; Ellouz-Chaabouni, S.; Bougatef, A.; Balti, R. Chitin and chitosan from the Norway lobster by-products: Antimicrobial and anti-proliferative activities. *Int. J. Biol. Macromol.* **2016**, *87*, 163–171. [CrossRef] [PubMed]
2. Croisier, F.; Jérôme, C. Chitosan-based biomaterials for tissue engineering. *Eur. Polym. J.* **2013**, *49*, 780–792. [CrossRef]
3. Thapa, B.; Narain, R. Mechanism, current challenges and new approaches for non viral gene delivery. *Polym. Nanomater. Gene Ther.* **2016**, 1–27. [CrossRef]
4. Rodríguez-Vázquez, M.; Vega-Ruiz, B.; Ramos-Zúñiga, R.; Saldaña-Koppel, D.A.; Quiñones-Olvera, L.F. Chitosan and Its Potential Use as a Scaffold for Tissue Engineering in Regenerative Medicine. *Biomed. Res. Int.* **2015**, *2015*, 1–15. [CrossRef] [PubMed]

5. Levengood, S.K.L.; Zhang, M. Chitosan-based scaffolds for bone tissue engineering. *J. Mater. Chem. B* **2014**, *2*, 3161–3184. [CrossRef] [PubMed]
6. Shukla, S.K.; Mishra, A.K.; Arotiba, O.A.; Mamba, B.B. Chitosan-based nanomaterials: A state-of-the-art review. *Int. J. Biol. Macromol.* **2013**, *59*, 46–58. [CrossRef]
7. Peña, A.; Sánchez, N.S.; Calahorra, M. Effects of chitosan on Candida albicans: Conditions for its antifungal activity. *BioMed Res. Int.* **2013**, *2013*, 527549. [CrossRef]
8. Szymańska, E.; Winnicka, K. Stability of chitosan-a challenge for pharmaceutical and biomedical applications. *Mar. Drugs* **2015**, *13*, 1819–1846. [CrossRef]
9. Leithner, K.; Bernkop-Schnürch, A. Chitosan and Derivatives for Biopharmaceutical Use: Mucoadhesive Properties. *Chitosan-Based Syst. Biopharm. Deliv. Target. Polym. Ther.* **2012**, 159–180. [CrossRef]
10. Muzzarelli, R.A.A.; Muzzarelli, C. Chitosan Chemistry: Relevance to the Biomedical Sciences. In *Polysaccharides I*; Springer: Berlin/Heidelberg, Germany, 2005; pp. 151–209. [CrossRef]
11. Prabaharan, M. Review Paper: Chitosan Derivatives as Promising Materials for Controlled Drug Delivery. *J. Biomater. Appl.* **2008**, *23*, 5–36. [CrossRef]
12. Yadav, H.K.S.; Joshi, G.B.; Singh, M.N.; Shivakumar, H.G. Naturally Occurring Chitosan and Chitosan Derivatives: A Review. *Curr. Drug Ther.* **2011**, *6*, 2–11. [CrossRef]
13. Zargar, V.; Asghari, M.; Dashti, A. A Review on Chitin and Chitosan Polymers: Structure, Chemistry, Solubility, Derivatives, and Applications. *ChemBioEng Rev.* **2015**, *2*, 204–226. [CrossRef]
14. Ahmed, J.; Roos, Y.H.; Rahman, S.; Ray, S.S. Glass Transition and Phase Transitions in Food and Biological Materials. n.d. Available online: https://www.wiley.com/en-us/Glass+Transition+and+Phase+Transitions+in+Food+and+Biological+Materials-p-9781118935729 (accessed on 6 July 2018).
15. Ball, R.; Bajaj, P.; Whitehead, K. Achieving long-term stability of lipid nanoparticles: Examining the effect of pH, temperature, and lyophilization. *Int. J. Nanomed.* **2016**, *12*, 305–315. [CrossRef] [PubMed]
16. Ahmed, T.; Aljaeid, B. Preparation, characterization, and potential application of chitosan, chitosan derivatives, and chitosan metal nanoparticles in pharmaceutical drug delivery. *Drug Des. Dev. Ther.* **2016**, *10*, 483–507. [CrossRef]
17. Jana, S.; Jana, S. *Particulate Technology for Delivery of Therapeutics*; Springer: New York, NY, USA, 2017. Available online: https://books.google.ru/books?id=xng5DwAAQBAJ&dq=Sougata,+and+Subrata+Jana,+eds.+Particulate+Technology+for+Delivery+of+Therapeutics.+Springer,+2017&hl=ru&source=gbs_navlinks_s (accessed on 6 July 2018).
18. James, S.L.; Adams, C.J.; Bolm, C.; Braga, D.; Collier, P.; Friščić, T.; Grepioni, F.; Harris, K.D.M.; Hyett, G.; Jones, W.; et al. Mechanochemistry: Opportunities for new and cleaner synthesis. *Chem. Soc. Rev.* **2012**, *41*, 413–447. [CrossRef] [PubMed]
19. Lyakhov, N.Z.; Grigorieva, T.F.; Barinova, A.P.; Vorsina, I.A. Mechanochemical synthesis of organic compounds and composites with their participation. *Russ. Chem. Rev.* **2010**, *79*, 189–203. [CrossRef]
20. Prut, E.V.; Zelenetskii, A.N. Chemical modification and blending of polymers in an extruder reactor. *Russ. Chem. Rev.* **2001**, *70*, 65–79. [CrossRef]
21. Akopova, T.A.; Demina, T.S.; Zelenetskii, A.N. Amphiphilic systems based on polysaccharides produced by solid-phase synthesis—A review. *Fibre Chem.* **2012**, *44*, 217–220. [CrossRef]
22. Ferguson, A.N.; O'Neill, A.G. *Focus on Chitosan Research*; Nova Science Publishers: Hauppauge, NY, USA, 2011. Available online: https://www.novapublishers.com/catalog/product_info.php?products_id=33937 (accessed on 19 July 2018).
23. Crawford, D.E.; Casaban, J. Recent Developments in Mechanochemical Materials Synthesis by Extrusion. *Adv. Mater.* **2016**, *28*, 5747–5754. [CrossRef]
24. Timashev, P.S.; Bardakova, K.N.; Minaev, N.V.; Demina, T.S.; Mishchenko, T.A.; Mitroshina, E.V.; Akovantseva, A.A.; Koroleva, A.V.; Asyutin, D.S.; Pimenova, L.F.; et al. Compatibility of cells of the nervous system with structured biodegradable chitosan-based hydrogel matrices. *Appl. Biochem. Microbiol.* **2016**, *52*, 508–514. [CrossRef]
25. Demina, T.S.; Bardakova, K.N.; Minaev, N.V.; Svidchenko, E.A.; Istomin, A.V.; Goncharuk, G.P.; Vladimirov, L.V.; Grachev, A.V.; Zelenetskii, A.N.; Timashev, P.S.; et al. Two-photon-induced microstereolithography of chitosan-g-oligolactides as a function of their stereochemical composition. *Polymers* **2017**, *9*, 302. [CrossRef]

26. Timashev, P.S.; Bardakova, K.N.; Demina, T.S.; Pudovkina, G.I.; Novikov, M.M.; Markov, M.A.; Asyutin, D.S.; Pimenova, L.F.; Svidchenko, E.M.; Ermakov, A.M.; et al. Novel biocompatible material based on solid-state modified chitosan for laser stereolithography. *Sovrem. Tehnol. Med.* **2015**, *7*. [CrossRef]
27. Akopova, T.A.; Demina, T.S.; Bagratashvili, V.N.; Bardakova, K.N.; Novikov, M.M.; Selezneva, I.I.; Istomin, A.V.; Svidchenko, E.A.; Cherkaev, G.V.; Surin, N.M.; et al. Solid state synthesis of chitosan and its unsaturated derivatives for laser microfabrication of 3D scaffolds. *IOP Conf. Ser. Mater. Sci. Eng.* **2015**, *87*, 012079. [CrossRef]
28. Nud'ga, L.A.; Petrova, V.A.; Lebedeva, M.F. Effect of Allyl Substitution in Chitosan on the Structure of Graft Copolymers. *Russ. J. Appl. Chem.* **2003**, *76*, 1978–1982. [CrossRef]
29. VPhilippova, I.; Andreeva, O.E.; Khokhlov, A.S.; Islamov, A.R.; Kuklin, A.K.; Gordeliy, A.I. Charge-Induced Microphase Separation in Polyelectrolyte Hydrogels with Associating Hydrophobic Side Chains: Small-Angle Neutron Scattering Study. *Langmuir* **2003**, *19*, 7240–7248. [CrossRef]
30. Kurisawa, M.; Yokoyama, M.; Okano, T. Transfection efficiency increases by incorporating hydrophobic monomer units into polymeric gene carriers. *J. Control. Release* **2000**, *68*, 1–8. [CrossRef]
31. Popa-Nita, S.; Alcouffe, P.; Rochas, C.; David, L.; Domard, A. Continuum of structural organization from chitosan solutions to derived physical forms. *Biomacromolecules* **2010**, *11*, 6–12. [CrossRef]
32. Ottøy, M.H.; Vårum, K.M.; Christensen, B.E.; Anthonsen, M.W.; Smidsrød, O. Preparative and analytical size-exclusion chromatography of chitosans. *Carbohydr. Polym.* **1996**, *31*, 253–261. [CrossRef]
33. Schatz, C.; Pichot, C.; Delair, T.; Viton, C.; Domard, A. Static Light Scattering Studies on Chitosan Solutions: From Macromolecular Chains to Colloidal Dispersions. *Langmuir* **2003**, *19*, 9896–9903. [CrossRef]
34. Sogias, I.A.; Khutoryanskiy, V.V.; Williams, A.C. Exploring the Factors Affecting the Solubility of Chitosan in Water. *Macromol. Chem. Phys.* **2010**, *211*, 426–433. [CrossRef]
35. Qin, C.; Li, H.; Xiao, Q.; Liu, Y.; Zhu, J.; Du, Y. Water-solubility of chitosan and its antimicrobial activity. *Carbohydr. Polym.* **2006**, *63*, 367–374. [CrossRef]
36. Souza, B.W.S.; Cerqueira, M.A.; Martins, J.T.; Casariego, A.; Teixeira, J.A.; Vicente, A.A. Influence of electric fields on the structure of chitosan edible coatings. *Food Hydrocoll.* **2010**, *24*, 330–335. [CrossRef]
37. Khan, M.A.; Ferdous, S.; Mustafa, A.I. Improvement of physico-mechanical properties of chitosan films by photocuring with acrylic monomers. *J. Polym. Environ.* **2005**, *13*, 193–201. [CrossRef]
38. Martins, J.T.; Cerqueira, M.A.; Vicente, A.A. Influence of α-tocopherol on physicochemical properties of chitosan-based films. *Food Hydrocoll.* **2012**, *27*, 220–227. [CrossRef]
39. Kim, K.M.; Son, J.H.; Kim, S.-K.; Weller, C.L.; Hanna, M.A. Properties of Chitosan Films as a Function of pH and Solvent Type. *J. Food Sci.* **2006**, *71*, E119–E124. [CrossRef]
40. Dong, Y.; Sakurai, K.; Wu, Y.; Kondo, Y. Multiple crystalline morphologies of N-Alkyl chitosan solution cast films. *Polym. Bull.* **2002**, *49*, 189–195. [CrossRef]
41. Rivero, S.; García, M.A.; Pinotti, A. Correlations between structural, barrier, thermal and mechanical properties of plasticized gelatin films. *Innov. Food Sci. Emerg. Technol.* **2010**, *11*, 369–375. [CrossRef]
42. Bangyekan, C.; Aht-Ong, D.; Srikulkit, K. Preparation and properties evaluation of chitosan-coated cassava starch films. *Carbohydr. Polym.* **2006**, *63*, 61–71. [CrossRef]
43. Rotta, J.; Minatti, E.; Barreto, P.L.M. Determination of structural and mechanical properties, diffractometry, and thermal analysis of chitosan and hydroxypropylmethylcellulose (HPMC) films plasticized with sorbitol. *Food Sci. Technol.* **2011**, *31*, 450–455. [CrossRef]
44. Modrzejewska, Z.; Maniukiewicz, W.; Wojtasz-Pająk, A. Determination of hydrogel chitosan membrane structure. *Pol. Chitin Soc. Monogr. XI* **2006**, 113–121.
45. Wan, D.; Wu, Y.; Yu, H.; Wen, A. Biodegradable Polylactide/Chitosan Blend Membranes. *Biomacromolecules* **2006**, *7*, 1362–1372. [CrossRef] [PubMed]
46. Yahya, M.Z.; Harun, M.K.; Ali, A.M.; Mohammat, M.F.; Hanafiah, M.A.; Ibrahim, S.C.; Mustaffa, M.; Darus, Z.M.; Latif, F. XRD and Surface Morphology Studies on Chitosan-Based Film Electrolytes. *J. Appl. Sci.* **2006**, *6*, 3150–3154. [CrossRef]
47. Dai, Z.; Ronholm, J.; Tian, Y.; Sethi, B.; Cao, X. Sterilization techniques for biodegradable scaffolds in tissue engineering applications. *J. Tissue Eng.* **2016**, *7*, 2041731416648810. [CrossRef] [PubMed]
48. Chung, K.; Wallace, J.; Kim, S.Y.; Kalyanasundaram, S.; Andalman, A.S.; Davidson, T.J.; Mirzabekov, J.J.; Zalocusky, K.A.; Mattis, J.; Denisin, A.K.; et al. Structural and molecular interrogation of intact biological systems. *Nature* **2013**, *497*, 332–337. [CrossRef] [PubMed]

49. Do, A.; Khorsand, B.; Geary, S.M.; Salem, A.K.; Therapeutics, E.; City, I. 3D Printing of Scaffolds for Tissue Regeneration Applications. *Adv. Healthc. Mater.* **2015**, *4*, 1742–1762. [CrossRef] [PubMed]
50. Loh, Q.L.; Choong, C. Three-Dimensional Scaffolds for Tissue Engineering Applications: Role of Porosity and Pore Size. *Tissue Eng. Part B Rev.* **2013**, *19*, 485–502. [CrossRef] [PubMed]
51. Bencherif, S.A.; Sands, R.W.; Bhatta, D.; Arany, P.; Verbeke, C.S.; Edwards, D.A. Injectable preformed scaffolds with shape-memory properties. *Proc. Natl. Acad. Sci. USA* **2012**, *109*, 19590–19595. [CrossRef]
52. Zhang, H.; Hussain, I.; Brust, M.; Butler, M.F.; Rannard, S.P.; Cooper, A.I. Aligned two- and three-dimensional structures by directional freezing of polymers and nanoparticles. *Nat. Mater.* **2005**, *4*, 787–793. [CrossRef]
53. Farrugia, B.L.; Whitelock, J.M.; Jung, M.; McGrath, B.; O'Grady, R.L.; McCarthy, S.J.; Lord, M.S. The localisation of inflammatory cells and expression of associated proteoglycans in response to implanted chitosan. *Biomaterials* **2014**, *35*, 1462–1477. [CrossRef]
54. Kwak, B.K.; Shim, H.J.; Han, S.-M.; Park, E.S. Chitin-based Embolic Materials in the Renal Artery of Rabbits: Pathologic Evaluation of an Absorbable Particulate Agent. *Radiology* **2005**, *236*, 151–158. [CrossRef]
55. VandeVord, P.J.; Matthew, H.W.T.; DeSilva, S.P.; Mayton, L.; Wu, B.; Wooley, P.H. Evaluation of the biocompatibility of a chitosan scaffold in mice. *J. Biomed. Mater. Res.* **2002**, *59*, 585–590. [CrossRef] [PubMed]
56. Kim, H.; Tator, C.H.; Shoichet, M.S. Chitosan implants in the rat spinal cord: Biocompatibility and biodegradation. *J. Biomed. Mater. Res. Part A* **2011**, *97*, 395–404. [CrossRef]
57. Peluso, G.; Petillo, O.; Ranieri, M.; Santin, M.; Ambrosic, L.; Calabró, D.; Avallone, B.; Balsamo, G. Chitosan-mediated stimulation of macrophage function. *Biomaterials* **1994**, *15*, 1215–1220. [CrossRef]
58. Tomihata, K.; Ikada, Y. In vitro and in vivo degradation of films of chitin and its deacetylated derivatives. *Biomaterials* **1997**, *18*, 567–575. [CrossRef]
59. Barbosa, J.N.; Amaral, I.F.; Águas, A.P.; Barbosa, M.A. Evaluation of the effect of the degree of acetylation on the inflammatory response to 3D porous chitosan scaffold. *J. Biomed. Mater. Res. Part A* **2009**, *93*, 20–28. [CrossRef]
60. Hartl, L.; Zach, S.; Seidl-Seiboth, V. Fungal chitinases: Diversity, mechanistic properties and biotechnological potential. *Appl. Microbiol. Biotechnol.* **2012**, *93*, 533–543. [CrossRef]
61. Park, C.J.; Gabrielson, N.P.; Pack, D.W.; Jamison, R.D.; Johnson, A.J.W. The effect of chitosan on the migration of neutrophil-like HL60 cells, mediated by IL-8. *Biomaterials* **2009**, *30*, 436–444. [CrossRef]
62. Simard, P.; Galarneau, H.; Marois, S.; Rusu, D.; Hoemann, C.D.; Poubelle, P.E.; El-Gabalawy, H.; Fernandes, M.J. Neutrophils exhibit distinct phenotypes toward chitosans with different degrees of deacetylation: Implications for cartilage repair. *Arthritis Res. Ther.* **2009**, *11*, R74. [CrossRef]
63. Nishimura, K.; Nishimura, S.; Nishi, N.; Saiki, I.; Tokura, S.; Azuma, I. Immunological activity of chitin and its derivatives. *Vaccine* **1984**, *2*, 93–99. [CrossRef]
64. Hwang, H.-G.; Choi, H.-J.; Lee, B.-I.; Yoon, H.-K.; Nam, S.-H.; Choi, H.-K. Multi-resolution wavelet-transformed image analysis of histological sections of breast carcinomas. *Anal. Cell. Oncol.* **2005**, *27*, 237–244.
65. Astaf'eva, N.M. Wavelet analysis: Basic theory and some applications. *Uspekhi Fizicheskikh Nauk* **1996**, *166*, 1145–1170. [CrossRef]
66. Park, H.; Choi, B.; Nguyen, J.; Fan, J.; Shafi, S.; Klokkevold, P.; Lee, M. Anionic carbohydrate-containing chitosan scaffolds for bone regeneration. *Carbohydr. Polym.* **2013**, *97*, 587–596. [CrossRef] [PubMed]
67. Rogovina, S.Z.; Akopova, T.A.; Vikhoreva, G.A. Investigation of properties of chitosan obtained by solid-phase and suspension methods. *J. Appl. Polym. Sci.* **1998**, *70*, 927–933. [CrossRef]
68. Aleksandrov, A.I.; Akopova, T.A.; Shevchenko, V.G.; Cherkaev, G.V.; Degtyarev, E.N. A Biocompatible Nanocomposite Based on Allyl Chitosan and Vinyltriethoxysilane for Tissue Engineering. *Popym. Sci. Ser. B* **2017**, *59*, 97–108. [CrossRef]
69. Serra, J.P. *Image Analysis and Mathematical Morphology*; Academic Press: Cambridge, MA, USA, 1982. Available online: https://dl.acm.org/citation.cfm?id=1098652 (accessed on 15 July 2018).
70. Schneider, O.D.; Mohn, D.; Fuhrer, R.; Klein, K.; Kämpf, K.; Nuss, K.M.; Sidler, M.; Zlinszky, K.; von Rechenberg, B.; Stark, W.J. Biocompatibility and Bone Formation of Flexible, Cotton Wool-like PLGA/Calcium Phosphate Nanocomposites in Sheep. *Open Orthop. J.* **2011**, *5*, 63–71. [CrossRef] [PubMed]

71. Melman, L.; Jenkins, E.D.; Hamilton, N.A.; Bender, L.C.; Brodt, M.D.; Deeken, C.R.; Greco, S.C.; Frisella, M.M.; Matthews, B.D. Histologic and biomechanical evaluation of a novel macroporous polytetrafluoroethylene knit mesh compared to lightweight and heavyweight polypropylene mesh in a porcine model of ventral incisional hernia repair. *Hernia* **2011**, *15*, 423–431. [CrossRef] [PubMed]
72. Bagratashvili, V.N.; Rybaltovsky, A.O.; Minaev, N.V.; Timashev, P.S.; Firsov, V.V.; Yusupov, V.I. Laser-induced atomic assembling of periodic layered nanostructures of silver nanoparticles in fluoro-polymer film matrix. *Laser Phys. Lett.* **2010**, *7*, 401–404. [CrossRef]

© 2019 by the authors. Licensee MDPI, Basel, Switzerland. This article is an open access article distributed under the terms and conditions of the Creative Commons Attribution (CC BY) license (http://creativecommons.org/licenses/by/4.0/).

marine drugs
MDPI

Article

Novel Efficient Bioprocessing of Marine Chitins into Active Anticancer Prodigiosin

Van Bon Nguyen [1,2], Shan-Ping Chen [3], Thi Hanh Nguyen [4], Minh Trung Nguyen [5], Thi Thanh Thao Tran [5], Chien Thang Doan [5], Thi Ngoc Tran [5], Anh Dzung Nguyen [4], Yao-Haur Kuo [6] and San-Lang Wang [3,7,*]

1 Division of Computational Mathematics and Engineering, Institute for Computational Science, Ton Duc Thang University, Ho Chi Minh City 700000, Vietnam; nguyenvanbon@tdtu.edu.vn
2 Faculty of Applied Sciences, Ton Duc Thang University, Ho Chi Minh City 700000, Vietnam
3 Department of Chemistry, Tamkang University, New Taipei City 25137, Taiwan; peter831119@gmail.com
4 Institute of Biotechnology and Environment, Tay Nguyen University, Buon Ma Thuot 630000, Vietnam; nguyenhanh2208.tn@gmail.com (T.H.N.); nadzungtaynguyenuni@yahoo.com.vn (A.D.N.)
5 Department of Science and Technology, Tay Nguyen University, Buon Ma Thuot 630000, Vietnam; nguyenminhtrung2389@gmail.com (M.T.N.); thanhthaotnu@gmail.com (T.T.T.T.); doanthng@gmail.com (C.T.D.); tranngoctnu@gmail.com (T.N.T.)
6 Division of Chinese Materia Medica Development, National Research Institute of Chinese Medicine, Taipei 11221, Taiwan; kuoyh@nricm.edu.tw
7 Department of Chemical and Materials Engineering, Tamkang University, New Taipei City 25137, Taiwan
* Correspondence: sabulo@mail.tku.edu.tw; Tel.: +886-2-2621-5656; Fax: +886-2-2620-9924

Received: 6 December 2019; Accepted: 20 December 2019; Published: 23 December 2019

Abstract: Marine chitins (MC) have been utilized for the production of vast array of bioactive products, including chitooligomers, chitinase, chitosanase, antioxidants, anti-NO, and antidiabetic compounds. The aim of this study is the bioprocessing of MC into a potent anticancer compound, prodigiosin (PG), via microbial fermentation. This bioactive compound was produced by *Serratia marcescens* TKU011 with the highest yield of 4.62 mg/mL at the optimal conditions of liquid medium with initial pH of 5.65–6.15 containing 1% α-chitin, 0.6% casein, 0.05% K_2HPO_4, and 0.1% $CaSO_4$. Fermentation was kept at 25 °C for 2 d. Notably, α-chitin was newly investigated as the major potential material for PG production via fermentation; the salt $CaSO_4$ was also found to play the key role in the enhancement of PG yield of *Serratia marcescens* fermentation for the first time. PG was qualified and identified based on specific UV, MALDI-TOF MS analysis. In the biological activity tests, purified PG demonstrated potent anticancer activities against A549, Hep G2, MCF-7, and WiDr with the IC_{50} values of 0.06, 0.04, 0.04, and 0.2 μg/mL, respectively. Mytomycin C, a commercial anti-cancer compound was also tested for comparison purpose, showing weaker activity with the IC_{50} values of 0.11, 0.1, 0.14, and 0.15 μg/mL, respectively. As such, purified PG displayed higher 2.75-fold, 1.67-fold, and 3.25-fold efficacy than Mytomycin C against MCF-7, A549, and Hep G2, respectively. The results suggest that marine chitins are valuable sources for production of prodigiosin, a potential candidate for cancer drugs.

Keywords: α-Chitin; prodigiosin; anti-tumors; *Serratia marcescens*; bioprocessing

1. Introduction

Chitin, an abundant material, has been widely produced from fishery processing byproducts. Of the natural chitin-containing materials, shrimp shells, squid pens, and crab shells have the highest chitin content [1], and as such, are used for chitin production. Chitin and its derivatives display great economic value thanks to their versatile activities and potential biotechnological applications, and chitin-containing materials have been reported to be used for the production of a vast array of bioactive products, such as exopolysaccharides [2–4], chitooligomers [5], antioxidants [6,7], biofertilizers [8] insecticidal materials [9,10], and biosorbents [11,12]. Recently, these chitin-containing materials were extensively used for the production of antidiabetic drugs [13–18]. In this study, chitinous materials were utilized for the production of prodigiosin, an active anticancer compound, via microbial fermentation.

Prodigiosin (PG), a red pigment is a typical alkaloid constituent produced by several bacterial genus, *Serratia marcescens* and some other Gram-negative bacterial strains [19]. PGs have been recognized as bioactive bacterial metabolites with vast reported valuable bioactivities, including antibacterial, cytotoxic, antifungal, algicidal, antiprotozoal, antimalarial, antiproliferative, anticancer [19–22], antioxidant, and immunosuppressant [23] activities. PG also has been uniquely used as a natural based dye for textiles and olefins [24].

Due to the wild range of unique applications of PG, the production studies on this bioactive compound have been received with great interest [13,24], and many types and selective media have been investigated for PG production via microbial fermentation, such as a medium containing 2% sodium oleate [25], maltose broth, nutrient broth containing sesame seeds, peptone glycerol broth [26], nutrient broth, nutrient broth with 0.5% maltose or 0.5% glucose, powdered peanut seed broth [27], corn steep mannitol medium, mannitol medium, corn steep medium, Cassava waste mannitol medium, cassava waste medium, and luria bertani glucose medium [23]. For low cost production of PG, we established the PG production from marine chitinous wastes [9–11]. In these studies, various marine chitinous materials, including crab shells, shrimp shells, shrimp heads and squid pens were used as the sole carbon/nitrogen source; squid pens were found to be the most effective material for PG production by *S. marcescens*. However, numerous scientific parameters were not investigated in our previous studies, such as the kind of marine chitin (α or β), protein sources, chitin/protein ratio, and supplementary minerals for the best PG productivity production by *S. marcescens*. All those previously unknown items were newly investigated in this study, and the PG produce from the medium containing marine chitin was also evaluated for its effect on four cancerous cell lines—A549, Hep G2, MCF-7, and WIDR—in this report.

2. Results and Discussion

2.1. *New Records of Marine α-Chitin as the Potential Carbon Source for Prodigiosin Synthesis by Serratia marcescens*

Carbon source has been proven to play an important role in PG production via microbial fermentation [19]. In previous studies, squid pens powder (SPP) was found to be cost-effective material for the production of PG by *Serratia marcescens* TKU011, compared to other materials; SPP was reported to contain approximately 60% chitin and 40% protein [13]. Thus, chitin contained in SPP may prove a significant factor in PG production. To investigate the role of chitin as well as its combination with free protein in different ratios on the PG production by *S. marcescens*, the chitins obtained from SPP (β-chitin) and shrimp shells (α-chitin) by using the method reported by Wang et al., 2006 [28] were mixed with free protein (casein) with the ratio (chitin/casein) of 7/1, 6/2, 5/3, 4/4, 2/6, and 1/7 (*w/w*) and used as the sole carbon and nitrogen source for fermentation by *S. marcescens* TKU011; SPP was also used as the control for comparison purpose. The results in Figure 1 show that β-chitin mixed with casein with the ratio of 2/6 (*w/w*) give higher PG yield production (2.73 mg/mL) than that of SPP (2.45 mg/mL) fermented by *S. marcescens* TKU011, while α-chitin mixed with free protein at the ratio of 5/3 (*w/w*) reach the greatest PG yield production of 3.23 mg/mL. In addition to the use of α-chitin providing higher PG yield, and α-chitin could be more abundantly obtained from vast resources (crab shells, shrimp shells, etc.) than β-chitin (mainly obtained from squid pens); thus, α-chitin was chosen for our further investigation. Based on the recent literature review, PG has been produced by *S. marcescens* with various types of carbon/nitrogen sources [9–11,13,14,25–33]; however, very few studies report on the use of chitinous materials (squid pens) [19] as the carbon/nitrogen source for PG production; for the first time in this study, α-chitin obtained from marine resources were investigated as a potent carbon source for high scale PG production via microbial fermentation.

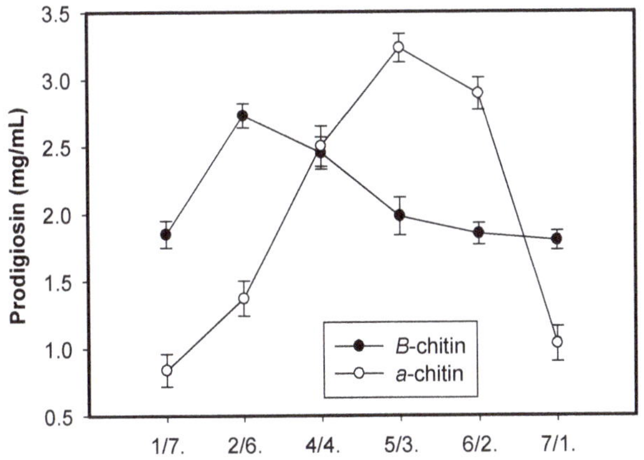

Figure 1. The effect of chitin/protein ratio. The chitin including two forms of α-chitin and β-chitin were mixed with free protein (casein) with six ratios of 1/7, 2/6, 4/4, 5/3, 6/2, and 7/1 (*w/w*) and used as the sole carbon and nitrogen source with the concentration of 1.5% (*w/v*). The fermentation was performed at the conditions at 30 °C in 1 d, and then at 25 °C in next 2 d, shaking speed of 150 rpm, and a ratio volume of medium: flask of 1:2.5 (*v/v*).

For the comparison of the PG producing by different *S. marcescens* strains, a total four strains including *S. marcescens* TKU011, *S. marcescens* CC17, *S. marcescens* TNU01, and *S. marcescens* TNU02 were conducted for fermentation. As shown in the Table 1, *S. marcescens* TKU01, *S. marcescens* TNU01, and *S. marcescens* TNU02 showed their same level in PG production with the PG yield of 325–335 mg/100mL, and 236–243 mg/100mL when the medium contained newly designed C/N source (0.94% α-chitin and 0.56% Casein), and 1.5% squid pens, respectively. *S. marcescens* CC17 demonstrated the lowest production of PG yield.

Table 1. Comparison of the prodigiosin yield (mg/100mL) produced by different *Serratia marcescens* strains.

PG – Producing Strains	C/N Source	
	0.94% α-Chitin + 0.56% Casein	1.5% Squid Pens
S. marcescens TKU011	335 ± 14.4 [a]	243 ± 24.8 [b]
S. marcescens CC17	227 ± 2.93 [b]	150 ± 5.77 [c]
S. marcescens TNU01	329 ± 16.7 [a]	240 ± 17.3 [b]
S. marcescens TNU02	325 ± 14.4 [a]	236 ± 20.8 [b]
No bacteria	-	-

Means of prodigiosin yield (mg/100mL) values with the same letter are not significantly different based on Duncan's multiple range test (alpha = 0.01). CV% = 4.271394. (-): no prodigiosin was detected.

To date, PG has been produced from many carbon sources with multiple designed media [9–11,13,14,25–33]. As summarized in Table 2, the designed medium gave the PG productivity in the scale of 0 up to around 200 (mg/100mL). With the medium containing 0.94% α-chitin + 0.56% Casein, PG produced by *S. marcescens* TKU011 strain reached 335 (mg/100mL). However, two previous studies reported that with 2.0% sesame seed [26] and the medium containing 6.97 g/L of peanut powder, 11.29 mL/L of olive oil and 16.02 g/L of beef extract [33] even reached the PG yield of 1668 and 1362.2 mg/100mL, respectively. These are cases with 4.979-fold and 4.066-fold higher yield than PG yield produced by *S. marcescens* TKU011 in this study. In these above cited reports [26,33], the PG-producing bacteria may be unique strains and the qualification of PG in these studies were not described in detail.

Table 2. Comparison of the prodigiosin yield produced by *S. marcescens* in different reports.

PG – Producing Strains	C/N Source	Prodigiosin (mg/100mL)	Reference
S. marcescens TKU011	0.94% α-chitin + 0.56% Casein	335	This study
S. marcescens TKU011	1.5% squid pens	97.8	[9]
S. marcescens TKU011	1.5% peanut powder	116.8	[9]
S. marcescens TKU011	1.0% shrimp shells powders	19	[9]
S. marcescens TKU011	1.0% crab shells powders	11	[9]
S. marcescens TKU011	1.0% shrimp heads powders	3	[9]
S. marcescens TKU011	1.5% squid pens	248	[28]
S. marcescens	2.0% peanut seed	387.5	[26]
S. marcescens	2.0% peanut oil	289	[26]
S. marcescens	2.0% sesame seed	1668	[26]
S. marcescens	2.0% sesame oil	100.6	[26]
S. marcescens	2.0% copra seed	194	[26]
S. marcescens	2.0% coconut oil	142	[26]
S. marcescens SMΔR	Modified Luria-Bertani broth, 6.0% sunflower oil	79	[29]
S. marcescens SS-1	5 g/L yeast extract as sole N/C source	69	[30]
S. marcescens Nima	2% tryptone/glycerol (1/1)	12.5	[31]
S. marcescens Nima	100 mM 3-[*N*-morpholino]-ethanesulphonic acid	47.5	[32]
S. marcescens FZSF02	6.97 g/L of peanut powder, 11.29 mL/L of olive oil and 16.02 g/L of beef extract	1362.2	[33]
S. marcescens FZSF02	1% Soya peptone	117.4	[33]
S. marcescens FZSF02	1% Tryptone	35.3	[33]
S. marcescens FZSF02	1% Yeast extract	38.02	[33]
S. marcescens FZSF02	1% Fish meal	0	[33]
S. marcescens FZSF02	1% Soybean powder	0	[33]
S. marcescens FZSF02	1% Corn steep liquor	0	[33]

2.2. Optimization of Culture Conditions for Enhancement of Prodigiosin Production by *Serratia marcescens*

To investigate the effect of C/N sources on PG production by *S. marcescens* TKU011, some chitinous materials, including chitosan (a derivative of chitin), *N*-acetyl-glucosamine (monomer of chitin), glucosamine (mono of chitosan), and some other carbon sources, such as cellulose and starch, were used for fermentation. As shown in Figure 2a, among various tested carbon sources, α-chitin displayed the most suitable substrate for PG production by *S. marcescens* with the greatest yield of 3.21 mg/mL, followed by its monomer *N*-acetyl-glucosamine with the PG yield production of 1.81 mg/mL, and all other tested carbon source give low yield PG production (≤ 0.96 mg/mL). Thus, α-chitin was chosen as an excellent substrate for further investigation. To further investigate the effect of the combination of α-chitin and free protein source, a total of five protein sources—beef extract, casein, nutrient broth, yeast extract, and peptone—were combined with α-chitin used as sole C/N source for fermentation by *Serratia marcescens* to produce PG. The experimental results in Figure 2b showed that the combination of casein and α-chitin gave a significantly higher yield of PG (3.31 ± 0.142 mg/mL) than other combinations (≤ 1.73 ± 0.166 mg/mL); casein was chosen for combination with α-chitin and used as the sole C/N source in our nest experiments. Casein was also found to be a suitable nitrogen source for producing PG with high level yield in several previous studies, such as maltose/casein and sucrose/casein with ratio 1/1 leading to PG yield production of 2.354 and 3.12 mg/ml, respectively [34]; 2% oral casein was mixed with some salts and used as the medium for fermentation to produce a high yield of PG with 4.28 mg/mL [23]. Differing from previous studies, we established the novel medium with the combination of abundant chitinous material (α-chitin) and casein with the ratio of 5/3 (*w/w*). This designed medium also reached the high PGs yield of 3.21 mg/mL, and as such used for next investigation.

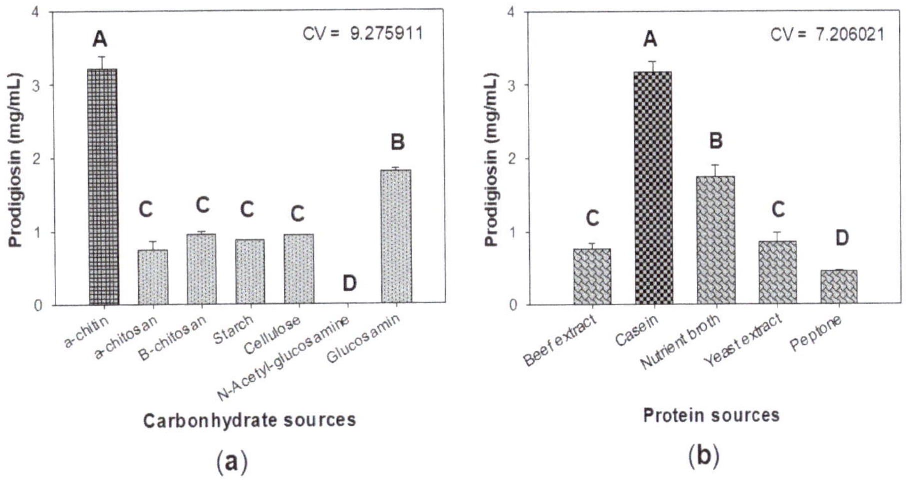

Figure 2. The effect of carbohydrate (**a**) and protein (**b**) sources on the prodigiosin production by *S. marcescens* TKU11. Carbohydrate and protein were mixed at the ratio of 5/3 and used as the C/N source. The culture medium contains 1.5% C/N source, 0.1% K_2HPO_4 and 0.1% $FeSO_4(NH_4)_2SO_4$. The fermentation was performed at the conditions at 30 °C in 1 d, and then at 25 °C over the next 2 d, shaking speed of 150 rpm, and a ratio volume of medium:flask of 1:2.5 (*v/v*). Means of prodigiosin yield (mg/100mL) values with the same letter in each figure are not significantly different based on Duncan's multiple range test (alpha = 0.01).

Some previous studies indicated that salt ingredients in medium, especially phosphate and sulfate salts, played a vital role in enhancing the yield of PG [9,19,35]. As shown in Figure 3a, among various tested salts, K_2HPO_4 was found to be the most suitable phosphate salt for PG biosynthesis by *S. marcescens*. Further experiments investigated the optimal added K_2HPO_4 was 0.05% (Figure 3b). This result is in agreement with the previous reports [19,36]. This added concentration of K_2HPO_4 was used to mix with various kinds of sulfate salts, including $FeSO_4(NH_4)_2SO_4$, $MgSO_4$, $CaSO_4$, $CuSO_4$, $(NH_4)_2SO_4$ as the basal salt solution. $CaSO_4$ demonstrated good effect on PG production with the highest yield of 4.32 mg/mL (Figure 3c). The final experiment (Figure 3d) found that $CaSO_4$ added at its of 0.1% to medium is the optimal concentration. Notably, $CaSO_4$ was newly investigated as potent salt added to significantly enhance PG production by *S. marcescens*.

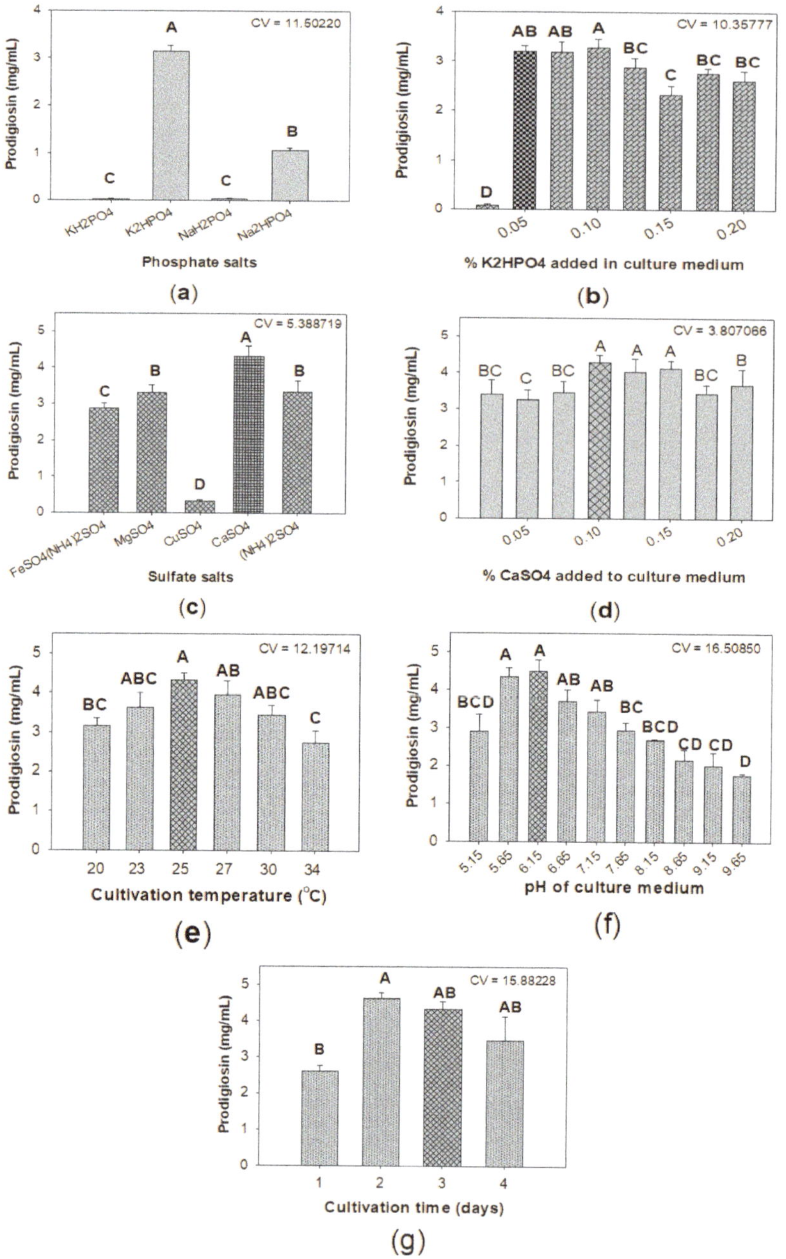

Figure 3. The effect of phosphate salts (**a**,**b**), sulfate salts (**c**,**d**), cultivation temperature (**e**), pH of culture medium (**f**), and cultivation time (**g**) on the prodigiosin production by *S. marcescens* TKU011. Medium with the combination of α-chitin and casein with the ratio of 5/3 (*w/w*). The culture medium containing 1.5% C/N source, 0.1% $FeSO_4(NH_4)_2SO_4$ (**a**,**b**), 0.05% K_2HPO_4 (**c**,**d**). The fermentation was performed at 30 °C in 1 d, and then at 25 °C in the next 2 d, shaking speed of 150 rpm, and a ratio volume of medium: flask of 1:2.5 (*v/v*). Means of prodigiosin yield (mg/100mL) values with the same letter in each figure are not significantly different based on Duncan's multiple range test (alpha = 0.01).

To achieve maximum production of prodigiosin, some parameters, including cultivation temperature (Figure 3e), initial pH of medium (Figure 3f), and period of cultivation time (Figure 3g), were also investigated for their effect on PG yield produced by *S. marcescens*. Overall, *S. marcescens* TKU011 produce highest PG (4.62 mg/mL) in liquid medium with initial pH of 5.65–6.15 containing 1% α-chitin, 0.6% casein, 0.05% K_2HPO_4, and 0.1% $CaSO_4$, fermentation was kept at 25 °C for 2 d.

2.3. Purification and Qualification of Prodigiosin from Fermented Medium Containing α-Chitin

α-chitin was mixed with casein with the ratio of 5/3 (*w/w*) and used as the sole C/N source at the concentration of 1.5% (*w/v*) for fermentation by *S. marcescens* TKU011. PG was primary extracted from the cultured broth by ethyl acetate. The PG from the cell pellet extracted with acetone was mixed with the ethyl acetate layer. After evaporation to dry crude PG, this compound was further purified via silica gel column, and then finally isolated by thin layer chromatography. The procedure is summarized in Figure 4.

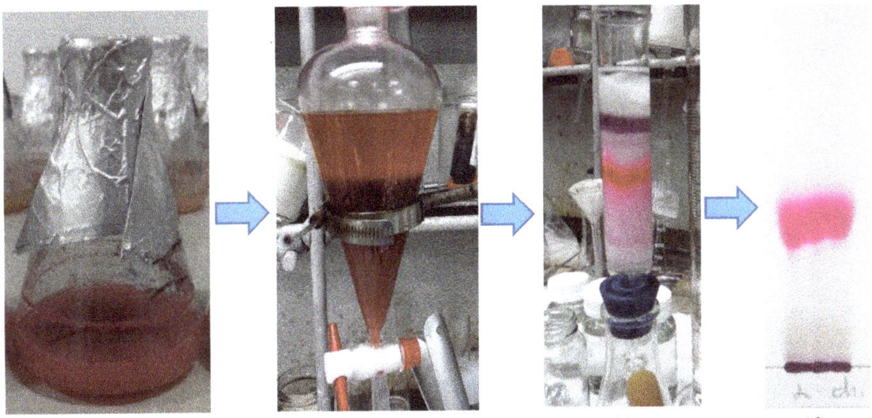

(a) (b) (c) (d)

Figure 4. The purification and isolation process of prodigiosin. The culture broth containing prodigiosin (**a**) was extract by ethyl acetate (**b**). The crude prodigiosin was further separated by silica gel column (**c**) and then isolated by thin layer chromatography (TLC) (**d**).

In our previous report [9], the *S. marcescens* TKU011 prodigiosin was identified via its UV absorption, molecular, and ^{1}H-NMR spectrum. Due to the prodigiosin produced by the same strain, in this study, we reconfirm this purified compound by some rapid method including UV spectra and MALDI-TOF MS analysis. The purified compound demonstrated significant absorption spectroscopy at 535 nm (Figure 5) and the MALDI-TOF MS revealed a molecular weight of 324 Da for the purified PG (Figure 6), which are the specific absorption weight length and molecular weight of prodigiosin [9,33].

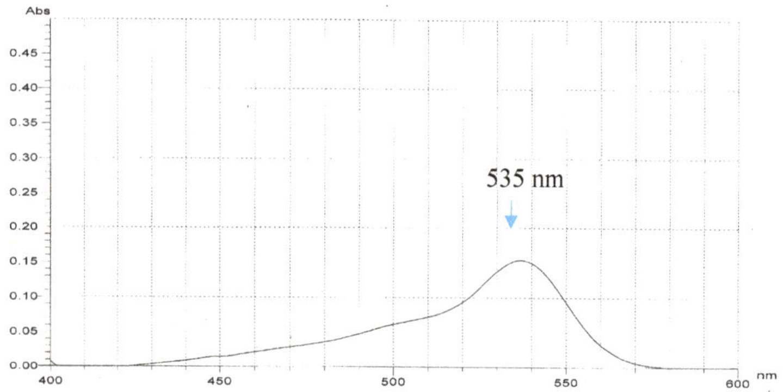

Figure 5. UV spectrum of purified prodigiosin newly biosynthesized from the novel designed substrate (α-chitin/casein = 5/3) by *S. marcescens* TKU011.

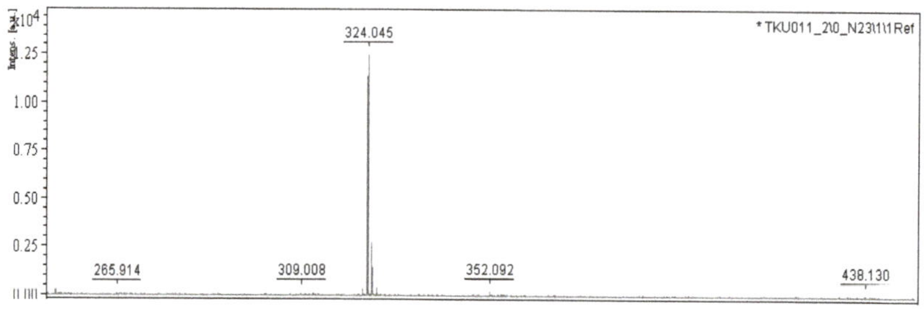

Figure 6. MALDI-TOF MS (Matrix-Assisted Laser Desorption Ionization - Time of Flight Mass Spectrometry) spectra of purified prodigiosin. 2,5-dihydroxybenzoic acid was used as a matrix in CAN-TFA-H_2O solution (50/0.1/50%, *v/v/v*) to separate the sample in the MALDI-TOF instrument (Bruker Daltonics, Bremen, Germany) with a nitrogen laser emitting at 337 nm, operating in linear mode. Each spectrum of mass was calculated based on the data of around 30–50 laser shots, and external calibration with three points was used for assignment of mass [36].

2.4. Evaluation of Inhibitory Effect of Prodigiosin against Cancerous Cell Lines Models

Prodigiosin has been investigated for its vast biological activities, including insecticidal, antioxidant, algicidal, antimicrobial, anti-inflammatory, antimalarial, anticancer, immunomodulatory, and anti-diabetic activities [19,37]. With the aim of evaluating the prodigiosin newly synthesized in this study for potential use in anticancer drugs, prodigiosin was tested for its inhibition against some cancerous cell lines, including A549, Hep G2, MCF-7, and WiDr. As presented in Table 3, prodigiosin produced from the novel medium with the combination of α-chitin and casein used as the C/N source demonstrated its highly effective inhibition against all tested cancerous cell lines with great inhibition values (%) in the range of 90.2–93.9% at the tested concentration at 10 μg/mL. These anticancer inhibition values of prodigiosin were comparable to those of Mitomycin C, a commercial anticancer compound (91.7–94.1%). The crude sample also showed potent activity with max inhibition values in the range of 79.4–93.2% at the concentration of at 10 μg/mL.

The samples were tested at their concentration of 10 μg/mL for their anticancer activity against MCF-7 (Human breast adenocarcinoma), A549 (Human lung carcinoma), Hep G2 (Human hepatocellular carcinoma), and WiDr (Human colon adenocarcinoma). The means of inhibition (%) with the same letter are not significantly different based on Duncan's multiple range test (alpha = 0.01). CV (%) = 1.979533.

Table 3. Max inhibition against cancerous cell lines of prodigiosin.

	Max Inhibition Against Cancerous Cell Lines (%)			
	MCF-7	**A549**	**Hep G2**	**WiDr**
Crude sample	91.6 ± 1.76 [a,b]	89.2 ± 1.43 [b]	93.2 ± 2.12 [a,b]	79.4 ± 1.72 [c]
Purified Prodigiosin	92.5 ± 1.4 [a,b]	92.6 ± 1.9 [a,b]	93.9 ± 2.0 [a]	90.2 ± 1.12 [a,b]
Mitomycin C	94.1 ± 1.61[a]	93.3 ± 1.54 [a,b]	91.7 ± 1.01 [a,b]	92.6 ± 1.02 [a,b]

The samples were tested at their concentration of 10 μg/mL for their anticancer activity against MCF-7 (Human breast adenocarcinoma), A549 (Human lung carcinoma), Hep G2 (Human hepatocellular carcinoma), and WiDr (Human colon adenocarcinoma). The means of inhibition (%) with the same letter are not significantly different based on Duncan's multiple range test (alpha = 0.01). CV (%) = 1.979533.

To clarify the potential effect of prodigiosin against these tested cancerous cells, the samples were diluted and tested in various concentrations; the result of anticancer activity was then calculated and presented as IC_{50} value. IC_{50} value is a concentration of sample that may reduce 50% of cancerous cells; therefore, the smallest this value of the sample, the strongest anticancer activity it displayed. As shown in Table 3, prodigiosin strongly inhibited all 4 tested cancerous cells with very low IC_{50} values of 0.04, 0.06, 0.04, and 0.20 against A549, Hep G2, MCF-7, and WiDr, respectively (Table 4). The anticancer activity of the purified prodigiosin is clearly higher than that of the crude sample with IC_{50} values in the range of 0.38–0.88 μg/mL. Mitomycin C was also tested in comparison and showed its inhibition against A549, Hep G2, MCF-7 and WiDr with IC50 values of 0.11, 0.10, 0.13, and 0.10 μg/mL, respectively. In comparison, prodigiosin displayed significantly higher inhibition against A549, Hep G2, and MCF-7 but weaker inhibition against WiDr than Mitomycin C.

Table 4. Anticancer activities of prodigiosin.

	Inhibition Against Cancerous Cell Lines (IC50, μg/mL)			
	MCF-7	**A549**	**Hep G2**	**WiDr**
Crude sample	0.44 ± 0.09 [c,b]	0.46 ± 0.01 [b]	0.38 ± 0.01 [c,b]	0.88 ± 0.05 [a]
Purified Prodigiosin	0.04 ± 0.01 [e]	0.06 ± 0.01 [e]	0.04 ± 0.01 [e]	0.20 ± 0.03 [d]
Mitomycin C	0.11 ± 0.01 [e]	0.10 ± 0.01 [e]	0.13 ± 0.01 [e]	0.10 ± 0.01 [e]

The samples were tested at their concentration range of 0.01–10 μg/mL for their anticancer activity against MCF-7 (Human breast adenocarcinoma), A549 (Human lung carcinoma), Hep G2 (Human hepatocellular carcinoma), and WiDr (Human colon adenocarcinoma). Means of IC_{50} (μg/mL) values with the same letter are not significantly different based on Duncan's multiple range test (alpha = 0.01). CV% = 12.9069.

To date, various prodigiosin compounds produced via fermentation reported anticancer activity against MCF-7 and A549. Prodigiosin was also reported showing inhibition against Hep G2 in several reports [38,39]. However, no available data report the potent inhibition of prodigiosin against human colon adenocarcinoma WiDr cell line. Specifically, the purified prodigiosin produced from marine chitin materials in the current study demonstrated high level anticancer activity. It displayed higher 2.75-, 1.67-, and 3.25-fold efficacy than commercial anticancer compounds against MCF-7, A549, and Hep G2, respectively.

Anticancer drugs have been extensively investigated for years. Commercially available anticancer drugs obtained from chemical synthesis show strong activity but result in various side effects [40]. Thus, the investigation of natural anticancer drugs has received much interest. Prodigiosin was investigated as a potent natural anticancer agent since it showed strong inhibition against a wide range of human cancer cell lines but lower toxicity toward normal cells [41]. The mechanisms of anticancer activity of prodigiosin were reported in previous studies [41–43]. Prodigiosin induces apoptosis in various human cancer cells [42], and some possible mechanisms were prosed that prodigiosin as mitogen-activated protein kinase regulators, cell cycle inhibitors, DNA cleavage agents, and pH modulators [43]. The results in this study contributed to announce the novel anticancer activity of prodigiosin against WiDr cell line and also reconfirmed that prodigiosin as effective anticancer agents.

3. Materials and Methods

3.1. Materials

Serratia marcescens TKU011 was obtained from our previous study [9]. *S. marcescens* CC17 obtained from the previous study [44], *S. marcescens* TNU01 and *S. marcescens* TNU02 were newly isolated from the soils of Buon Ma Thuot City, Vietnam, and identified based on 16S gene sequence in this study. Shrimp shell and squid pens were purchased from Fwu-Sow Industry (Taichung, Taiwan). Four cancerous cell lines—MCF-7 (Human breast adenocarcinoma), A549 (Human lung carcinoma), Hep G2 (Human hepatocellular carcinoma), and WiDr (Human colon adenocarcinoma)—were purchased from the Bioresources Collection and Research Centre (Hsinchu, Taiwan). Mitomycin C and Silicagel (Geduran® Si 60 for column chromatography, size: 0.040–0.063 mm) were obtained from Sigma Chemical Co. (St. Louis City, MO, USA) and Mitsubishi Chemical Co. (Tokyo, Japan), respectively. Reagents, solvents and common chemicals were used at the highest grade available.

16S gene sequence of *Serratia marcescens* TNU01:

TGGCTCAGATTGAACGCTGGCGGCAGGCTTAACACATGCAAGTCGAGCGGTAGCACAGGG GAGCTTGCTCCCTGGGTGACGAGCGGCGGACGGGTGAGTAATGTCTGGGAAACTGCCTGAT GGAGGGGGATAACTACTGGAAACGGTAGCTAATACCGCATAACGTCGCAAGACCAAAGAGG GGGACCTTCGGGCCTCTTGCCATCAGATGTGCCCAGATGGGATTAGCTAGTAGGTGGGGTAA TGGCTCACCTAGGCGACGATCCCTAGCTGGTCTGAGAGGATGACCAGCCACACTGGAACTG AGACACGGTCCAGACTCCTACGGGAGGCAGCAGTGGGGAATATTGCACAATGGGCGCAAGC CTGATGCAGCCATGCCGCGTGTGTGAAGAAGGCCTTCGGGTTGTAAAGCACTTTCAGCGAG GAGGAAGGTGGTGAACTTAATACGTTCATCAATTGACGTTACTCGCAGAAGAAGCACCGGC TAACTCCGTGC.

16S gene sequence of *Serratia marcescens* TNU02:

CTGGCTCAGATTGAACGCTGGCGGCAGGCTTAACACATGCAAGTCGAGCGGTAGCACAGG GGAGCTTGCTCCCCTGGGTGACGAGCGGCGGACGGGTGAGTAATGTCTGGGAAACTGCCTGA TGGAGGGGGATAACTACTGGAAACGGTAGCTAATACCGCATAACGTCGCAAGACCAAAGAG GGGGACCTTCGGGCCTCTTGCCATCAGATGTGCCCAGATGGGATTAGCTAGTAGGTGGGGTA ATGGCTCACCTAGGCGACGATCCCTAGCTGGTCTGAGAGGATGACCAGCCACACTGGAACT GAGACACGGTCCAGACTCCTACGGGAGGCAGCAGTGGGGAATATTGCACAATGGGCGCAA GCCTGATGCAGCCATGCCGCGTGTGTGAAGAAGGCCTTCGGGTTGTAAAGCACTTTCAGCG AGGAGGAAGGTGGTGAACTTAATACGTTCATCAATTGACGTTACTCGCAGAAGAAGCACCG GCTAACTCCGTG C.

3.2. Fermentation for Prodigiosin Biosynthesis by S. marcescens TKU011

α-chitin and β-chitin obtained from shrimp shells and squid pens were mixed with casein with 6 ratios of 1/7, 2/6, 4/4, 5/3, 6/2, and 7/1 (*w/w*) and used as the sole carbon and nitrogen source with the concentration of 1.5% (*w/v*) for fermentation. The medium containing 1.5% carbon and nitrogen source, 0.1% K_2HPO_4 and 0.1% $FeSO_4(NH_4)_2SO_4$ was fermented by *S. marcescens* TKU011 at 30 °C in 1 d, and then 25 °C over the next 2 d, shaking speed of 150 rpm, and a ratio volume of medium:flask of 1:2.5 (*v/v*). α-chitin mixed with casein at the ratio of 5/3 (*w/w*) reached the greatest PG yield production; as such, α-chitin/casein was used for comparison in the following experiments evaluating other carbohydrate sources (chitosan, *N*-acetyl-glucosamine, glucosamine, cellulose and starch) and proteinous sources. α-chitin/casein at the ratio of 5/3 (*w/w*) finally proved best and was used for fermentation in the subsequent investigation, including the effect of added salts and some parameters.

The effect of phosphate salts and its optimal concentration added to culture medium on PG production: four kinds of phosphate salts—KH_2PO_4, K_2HPO_4, NaH_2PO_4, and Na_2HPO_4—were used. The medium containing 0.1% $FeSO_4(NH_4)_2SO_4$, 0.1% phosphate salt, and 1.5% C/N source were fermented at 30 °C in 1 d, and then at 25 °C over the next 2 d, shaking speed of 150 rpm, and a ratio volume of medium:flask of 1:2.5 (*v/v*). KH_2PO_4 was found to be the most suitable phosphate salt; as such, it was used to investigate its optimal concentration added to the medium. 0.025, 0.05, 0.1, 0.125, 0.15, 0.175, and 0.2% K_2HPO_4 and combined with 0.1% $FeSO_4(NH_4)_2SO_4$; the fermentation procedure was conducted at 30 °C in 1 d, and then 25 °C over the next 2 d, shaking speed of 150 rpm, and a ratio volume of medium:flask of 1:2.5 (*v/v*).

The effect of sulfate salts and its optimal concentration added to culture medium on PG production: $FeSO_4(NH_4)_2SO_4$, $MgSO_4$, $CaSO_4$, $CuSO_4$, and $(NH_4)_2SO_4$ were used as sulfate salts. The medium containing 0.05% K_2HPO_4 and 0.1% sulfate salt, 1.5% C/N source were fermented at 30 °C in 1 d, and then 25 °C over the next 2 d, shaking speed of 150 rpm, and a ratio volume of medium:flask of 1:2.5 (*v/v*). $CaSO_4$ was found to be the most suitable sulfate salt; as such, it was used to investigate its optimal concentration added to the medium. 0.025, 0.05, 0.1, 0.125, 0.15, 0.175, and 0.2% $CaSO_4$ and combined with 0.1% K_2HPO_4; the fermentation was conducted at 30 °C in 1 d, and then 25 °C over the next 2 d, shaking speed of 150 rpm, and a ratio volume of medium:flask of 1:2.5 (*v/v*).

The effect of some parameters on PG production: some parameters including temperature programs (activated at 20, 23, 25, 27, 30, and 34 °C, and then fermented at 25 °C over the next 2 d), initial pH (5.15, 5.65, 6.15, 6.65, 7.15, 7.65, 8.15, 8.65, 9.15, 9.65) and period of cultivation time (0, 1, 2, 3, and 4 d).

3.3. Prodigiosin Quilification and Purification

PG concentration was determined according to the method previously described by Wang et al., 2012 [36]. A mixture including 0.5 mL of fermented medium broth and 4 mL of methanol was vortexed. 2% (*w/v*) hydrated potassium aluminum sulfate was added into this mixture, mixed, and then centrifuged at 1400 g for 5 min. The harvested supernatant was then mixed with a solution of methanol/0.5 N HCl at the ratio of 1/9, *v/v*. The final solution optical density was measured at 535 nm. PG purified from the culture broth was used as the standard to convert OD535 nm measurement to mass concentration via an appropriate calibration. PG was purified by the method previously described [36] with modification. The culture broth was centrifugated at 10000× *g* for 15 min. The supernatant was collected and mixed with ethyl acetate with the ratio 1/1. The mixture was kept in a funnel for 3 h and immediately shaken every 30 min. The PG dissolved in ethyl acetate layer was collected. The PG from the cell pellet was extracted with acetone, and centrifugated at 10000× *g* for 15 min. The ethyl acetate layer and acetone containing PG were mixed, concentrated by evaporation of the solvent and then dissolved in ethyl acetate for further air oven drying at 55 °C to get dry crude PG powder. The crude PG was further purified by loading onto a silica open column (Geduran® Si 60 (Merck KGaA, Darmstadt, Germany) for column chromatography, size: 0.040–0.063 mm) and eluted with methanol in chloroform with a ratio of 0/10–2/8 (*v/v*). The PG was finally isolated by thin layer chromatography (TLC) with the mobile phase system using methanol in chloroform with a ratio of 2/8 (*v/v*). After TLC separation, the lane contained PG was cut into small pieces, and methanol was used to dissolve PG. Then PG was concentrated in a rotary evaporator (IKA, Staufen, Germany) at 60 °C under vacuum. Finally, all the residue solvent was removed by keeping the sample in the oil pump in 12 h at 60 °C. The isolated PG was used to detect UV, MALDI-TOF MS and biological activities.

3.4. Biological Activity Assays

Four cancerous cell lines: A549, Hep G2, MCF-7, and WIDR were conducted to evaluate the anticancer activities. The bioassay was done according to the methods described in detail in our previous report [6]. The significant differences of anticancer activity, including inhibition (%) and IC_{50} values, were analyzed with the use of Statistical Analysis Software (SAS-9.4) provided by the SAS Institute Taiwan Ltd. (Taipei City, Taiwan).

4. Conclusions

The current study established the novel designed medium containing 1% α-chitin, 0.6% casein, 0.05% K_2HPO_4, and 0.1% $CaSO_4$ for efficient biosynthesis of bioactive prodigiosin. The fermentation was maintained at 25 °C for 2 d. The prodigiosin was purified, qualified via UV and Mass. The purified prodigiosin was also evaluated for its anticancer properties. Notably, the purified PG displayed high inhibition on four cancerous cell lines. The results in this study suggest that the purified prodigiosin newly biosynthesized may be a potential candidate for cancer drugs.

Author Contributions: Conceptualization, V.B.N. and S.-L.W.; methodology, S.-L.W. and V.B.N.; software, V.B.N.; validation, S.-L.W., Y.-H.K., and T.H.N.; formal analysis, V.B.N., A.D.N., T.T.T.T., M.T.N., C.T.D., and T.N.T.; investigation, V.B.N., S.-P.C., and T.H.N.; resources, S.-L.W. and V.B.N.; data curation, S.-L.W.; writing—original draft preparation, V.B.N.; writing—review and editing, S.-L.W. and V.B.N.; visualization, V.B.N., S.-L.W.; supervision, V.B.N. and S.-L.W.; project administration, S.-L.W. and V.B.N. All authors have read and agreed to the published version of the manuscript.

Funding: This study was supported in part by a grant from the Ministry of Science and Technology, Taiwan (MOST 106-2320-B-032-001-MY3).

Acknowledgments: We express great thanks to the Department of Chemistry, Tamkang University, New Taipei City 25137; Taiwan and Division of Chinese Materia Medica Development, National Research Institute of Chinese Medicine for the kind provision of some analysis tools for this study.

Conflicts of Interest: The authors declare no conflict of interest

References

1. Nguyen, V.B.; Wang, S.L. Reclamation of marine chitinous materials for the production of α-glucosidase inhibitors via microbial conversion. *Mar. Drugs* **2017**, *15*, 350. [CrossRef] [PubMed]
2. Liang, T.W.; Tseng, S.C.; Wang, S.L. Production and characterization of antioxidant properties of exopolysaccharides from *Paenibacillus mucilaginosus* TKU032. *Mar. Drugs* **2016**, *14*, 40. [CrossRef] [PubMed]
3. Liang, T.W.; Wang, S.L. Recent advances in exopolysaccharides from *Paenibacillus* spp.: Production, isolation, structure, and bioactivities. *Mar. Drugs* **2015**, *13*, 1847–1863. [CrossRef] [PubMed]
4. Liang, T.W.; Wu, C.C.; Cheng, W.T.; Chen, Y.C.; Wang, C.L.; Wang, I.L.; Wang, S.L. Exopolysaccharides and antimicrobial biosurfactants produced by *Paenibacillus macerans* TKU029. *Appl. Biochem. Biotechnol.* **2014**, *172*, 933–950. [CrossRef]
5. Liang, T.W.; Chen, W.T.; Lin, Z.H.; Kuo, Y.H.; Nguyen, A.D.; Pan, P.S.; Wang, S.L. An amphiprotic novel chitosanase from *Bacillus mycoides* and its application in the production of chitooligomers with their antioxidant and anti-inflammatory evaluation. *Int. J. Mol. Sci.* **2016**, *17*, 1302. [CrossRef]
6. Kuo, Y.H.; Liang, T.W.; Liu, K.C.; Hsu, Y.W.; Hsu, H.C.; Wang, S.L. Isolation and identification of a novel antioxidant with antitumor activity from *Serratia ureilytica* using squid pen as fermentation substrate. *Mar. Biotechnol.* **2011**, *13*, 451–461. [CrossRef]
7. Nguyen, V.B.; Nguyen, T.H.; Doan, C.T.; Tran, T.N.; Nguyen, A.D.; Kuo, Y.-H.; Wang, S.-L. Production and bioactivity-guided isolation of antioxidants with α-glucosidase inhibitory and anti-NO properties from marine chitinous materials. *Molecules* **2018**, *23*, 1124. [CrossRef]
8. Wang, S.L.; Huang, T.Y.; Wang, C.Y.; Liang, T.W.; Yen, Y.H.; Sakata, Y. Bioconversion of squid pen by *Lactobacillus paracasei* subsp *paracasei* TKU010 for the production of proteases and lettuce enhancing biofertilizers. *Bioresour. Technol.* **2008**, *99*, 5436–5443. [CrossRef]
9. Wang, S.L.; Wang, C.Y.; Yen, Y.H.; Liang, T.W.; Chen, S.Y.; Chen, C.H. Enhanced production of insecticidal prodigiosin from *Serratia marcescens* TKU011 in media containing squid pen. *Process Biochem.* **2012**, *47*, 1684–1690. [CrossRef]
10. Liang, T.W.; Chen, C.H.; Wang, S.L. Production of insecticidal materials from *Pseudomonas tamsuii*. *Res. Chem. Intermed.* **2015**, *41*, 7965–7971. [CrossRef]
11. Wang, S.L.; Chen, S.Y.; Yen, Y.H.; Liang, T.W. Utilization of chitinous materials in pigment adsorption. *Food Chem.* **2012**, *135*, 1134–1140. [CrossRef] [PubMed]
12. Liang, T.W.; Lo, B.C.; Wang, S.L. Chitinolytic bacteria-assisted conversion of squid pen and its effect on dyes and adsorption. *Mar. Drugs* **2015**, *13*, 4576–4593. [CrossRef] [PubMed]
13. Nguyen, V.B.; Nguyen, A.D.; Wang, S.L. Utilization of fishery processing by-product squid pens for α-glucosidase inhibitors production by *Paenibacillus* sp. *Mar. Drugs* **2017**, *15*, 274. [CrossRef] [PubMed]
14. Doan, C.T.; Tran, T.N.; Nguyen, M.T.; Nguyen, V.B.; Nguyen, A.D.; Wang, S.-L. Anti-α-glucosidase activity by a protease from *Bacillus licheniformis*. *Molecules* **2019**, *24*, 691. [CrossRef] [PubMed]

15. Wang, S.L.; Su, Y.C.; Nguyen, V.B.; Nguyen, A.D. Reclamation of shrimp heads for the production of α-glucosidase inhibitors by *Staphylococcus* sp. TKU043. *Res. Chem. Intermed.* **2018**, *44*, 4929–4937. [CrossRef]
16. Hsu, C.H.; Nguyen, V.B.; Nguyen, A.D.; Wang, S.L. Conversion of shrimp heads to α-glucosidase inhibitors via co-culture of *Bacillus mycoides* TKU040 and *Rhizobium* sp. TKU041. *Res. Chem. Intermed.* **2017**, *44*, 4597–4607. [CrossRef]
17. Nguyen, V.B.; Nguyen, A.D.; Kuo, Y.-H.; Wang, S.-L. Biosynthesis of α-glucosidase inhibitors by a newly isolated bacterium, *Paenibacillus* sp. TKU042 and Its effect on reducing plasma glucose in a mouse model. *Int. J. Mol. Sci.* **2017**, *18*, 700. [CrossRef]
18. Nguyen, V.B.; Wang, S.L. Production of potent antidiabetic compounds from shrimp head powder via *Paenibacillus* conversion. *Process Biochem.* **2019**, *76*, 18–24. [CrossRef]
19. Liang, T.W.; Chen, S.Y.; Chen, Y.C.; Chen, Y.C.; Yen, Y.H.; Wang, S.L. Enhancement of prodigiosin production by *Serratia marcescens* TKU011 and its insecticidal activity relative to food colourants. *J. Food Sci.* **2013**, *78*, 1743–1751. [CrossRef]
20. Furstner, A. Chemistry and biology of roseophilin and the prodigiosin alkaloids: A survey of the last 2500 years. *Chem. Int. Ed. Engl.* **2003**, *42*, 3582–3603. [CrossRef]
21. Cerdeno, A.M.; Bibb, M.J.; Challis, G.L. Analysis of the prodiginine biosynthesis gene cluster of *Streptomyces coelicolor* A3(2): New mechanisms for chain initiation and termination in modular multienzymes. *Chem. Biol.* **2001**, *8*, 817–829. [CrossRef]
22. Samrot, A.V.; Chandana, K.; Senthilkumar, P.; Narendra, K.G. Optimization of prodigiosin production by *Serratia marcescens* SU-10 and evaluation of its bioactivity. *Int. Res. J. Biotechnol.* **2011**, *2*, 128–133.
23. de Casullo Araújo, H.W.; Fukushima, K.; Campos Takaki, G.M. Prodigiosin production by *Serratia marcescens* UCP 1549 using renewable-resources as a low-cost substrate. *Molecules* **2010**, *15*, 6931–6940. [CrossRef] [PubMed]
24. Gulani, C.; Bhattacharya, S.; Das, A. Assessment of process parameters influencing the enhanced production of prodigiosin from *Serratia marcescens* and evaluation of its antimicrobial, antioxidant and dyeing potentials. *Malays. J. Microbiol.* **2012**, *8*, 116–122.
25. Nakamura, K.; Kitamura, K. Process for Preparation of Prodigiosin. U.S. Patent 4,266,028A, 5 May 1981.
26. Giri, A.V.; Anandkumar, N.; Muthukumaran, G.; Pennathur, G. A novel medium for the enhanced cell growth and production of prodigiosin from *Serratia marcescens* isolated from soil. *BMC Microbiol.* **2004**, *4*, 11–18. [CrossRef]
27. Shahitha, S.; Poornima, K. Enhanced production of prodigiosin production in *Serratia marcescens*. *J. Appl. Pharm. Sci.* **2012**, *2*, 138–140. [CrossRef]
28. Wang, S.L.; Kao, D.Y.; Wang, C.L.; Yen, Y.H.; Chern, M.K.; Chen, Y.H. A solvent stable metalloprotease produced by *Bacillus* sp. TKU004 and its application in the deproteinization of squid pen for beta-chitin preparation. *Enzyme Microb. Technol.* **2006**, *39*, 724–731. [CrossRef]
29. Wei, Y.H.; Chen, W.C. Enhanced production of prodigiosin-like pigment from *Serratia marcescens* SMdeltaR by medium improvement and oil-supplementation strategies. *J. Biosci. Bioeng.* **2005**, *99*, 616–622. [CrossRef]
30. Wei, Y.H.; Yu, W.J.; Chen, W.C. Enhanced undecylprodigiosin production from *Serratia marcescens* SS-1 by medium formulation and amino-acid supplementation. *J. Biosci. Bioeng.* **2005**, *100*, 466–471. [CrossRef]
31. Wang, X.; Tao, J.; Wei, D.; Shen, Y.; Tong, W. Development of an adsorption procedure for the direct separation and purification of prodigiosin from culture broth. *Biotechnol. Appl. Biochem.* **2004**, *40*, 277–280.
32. Solé, M.; Rius, N.; Francia, A.; Lorén, J.G. The effect of pH on prodigiosin production by non-proliferating cells of *Serratia marcescens*. *Lett. Appl. Microbiol.* **1994**, *19*, 341–344. [CrossRef] [PubMed]
33. Lin, C.; Jia, X.; Fang, Y.; Chen, L.; Zhang, H.; Lin, R.; Chen, J. Enhanced production of prodigiosin by *Serratia marcescens* FZSF02 in the form of pigment pellets. *Electron. J. Biotechnol.* **2019**, *40*, 58–64. [CrossRef]
34. Sumathi, C.; MohanaPriya, D.; Swarnalatha, S.; Dinesh, M.G.; Sekaran, G. Production of prodigiosin using tannery fleshing and evaluating its pharmacological effects. *SCI World J.* **2014**, *2014*, 290327. [CrossRef] [PubMed]
35. Holly, S.; Matthew, C.; Lee, E.; George, P.C.S. Phosphate availability regulates biosynthesis of two antibiotics, prodigiosin and carbapenem, in *Serratia* via both quorum-sensing-dependent and -independent pathways. *Mol. Microbiol.* **2003**, *47*, 303–320.

36. Doan, C.T.; Tran, T.N.; Nguyen, V.B.; Nguyen, A.D.; Wang, S.-L. Reclamation of marine chitinous materials for chitosanase production via microbial conversion by *Paenibacillus macerans*. *Mar. Drugs* **2018**, *16*, 429. [CrossRef]
37. Arivizhivendhan, K.V.; Mahesh, M.; Boopathy, R.; Swarnalatha, S.; Regina Mary, R.; Sekaran, G. Antioxidant and antimicrobial activity of bioactive prodigiosin produces from *Serratia marcescens* using agricultural waste as a substrate. *J. Food Sci. Technol.* **2018**, *55*, 2661. [CrossRef]
38. Yenkejeh, R.A.; Sam, M.R.; Esmaeillou, M. Targeting survivin with prodigiosin isolated from cell wall of *Serratia marcescens* induces apoptosis in hepatocellular carcinoma cells. *Hum. Exp. Toxicol.* **2017**, *36*, 402–411. [CrossRef]
39. Chen, J.; Li, Y.; Liu, F.; Hou, D.-X.; Xu, J.; Zhao, X.; Yang, F.; Feng, X. Prodigiosin promotes Nrf2 activation to inhibit oxidative stress induced by microcystin-LR in HepG2 cells. *Toxins* **2019**, *11*, 403. [CrossRef]
40. Orlikova, B.; Legrand, N.; Panning, J.; Dicato, M.; Diederich, M. Anti-inflammatory and anticancer drugs from nature. *Cancer Res. Treat.* **2014**, *159*, 123–143.
41. Li, D.; Liu, J.; Wang, X.; Kong, D.; Du, W.; Li, H.; Hse, C.-Y.; Shupe, T.; Zhou, D.; Zhao, K. Biological potential and mechanism of prodigiosin from *Serratia marcescens* subsp. *lawsoniana* in human choriocarcinoma and prostate cancer cell lines. *Int. J. Mol. Sci.* **2018**, *19*, 3465.
42. Dalili, D.; Fouladdel, S.; Rastkari, N.; Samadi, N.; Ahmadkhaniha, R.; Ardavan, A.; Azizi, E. Prodigiosin, the red pigment of *Serratia marcescens*, shows cytotoxic effects and apoptosis induction in HT-29 and T47D cancer cell lines. *Nat. Prod. Res.* **2011**, *26*, 2078–2083. [PubMed]
43. Perez-Tomas, R.; Montaner, B.; Llagostera, E.; Soto-Cerrato, V. The prodigiosins, proapoptotic drugs with anticancer properties. *Biochem. Pharmacol.* **2003**, *66*, 1447–1452. [CrossRef]
44. Nguyen, V.B.; Wang, S.L.; Nguyen, T.H.; Nguyen, T.H.; Trinh, T.H.T.; Nong, T.T.; Nguyen, T.U.; Nguyen, V.N.; Nguyen, A.D. Reclamation of rhizobacteria newly isolated from black pepper plant roots as potential biocontrol agents of root-knot nematodes. *Res. Chem. Intermed.* **2019**. [CrossRef]

© 2019 by the authors. Licensee MDPI, Basel, Switzerland. This article is an open access article distributed under the terms and conditions of the Creative Commons Attribution (CC BY) license (http://creativecommons.org/licenses/by/4.0/).

marine drugs

MDPI

Article

Identification, Purification and Molecular Characterization of Chondrosin, a New Protein with Anti-tumoral Activity from the Marine Sponge *Chondrosia Reniformis* Nardo 1847

Sonia Scarfì [1,2], Marina Pozzolini [1], Caterina Oliveri [1], Serena Mirata [1], Annalisa Salis [3], Gianluca Damonte [3,4], Daniela Fenoglio [3,4], Tiziana Altosole [3], Micha Ilan [5], Marco Bertolino [1] and Marco Giovine [1,*]

1 Department of Earth, Environment and Life Sciences (DISTAV), University of Genova, Via Pastore 3, 16132 Genova, Italy; soniascarfi@unige.it (S.S.); marina.pozzolini@unige.it (M.P.); Caterina.oliveri@unige.it (C.O.); serena.mirata@edu.unige.it (S.M.); marco.bertolino@unige.it (M.B.)
2 Centro 3R, Interuniversitary Center for the Promotion of the Principles of the 3Rs in Teaching and Research, Via Caruso 16, 56122 Pisa, Italy
3 Department of Experimental Medicine (DIMES), Biochemistry Section, University of Genova, Viale Benedetto XV 1, 16132 Genova, Italy; annalisa.salis@unige.it (A.S.); gianluca.damonte@unige.it (G.D.); Daniela.fenoglio@unige.it (D.F.); tiziana.alto@gmail.com (T.A.)
4 Centre of Excellence for Biomedical Research (CEBR), University of Genova, Viale Benedetto XV 9, 16132 Genova, Italy
5 School of Zoology, Tel Aviv University, Tel Aviv 69978, Israel; milan@tauex.tau.ac.il
* Correspondence: mgiovine@unige.it; Tel.: +39-010-3533-8221

Received: 6 July 2020; Accepted: 30 July 2020; Published: 2 August 2020

Abstract: *Chondrosia reniformis* is a common marine demosponge showing many peculiarities, lacking silica spicules and with a body entirely formed by a dense collagenous matrix. In this paper, we have described the identification of a new cytotoxic protein (chondrosin) with selective activity against specific tumor cell lines, from *C. reniformis*, collected from the Liguria Sea. Chondrosin was extracted and purified using a salting out approach and molecular weight size exclusion chromatography. The cytotoxic fractions were then characterized by two-dimensional gel electrophoresis and mass spectrometry analysis and matched the results with *C. reniformis* transcriptome database. The procedure allowed for identifying a full-length cDNA encoding for a 199-amino acids (aa) polypeptide, with a signal peptide of 21 amino acids. The mature protein has a theoretical molecular weight of 19611.12 and an IP of 5.11. Cell toxicity assays showed a selective action against some tumor cell lines (RAW 264.7 murine leukemia cells in particular). Cell death was determined by extracellular calcium intake, followed by cytoplasmic reactive oxygen species overproduction. The in silico modelling of chondrosin showed a high structural homology with the *N*-terminal region of the ryanodine receptor/channel and a short identity with defensin. The results are discussed suggesting a possible specific interaction of chondrosin with the Cav 1.3 ion voltage calcium channel expressed on the target cell membranes.

Keywords: Chondrosin; *Chondrosia reniformis*; marine toxin; cytotoxic protein; Porifera

1. Introduction

The marine sponge *Chondrosia reniformis* Nardo 1847 is a common marine demosponge, widely distributed along all the Mediterranean Sea and East Atlantic Ocean, where it inhabits both shallow and deep-water environments [1]. This demosponge lacks siliceous spicules and its body is entirely formed by a dense collagenous matrix with peculiar molecular features [2–4] with finely-regulated production [5]. This sponge is also characterized by good regenerative properties [6] whose molecular mechanisms have recently been described [7]. *C. reniformis* collagens pose remarkable biotechnology potential: their successful use has been demonstrated in cosmetic preparations [8], in drug delivery [9,10], in biomembrane production [11] and in the production of active peptides with biomedical targets [12]. The well-known industrial value of this marine resource has pushed scientists to find sustainable methods of exploitation, whether through the production of sponge collagen by recombinant approaches [13,14] or by aquaculture attempts [15]. In particular, the current attempts at *C. reniformis* farming are promising, even if not yet optimised for a sustainable production of sponge biomass on a large scale, but in the next future relevant improvements in this field are expected. Some sporadic observations on this peculiar animal also document the release of unknown toxic compound(s) in the water hosting the specimens after collection, able to kill other animals in the same tank and to cause skin irritation in humans. On the other hand, it is also known that *C. reniformis* in some areas of the Adriatic Sea was usually eaten, after cooking, possibly implying a thermolability of this toxic compound(s) [16].

The aim of this study was to fill in the gap of knowledge on the toxic compounds produced by this common sponge, and to investigate their possible applicability in biomedicine, specifically in the field of anticancer therapy. Based on the above-mentioned evidences, a chemical purification procedure from a crude extract of *C. reniformis* specimens, collected in the Ligurian Sea was performed, and a cell cytotoxicity assay was set up to verify its activity and its possible anti-tumour effect on different cancer cell lines. Various experimental strategies were used to assess the compounds chemical nature, and to define the range of molecular weight (MW) of these toxic component(s). Chromatographic fractionation of the crude extract, mass spectrometry (MS) analysis and *C. reniformis* transcriptome data mining, were then performed to identify the active compound and its three-dimensional (3D) structure. Finally, the mechanism of toxicity on four cancer cell lines, representatives of different typologies of tumours, was also investigated, to define its mode of action that causes cell death preferentially in cancer cells.

2. Results and Discussion

2.1. The Cytotoxicity of a Crude Extract (CE) of *C. reniformis* is Due to a Protein Fraction

Preliminary experiments were performed on the crude hydrophilic extract (CE) of *C. reniformis* obtained by squeezing sponge specimens, collected in the Ligurian Sea. As shown in Figure 1A the RE exhibited a significant cytotoxic activity on L929 murine fibroblast cell line, where a 100-fold dilution of the CE caused 74.9 ± 4.5% cell death at 24 h incubation, analysed by the 3-(4,5-dimethylthiazol-2-yl)-2,5-diphenyltetrazolium bromide dye test (MTT) (CE-100 bar, $p < 0.0001$ compared to C). To determine if the cytotoxic activity of the CE was due to a small-molecule metabolite or to a protein, three different approaches were performed: a thermal sensitivity experiment, a 10,000 kDa cut-off dialysis of the CE (DE), and a trypsin digestion. Indeed, the CE cytotoxic component was sensitive to thermal treatment, as shown in Figure 1A (CE-therm bar), being completely inactivated after 10 min incubation at 100 °C. Conversely, the DE showed that the cytotoxic component was totally retained in the 10 kDa cut-off fraction (Figure 1A, DE-100 bar, 70.1 ± 9.7% cytotoxic activity compared to C, $p < 0.0001$). Finally, the trypsin digestion demonstrated a high degree of fragmentation into smaller peptides in the DE as shown in the gel electrophoresis analysis (Figure 1C lanes 3 and 4 compared to control lane 2) and L929 cells challenged with the trypsin-digested DE (Figure 1B, DE-Tryp20 and DE-Tryp50 bars) for 24 h showed a significant loss of the cytotoxic effect after the protease treatment compared to the untreated DE (Figure 1B, 57% loss of cytotoxic activity for DE-Tryp20 and 71% for DE-Tryp50, respectively, compared to DE-100, $p < 0.0001$ for both bars). These results clearly demonstrated that a significant cytotoxic activity on a mammalian cell viability of the DE fraction was due to one or more proteins. The production of toxic proteins is well known in marine sponges [17,18]. For biomedical applications, smaller molecules demonstrate a better exploitability than the larger ones [19], due to their easiness for in vitro and in vivo biological and pharmacological assays, even if there is not a true "dimensional" cut-off in the evaluation criteria for the pharmaceutical applicability of a polypeptide. Bioactivity, specificity of action, and low immunogenicity are the main keys for the successful use of a bioactive protein in therapy. The pharmacological target also plays a role, and like toxins of other marine and terrestrial organisms, the biomolecule's action could have different levels of specificity. Proteins and peptides with selective action against bacteria and viruses are topics of increasing interest, whereas the research for new proteins and peptides with anti-tumour activity is the most promising.

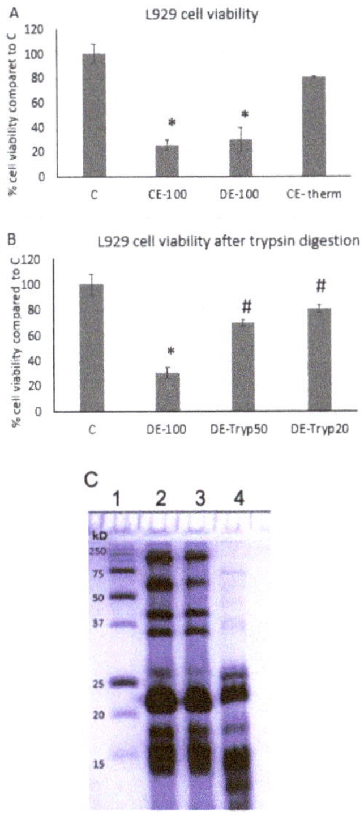

Figure 1. Cell toxicity evaluation. (**A**) L929 fibroblast cell growth quantitative evaluation, by the cell viability MTT test at 24 h, in the presence or absence of a 100-fold diluted crude extract (CE-100), of a 100-fold diluted dialysed extract (DE-100) and of a thermally-inactivated 100-fold diluted crude extract (CE-therm). Results are expressed as cell percentages relative to control cells (**C**) and are the mean ± Standard deviation (S.D). of three experiments performed in quadruplicate. Asterisks indicate significance in paired Tukey test (Analysis of Variance-ANOVA, $p < 0.000001$; Tukey vs. C: * $p < 0.0001$). (**B**) L929 fibroblast cell growth quantitative evaluation, by the cell viability MTT test at 24 h, in the presence or absence of a 100-fold diluted DE (DE-100) or of the same DE previously digested with two different concentrations of trypsin (DE-Tryp50 and DE-Tryp20, respectively). Results are expressed as cell percentages relative to control cells (C) and are the mean ± S.D. of three experiments performed in quadruplicate. Asterisks indicate significance in paired Tukey test (ANOVA, $p < 0.000001$; Tukey vs. C: * $p < 0.0001$; Tukey vs. DE-100: # $p < 0.0001$). (**C**) Sodium Dodecyl Sulphate-PolyAcrylamide Gel Electrophoresis (SDS-PAGE) of 20 µg of undiluted DE fraction after trypsin digestion for 24 h. Lane 1 molecular weight standards, Lane 2 untreated DE, lane 3 DE digested with tryspin 1:50 (*w:w*), lane 4 DE digested with trypsin 1:20 (*w:w*).

2.2. Identification and Characterization of Chondrosin

In initial results (Figure 1), the main cytotoxic activity was confined to the protein fraction of the *C. reniformis* crude extract, therefore a biochemical protocol of protein fractionation was designed and tested to purify and identify the active protein(s) (Scheme 1). Thus, the RE was subjected to the following step-by-step purification procedure: (i) a 10 kDa-cut-off dialysis to get rid of small molecules and metabolites, and to obtain a dialysed extract fraction (DE); (ii) an ammonium sulphate (AS) biochemical protein fractionation (salting out), giving active proteins in the precipitate fraction (ASP); (iii) a high-performance liquid chromatography (HPLC) separation by size-exclusion gel filtration to obtain a limited number of protein peaks (P1-P5). This procedure allowed us to obtain five different *C. reniformis* protein fractions, shown in the chromatogram of Figure 2A, with decreasing molecular weight, named P1 to P5, and in the range of: P1 480–250 kDa, P2 250–130 kDa, P3 130–75 kDa, P4 75–35 kDa and P5 35–15 kDa. As shown in the MTT tests in Figure 3, only P4 and P5 HPLC fractions retained a significant cytotoxic effect, thus, these two peaks were processed for the proteomic analysis. Both HPLC fractions were therefore dried and subsequently subjected to two-dimensional (2D) electrophoretic analysis. The results are summarized in Figure 2B, C where a very similar and well-defined row of spots in the same position in the 2D gels is evident (spots from 1 to 4), suggesting the presence of the same protein in both peaks. More specifically, peak 5 showed a purer composition, whereas peak 4 contained traces of other proteins together with the protein showing a cytotoxic activity. The HPLC analysis is coherent with the MS result, where the chromatogram obtained clearly suggests that peaks 4 and 5 are not completely resolved and the proteins eluted in peak 5 are also present in peak 4 (Figure 2A). The MS analysis of the proteins extracted from the four spots of the 2D gels of peaks 4 and 5 corresponds to a protein that we named chondrosin (see Tables 1 and 2). The row of spots is considered typical of post-translational modifications like that of different patterns of phosphorylation or glycosylation [20,21]. In all four spots, the same peptides were identified. Matches between the MS data and *C. reniformis* transcriptome database allowed us to identify a putative sequence corresponding to the one showed in Figure 2D. The MS analysis clearly identified the primary sequence of the protein, and the data mining of *C. reniformis* transcriptome database allowed to identify a full-length cDNA encoding for a 199-aa polypeptide, with a signal peptide of 21 aa (Figure 2D, underlined in red). The cleavage site of the signal peptide is positioned between amino acids (aa) AEA and SK, with 0.963% of probability (see methods). The mature protein consists of 178 aa (Figure 2C in black), with a theoretical Molecular weight (MW) of 19611.12 and an Isoelectric point (IP) of 5.11. MS analysis confirmed the primary sequence of chondrosin with a 65.17% of coverage (Figure 2D, MS-identified peptides highlighted in yellow). The uncovered part of the sequence is probably the site of post-translational modifications. The in silico predicted structure analysis (Figure 2E) evidenced a clear homology with the *N*-terminal region of the ryanodine receptor/channel and with a small region found in the defensin beta sheet domain (Supplementary Materials, File S1). Many toxins contain defensin-like domains conjugated with different types of protein domains. The genetic toxin evolution, in these cases, starts from a gene encoding a non-toxic protein subjected to mutation by duplication and/or exon shuffling phenomena, and/or specific point mutations, to give rise to the final toxic protein [22,23]. The absence of *C. reniformis* genome database does not allow more specific considerations about the genetic origin of chondrosin, but the presence of this short defensin domain might be explained by a related evolutionary process. More intriguing and peculiar is the presence of a larger domain with high structural homology with the ryanodine receptor. To the best of our knowledge, there has been no previous report for protein toxins, and the hypothesis of action discussed in the following sections is challenging.

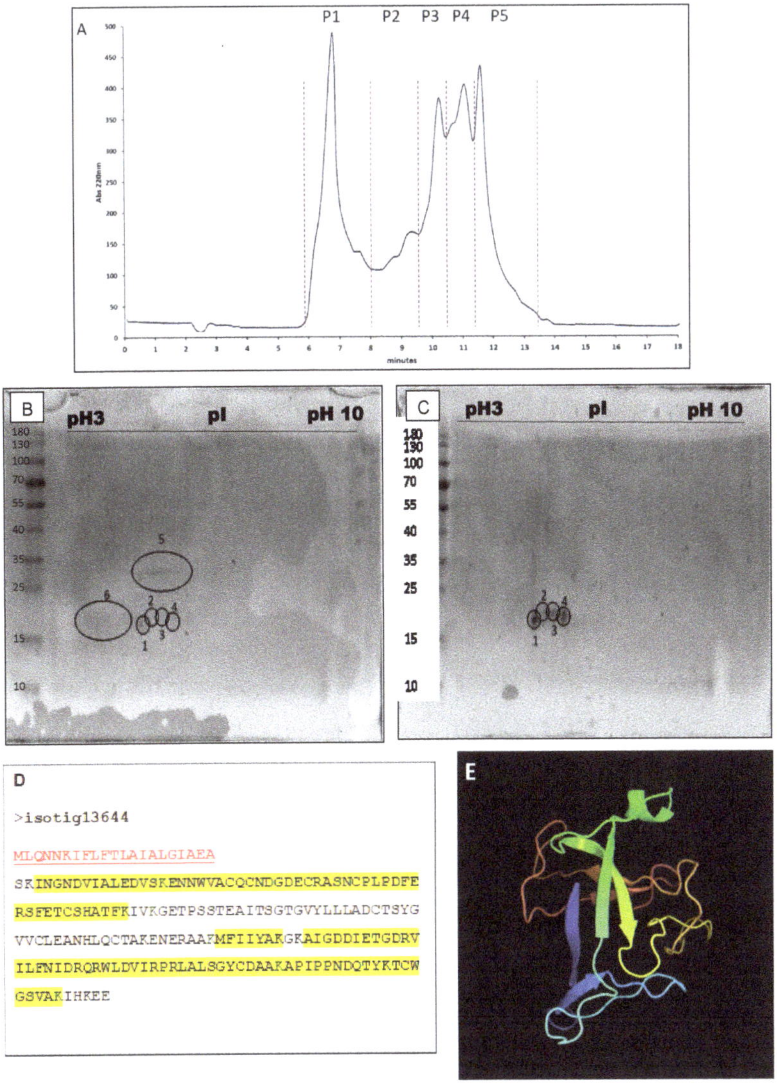

Figure 2. Identification by proteomic analysis. (**A**) Chromatogram at 220 nm absorbance obtained by HPLC (high-performance liquid chromatography) separation of the ammonium sulphate precipitate (ASP) fraction through a molecular weight size-exclusion column. The obtained peaks, from P1 to P5, were separately collected for further biological and chemical characterization. (**B**,**C**) Two-dimensional gel electrophoresis of *C. reniformis* HPLC purified P4 and P5 peaks, respectively. Samples were loaded in precast, 7-cm long, IPG strips with isoelectric focusing (IEF) pH 3–10. Spot protein identification (from spots 1 to 6) relative to peak 4 (**B**) and (from spot 1 to 4) relative to peak 5 (**C**), by MS analysis, are reported, respectively, in Tables 1 and 2. Spots (1–4) are present in the same position in both gels corresponding to the same protein. (**D**) Chondrosin protein primary amino acid sequence. The identified signal peptide is in red, while the protein peptide coverage identified by MS analysis is highlighted in yellow. (**E**) Chondrosin predicted 3D structure using the Phyre^2 web portal for protein modelling, prediction and analysis (http://www.sbg.bio.ic.ac.uk/phyre2/html/page.cgi?id=index © Structural Bioinformatics Group, Imperial College, London)

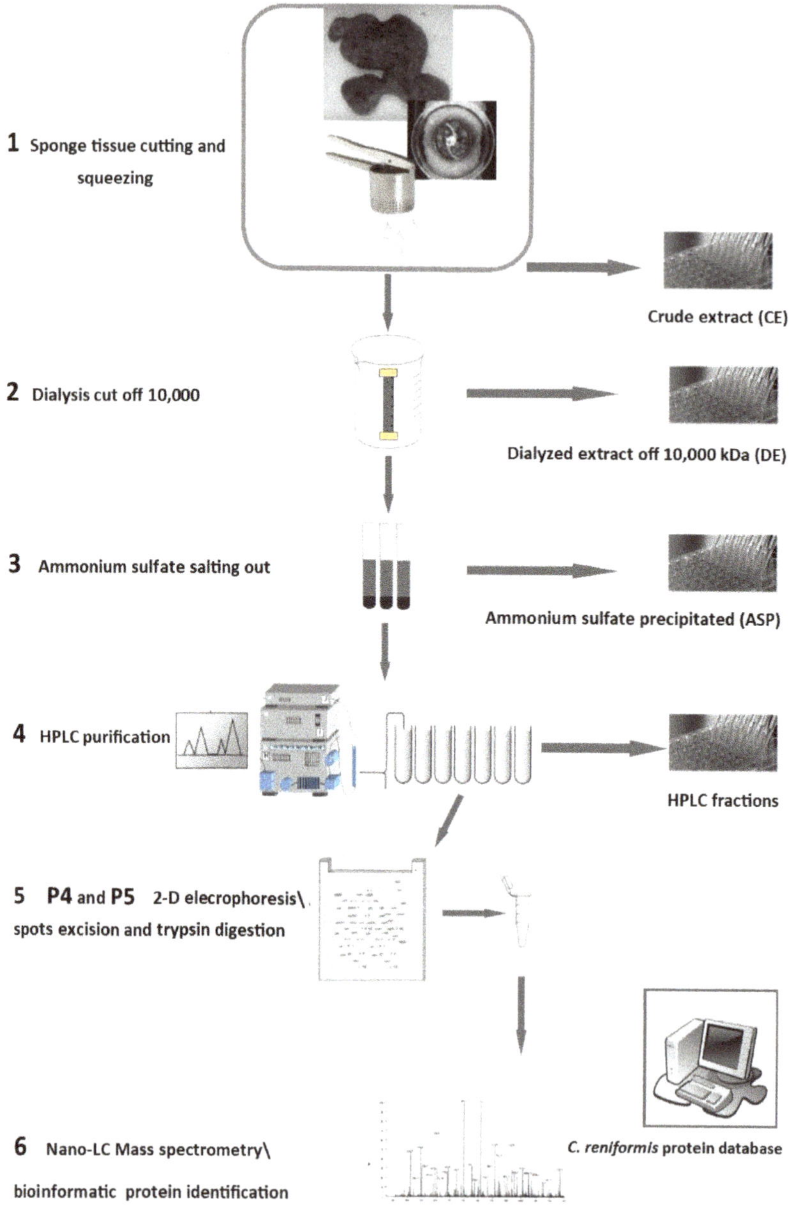

Scheme 1. Procedure flowchart for the step-by-step purification and characterization of the cytotoxic/anti-tumour protein chondrosin from the marine sponge *C. reniformis*.

Table 1. The proteins identified from 2D (two-dimensional) gel spots of peaks 4 and 5 by Q Exactive™ nano- electrospray ionization coupled with tandem mass spectrometry (ESI-MS/MS) and SEQUEST search engine. For each protein (isotig) the following details are reported: Score (Sequest), coverage (% of the protein sequence covered by identified peptides), unique peptides (unique peptides in the protein group), peptides (distinct peptides in the protein group).

			P4			
Spot	**C. R. Database Id**	**Score**	**Coverage**	**Proteins**	**Unique Peptides**	**Peptides**
1	isotig13644	207.90	58.29	1	10	11
2	isotig13644	133.15	58.29	1	8	11
3	isotig13644	137.50	58.29	1	8	11
4	isotig13644	237.20	58.29	1	11	11
5	isotig11703	66.86	37.37	1	4	10
6	isotig13644	19.68	45.23	1	7	8
6	isotig02770	74.19	45.81	2	2	6
6	isotig02771	47.81	45.81	2	2	6
			P5			
Spot	**C. R. Database Id**	**Score**	**Coverage**	**Proteins**	**Unique peptides**	**Peptides**
1	isotig13644	379.61	58.29	1	12	12
2	isotig13644	340.54	58.29	1	10	12
3	isotig13644	181.69	58.29	1	11	11
4	isotig13644	309.34	58.29	1	12	12

Table 2. Identified proteins. For each identified protein total amino acid number, theoretical MW and IP are given. Moreover, the table indicates the accession number, the protein description and the organism in which the proteins displaying the maximum alignment score (sorted by E-value), obtained by the National Center for Biotechnology Information (NCBI) Protein Blast analysis, are identified.

C. R. Database Id	aa	MW (kDa)	IP	Accession Number	Description	Organism	E Value
isotig13644	199	21.9	5.27	WP_142038611.1	DNA-binding response regulator	*Arthrobacter sp.*	5.9
isotig11703	281	31.9	5.76	ABR53885.1	Astrosclerin-1	*Astrosclera willeyana*	7.30×10^{-61}
isotig02770	203	23.3	4.59	XP_016993171.1	PREDICTED: ubiquitin-conjugating enzyme E2 H	*Drosophila takahashii*	4.4
isotig02771	203	23.3	4.55	XP_016993171.1	PREDICTED: ubiquitin-conjugating enzyme E2 H	*Drosophila takahashii*	4.4

2.3. *Anti-Tumour Activity of Protein Purified Fractions Derived from C. reniformis CE*

The cytotoxic action of CE was better characterized by purification of the active compounds responsible of the observed effects. At each purification step, the total protein content of each fraction was quantified (see Section 4), and the increasing concentration of the active protein(s) was monitored by testing its(their) cytotoxic/anti-tumour activity using the MTT test (Figure 3) on normal human dermal fibroblasts (NHDF) and on four cancer cell lines at 24 h incubation at various dilutions (1 to 100 μg/mL total protein content). The cytotoxicity test on NHDF at 24 h incubation showed no effect on the cell viability with respect to control cells in the presence of the DE fraction, at all concentrations tested (Figure 3A). At the same time the ASP fraction showed a weak cytotoxicity only at the highest concentrations (18.5 ± 7.5 and 14.7 ± 7.1% cell death at 100 and 10 μg/mL compared to the control, respectively, $p > 0.05$ for both). Finally, whereas P1 to P3 HPLC purified fractions exhibited no sign of toxicity in all cell lines tested from normal fibroblasts to cancer cell lines (data not shown), P4 and P5 fractions showed a significant cytotoxicity in all types of cells. In particular, in NHDF cells, both P4 and

P5 fractions manifested a significant cytotoxicity at the highest and the middle concentrations tested (100 and 10 μg/mL, respectively), namely 73.1 ± 3.7 and 42.1 ± 6.9% cell death were observed for P4 ($p < 0.0001$ vs. C for both bars, respectively), while 81.1 ± 6.3 and 44.2 ± 8.2% cell death were recorded for P5 ($p < 0.0001$ vs. C for both bars, respectively). Finally, at the lowest concentration (1 μg/mL) both P4 and P5 showed no sign of cytotoxicity on NHDF cells. Subsequently, the cytotoxic test was performed on four different cancer cell lines: L929 murine fibroblasts (tumorigenic in immunocompromised mice), RAW 264.7 (murine leukemic macrophages), MDA-MB-468 (human breast carcinoma) and HeLa (human cervical carcinoma). L929 and RAW 264.7 cells showed the highest sensitivity to the cytotoxic effects of the *C. reniformis* protein fractions, whereas the MDA and HeLa cells were the less sensitive, although also in these cell lines a significant effect was observed. Concerning L929 cells, all *C. reniformis* protein fractions i.e., from DE to ASP and from P4 and P5 showed a relevant cytotoxic effect (Figure 3B). DE fraction was dramatically effective both at 100 and 10 μg/mL concentrations while at 1 μg/mL concentration cell death percentage reached 82.8 ± 3.3% compared to control cells ($p < 0.0001$). A similar pattern was observed also for ASP toxicity test where the highest concentrations tested (100 and 10 μg/mL) showed a 94.9 ± 0.5 and 84.7 ± 2.3% cell death while the lowest (1 μg/mL) a 30 ± 4.2% mortality compared to the control ($p < 0.01$). Finally, the cytotoxicity of P4 and P5 HPLC fractions was very high at the highest and middle concentrations tested (87.7 ± 4.2 and 74.6 ± 1.2% for P4 and 80.2 ± 3.1 and 74 ± 2.5% for P5, respectively, $p < 0.0001$ vs. C for both concentrations and both purified peaks) but completely ineffective at the lowest concentration. RAW 264.7 murine leukemic macrophages revealed the highest sensitivity to the *C. reniformis* protein fractions cytotoxic effect. In fact, all fractions from DE to ASP and to P4 and P5, at the highest and middle concentrations tested, showed a cell mortality close to 100% (Figure 3C) and the lowest concentration was still able to significantly affect cell viability vs. control, with a mortality of 76.7 ± 4.4% for DE 1($p < 0.0001$), 53.9 ± 10.5% for ASP 1 ($p < 0.0001$), 18 ± 9.5% for P4 1 ($p < 0.05$) and 36.7 ± 9.3% for P5 1 ($p < 0.0005$). In MDA-MB-468 breast carcinoma cell line, a different behaviour was observed (Figure 3D). The *C. reniformis* protein fractions never reached a very high rate of mortality, except maybe for DE, ASP and P4 at 100 μg/mL where 79.7 ± 2.5%, 44.5 ± 6.1% and 54 ± 5.9% cell death were reached, respectively ($p < 0.0001$ vs. C for all conditions). Conversely, all the other tested concentrations showed a lower cell death varying from 30–35% yet significantly higher than the control (P5 all concentrations, P4 10 μg/mL, $p < 0.005$) to only 20% (DE 10 and 1 μg/mL, P4 1 μg/mL, $p < 0.005$). Similarly, HeLa cells (Figure 3E) showed a higher rate of mortality only at the highest concentration tested, with a percentage of cell death of 59.4 ± 3.8% for DE, 36.7 ± 1.8% for ASP, 65.7 ± 4.3% for P4 and 51.9 ± 8.1% for P5 compared to C ($p < 0.005$, for all bars), while at the middle and the lowest concentrations cell death rates were around 47.6 ± 2.1% and 29.7 ± 10.7% for DE, 45.6 ± 3.3% and 34.7 ± 10.4% for ASP, 30% for P4 and 35.7 ± 1.3% and 41.8 ± 8.1% for P5, respectively ($p < 0.05$ vs. C for all bars).

Overall, these data indicate that there is a higher cytotoxicity of the *C. reniformis* protein fractions to the cancer cell lines compared to the primary normal cells (Figure 2B–E vs. 2A) with a respective EC_{50} calculated for the P4 and P5 purified fractions of 17.8 and 14.6 μg/mL for NHDF, 3.56 and 4.9 μg/mL for L929, 1.99 and 1.12 μg/mL for RAW 264.7, 59.88 μg/mL for P4 in MDA-MB-468 and 17.7 μg/mL for P4 in HeLa cells. The EC_{50} of the P5 fraction for MDA and HeLa cells was not possible to calculate. Thus, we can conclude that the identified protein chondrosin, present in P4 and P5 fractions, seems to exert an anti-tumour effect on two of the four cancer cell lines (L929 and RAW 264.7) and a cytotoxic/anti-proliferative effect on the other two cell lines (MDA-MB-468 and HeLa). Furthermore, a different sensitivity to the *C. reniformis* anti-tumour protein chondrosin in the four cancer cell lines can be envisaged, probably due to some differences in the chondrosin specific interaction with these cells, as further discussed in Section 2.4. In particular, the two murine tumorigenic cell lines (panels B and C) showed the highest sensitivity to *C. reniformis* protein fractions, with the hematologic cancer cell line being the most affected of all, while the two human carcinomas (panels D and E) demonstrated a higher resilience to the cytotoxic effect, even at the lowest protein fraction concentration (1 μg/mL), cell viability was always significantly lower than the untreated control (in MDA between 20 and 30%

less cells, in HeLa between 30 and 40% less cells). These numbers could indicate that while a strong cell death mechanism could operate in L929 and RAW 264.7 murine cells, the effect in the human carcinoma cell lines could be more cytostatic, resulting in a lower cell death rate and a slow-down of cell growth whose cell death never reached the values of the untreated controls.

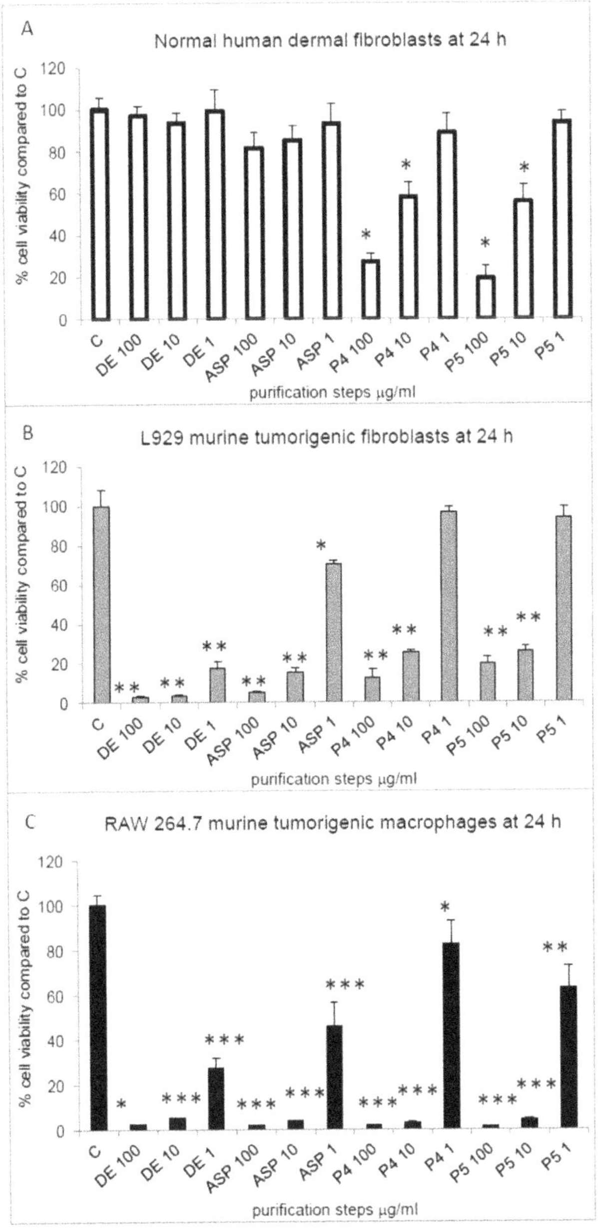

Figure 3. *Cont.*

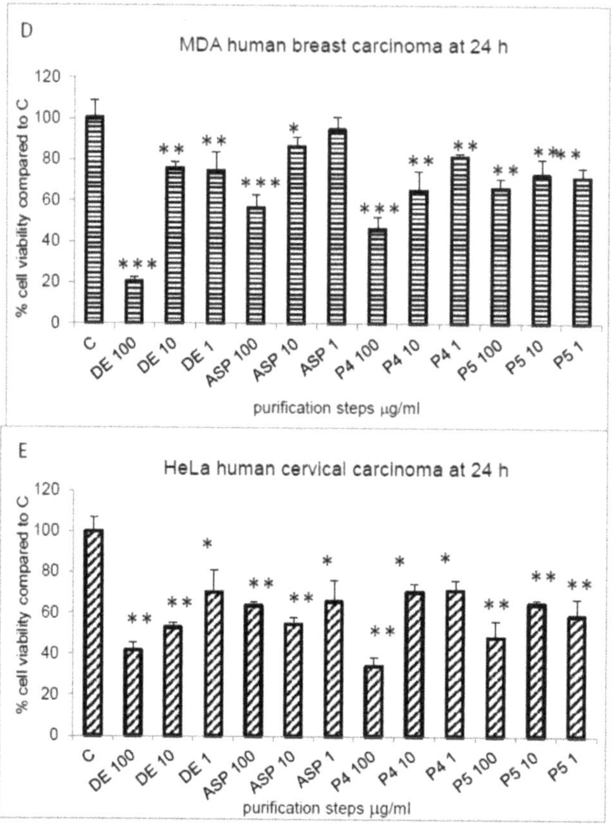

Figure 3. Cytotoxic/anti-tumour activity evaluation. (**A**) Normal human dermal fibroblast cell growth quantitative evaluation, by the cell viability MTT test at 24 h, in the presence or absence of various dilutions of *C. reniformis* purified fractions: dialysed extract (DE) from 1 to 100 μg/mL, ammonium sulfate precipitate extract (ASP) from 1 to 100 μg/mL, HPLC purified peak 4 (P4) and peak 5 (P5) from 1 to 100 μg/mL. Results are expressed as living cell percentages with respect to control cells (C) and are the mean ± S.D. of three experiments performed in quadruplicate. Asterisks indicate significance in paired Tukey test (ANOVA, $p < 0.000001$; Tukey vs. C: * $p < 0.0001$). (**B**) L929 murine tumorigenic fibroblasts cell growth quantitative evaluation in the same conditions as (A). Asterisks indicate significance in paired Tukey test (ANOVA, $p < 0.000001$; Tukey vs. C: ** $p < 0.0001$, * $p < 0.01$, respectively). (**C**) RAW 264.7 murine leukemia cell growth quantitative evaluation in the same conditions as (**A**). Asterisks indicate significance in paired Tukey test (ANOVA, $p < 0.000001$; Tukey vs. C: *** $p < 0.0001$, ** $p < 0.0005$, * $p < 0.05$, respectively). (**D**) MDA-MB-468 human breast carcinoma cell growth quantitative evaluation in the same conditions as (A). Asterisks indicate significance in paired Tukey test (ANOVA, $p < 0.000001$; Tukey vs. C: *** $p < 0.0001$, ** $p < 0.005$, * $p < 0.05$, respectively). (E) HeLa human cervical carcinoma cell growth quantitative evaluation in the same conditions as (A). Asterisks indicate significance in paired Tukey test (ANOVA, $p < 0.000001$; Tukey vs. C: ** $p < 0.005$, * $p < 0.05$, respectively).

2.4. *Mechanisms of Toxicity of Chondrosin on Tumour Cells*

2.4.1. Necrosis and Apoptosis Assessment

To investigate which type of cell death the four cancer cell lines were undergoing, two types of analyses were performed: the Lactate Dehydrogenase (LDH) assay, quantifying the enzyme leakage in the cell medium, in order to evaluate the level of cell death by necrosis in the cultures, and the annexin/propidium iodide positivity assay, analysed both by cytofluorimetry (FACS analysis), and by confocal microscopy in order to establish the level of apoptosis of the cancer cells. The LDH assay performed after 24 h of incubation revealed a certain rate of necrosis in the four cancer cell lines (Figure 4), but mainly in the presence of the DE fraction and not in the further purified fractions, and especially in the two murine cancer cell lines (L929 and RAW 264.7, panels A and B, respectively). In detail, L929 cells showed a significant cell necrosis in the DE fraction at both concentrations tested compared to control cells (44.6 ± 3.1% and 13.3 ± 1.4% at 100 and 10 μg/mL, $p < 0.001$ and $p < 0.05$, respectively), and also in the ASP fraction at the highest concentration (23.5 ± 3.8%, $p < 0.05$), while in the P4 fraction the percentage of necrosis was always below 10% and comparable to the control. RAW 264.7 cells showed a comparable behaviour with a significant necrosis with respect to that of the control, observable only in the DE fraction (36.2 ± 3.4% and 26.6 ± 4%, at 100 and 10 μg/mL, $p < 0.001$ and $p < 0.05$, respectively), while the ASP and P4 fractions always showed a necrosis percentage below 10% and comparable to that of the control. In MDA cells (Figure 4C) necrosis was only observable at the highest concentration of DE and P4 fractions in the range of 15% for both, compared to the control ($p < 0.05$), and finally in HeLa cells, the only protein fraction causing a slight but measurable rate of necrosis was the DE at both concentrations tested (13 ± 1.6% and 8.1 ± 0.6%, at 100 and 10 μg/mL, respectively, $p < 0.05$). Overall, the two human cell lines showed a very low level of necrosis, although still measurable, in their cultures. These data indicate that: (i) in the DE protein fraction there is a multifactorial cytotoxic activity provoking cell death partly by necrosis, as documented in Figure 4, but not only, and this is especially visible at 100 μg/mL DE protein fraction concentration where the rate of cell death measured by the MTT test (Figure 3) is significantly higher compared to the percentage of necrosis at the same time point (24 h) in all cancer cell lines; (ii) in the further purified *C. reniformis* protein fractions, namely the ASP and the P4, the necrotic component of the protein extract has been eliminated by the purification steps, and the still high rate of cytotoxicity measured in these fractions in all cancer cell lines at 24 h (MTT test in Figure 3) is probably due to an apoptotic mechanism. To test this hypothesis, the annexin/propidium iodide staining was used to evaluate the apoptotic state in all cancer cell lines and the cultures were analysed by both Fluorescence-activated cell sorting flow cytometry (FACS) and confocal microscopy for a quantitative and qualitative assessment, respectively. In particular, the FACS analysis was performed at 6 and 24h on the four tumour cell lines on the cells recovered after trypsin detachment from the wells where the treatment with the DE or P4 was performed. Thus, the results refer to the percentage of apoptotic cells observed in the population of cells still attached to the plate and, therefore, still alive in the plate. Results are shown in Figure 5 and exemplify one of the three experiments performed on the four cell lines. Concerning L929 (panel A) and RAW 264.7 cells (panel B) only the 6 h endpoint is shown since at 24h it was not possible to retrieve a sufficient number of manageable cells from the plates to perform the analysis, and for the same reason the concentrations of protein fractions used for these cells were of 10 and 1 μg/mL for both DE and P4 fractions. In both cell lines it was possible to observe, at the only time point analysed, a significant number of apoptotic cells (the percentage is the sum of early + late apoptotic) with respect to all the cells retrieved from the plates. The highest percentage of apoptotic cells in L929 cell line was observed in the sample treated with 10 μg/mL P4 (14.3%) and in the RAW 264.7 cell line treated with 1 μg/mL DE (26.4%), although in these cells also the P4 treatment, both at 10 and 1 μg/mL, showed a significant percentage of apoptosis relative to the total number of cells retrieved from the plate (18.8% and 18.1%, respectively). Interestingly, also in MDA (panel C) and HeLa cells (panel D–E), although the *C. reniformis* protein fractions were less cytotoxic (see Figure 3), it was possible to observe a significant number of apoptotic cells both at 6 and 24 h at 100 and 10 μg/mL concentrations for the DE and P4 treatments. In particular, in both MDA and HeLa cells, the highest percentage of apoptotic cells was observed in the P4 treatment at the highest concentration after 6 h incubation (23.3% and 39.3%, respectively), while at 24 h the percentage of apoptosis in the same sample was lower in both cell lines (12.6% and 31.8%, respectively). Furthermore, in the same cell lines the second highest apoptotic percentage was obtained by treatment with the DE at 100 µg/mL for 24 h, where in both cell lines the level of apoptosis was around 20% with respect to all cells retrieved from the plates (panels C, D and E). These data were also confirmed by a confocal microscopy analysis of the four cell lines, after treatment with P4, by annexin/propidium iodide staining of cells (Figure 6). In particular, L929 (panels A) and RAW 264.7 cells (panels B) images were acquired after 6 h treatment with 10 µg/mL P4. In both cell lines it was possible to observe numerous groups of cells showing signs of both early (only green positivity) and late (concomitant green/red positivity) apoptosis (panels A-III and B-III, respectively), being the second more prevalent than the first (i.e., more green/red cells than only green in both cell lines). Conversely, both in MDA (panels C) and HeLa cells (panels D) treated with 100 µg/mL P4 for 6 h, early apoptotic cells (only green positivity) were more prevalent than late apoptotic (concomitant green/red positivity) cells at this time point (panels C-III and D-III, respectively). Altogether, these data indicate that a significant phenomenon of apoptosis is observable in the four tumor cell lines treated with the *C. reniformis* protein fractions. Thus, we can infer that the cytotoxicity of chondrosin, a new protein identified as the main component of the P4 and P5 fractions, is likely due to a mechanism promoting apoptosis in the affected cells.

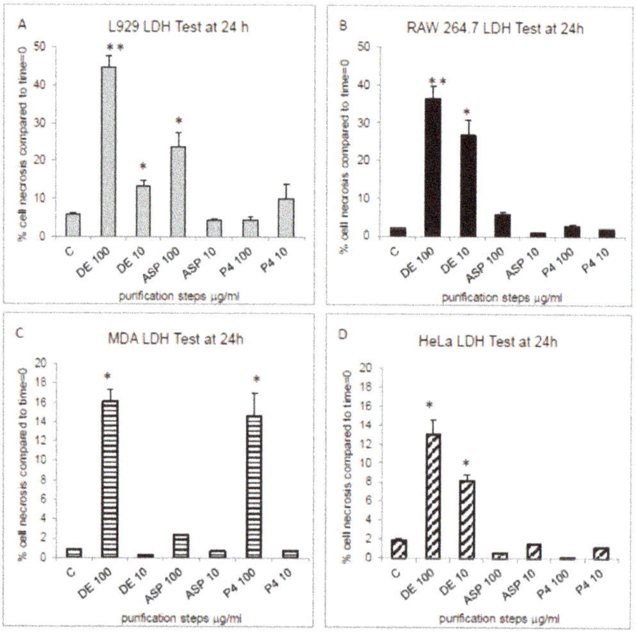

Figure 4. Cell necrosis assessment. (**A**) The percentage of necrotic cells measured by quantification of LDH release in the cell medium at 24 h in L929 murine tumorigenic fibroblasts after incubation in the presence or absence (Control, C) of DE, ASP and P4 (100 and 10 µg/mL, respectively). Results are expressed as percentage of dead cells with respect to the number of seeded cells at time = 0 and are the mean ± S.D. of three experiments performed in quadruplicate. Asterisks indicate significance in paired Tukey test (ANOVA, $p < 0.00001$; Tukey vs. C: ** $p < 0.001$, * $p < 0.05$, respectively). (**B**) The percentage of necrotic cells measured in the same conditions as (A) in RAW 264.7 murine leukemia cells. Asterisks indicate significance in a paired Tukey test (ANOVA, $p < 0.00001$; Tukey vs. C: ** $p < 0.001$, * $p < 0.05$, respectively). (**C**) The percentage of necrotic cells measured in the same conditions as (**A**) in MDA-MB-468 human breast carcinoma cells. Asterisks indicate significance in paired Tukey test (ANOVA, $p < 0.001$; Tukey vs. C: * $p < 0.05$). (**D**) The percentage of necrotic cells measured in the same conditions as (A) in HeLa human cervical carcinoma cells. Asterisks indicate significance in a paired Tukey test (ANOVA, $p < 0.001$; Tukey vs. C: * $p < 0.05$).

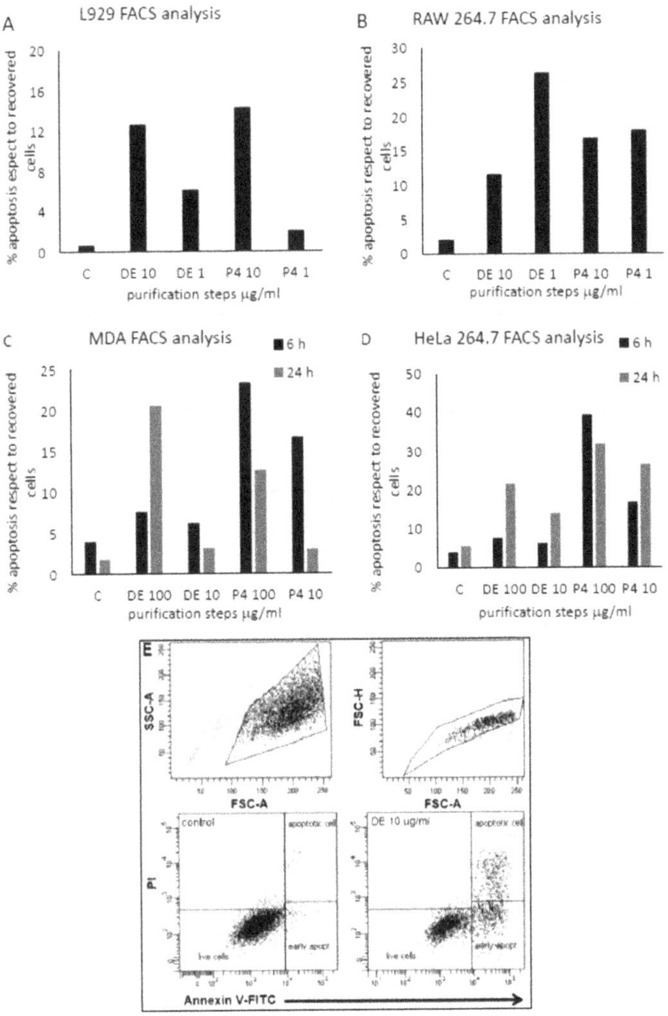

Figure 5. Cell apoptosis assessment by FACS analysis. (**A**) The percentage of annexin-positive, apoptotic cells measured by FACS analysis in trypsin-detached L929 murine tumorigenic fibroblasts after 6 h incubation in the presence or absence (**C**) of DE and P4 (10 and 1 µg/mL, respectively). Results are expressed as percentage of positive apoptotic cells compared to the total number of still living cells retrieved from the plate by trypsin detachment and are representatives of one of the two FACS acquisition experiments performed in duplicate. (**B**) The percentage of annexin-positive, apoptotic cells measured in the same conditions as cells in panel (**A**) in RAW 264.7 murine leukemia cells. (**C**) The percentage of annexin-positive, apoptotic cells measured by FACS analysis in trypsin-detached MDA-MB-468 cells after 6 (black bars) or 24 h (grey bars) incubation in the presence or absence (**C**) of DE and P4 (100 and 10 µg/mL, respectively). Results are expressed as percentage of positive apoptotic cells compared to the total number of still living cells retrieved from the plate by trypsin detachment and are representatives of one of the two FACS acquisition experiments performed in duplicate. (**D**) The percentage of annexin-positive, apoptotic cells measured in the same conditions as cells in panel (**C**) in HeLa human cervical carcinoma cells. (**E**) Representative image of FACS analysis raw data obtained in annexin/PI detection on HeLa cells at 6 h incubation in the absence (control) or presence of 10 µg/mL DE.

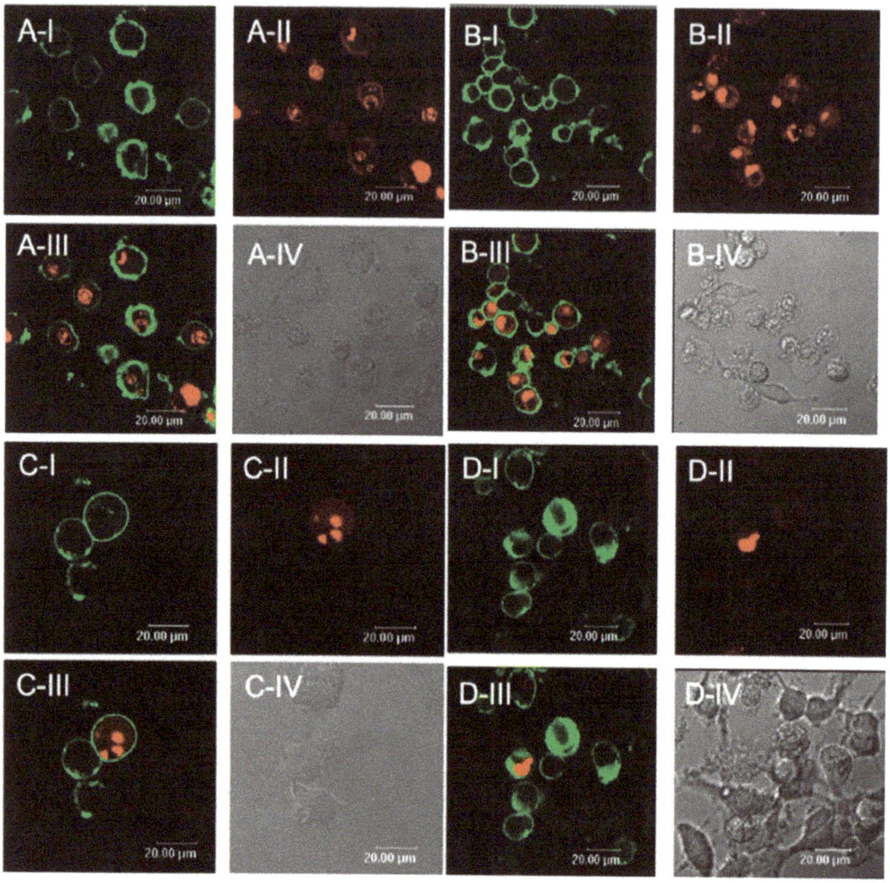

Figure 6. Cell apoptosis assessment by confocal microscopy analysis. (**A**) Visualization by confocal microscopy analysis (HCX PL APO CS 63.0 × 1.40 oil objective, 2 × digital zoom) of annexin-positive (green fluorescence) and/or propidium iodide-positive (red fluorescence) cells in L929 murine tumorigenic fibroblasts after 6 h incubation in the presence of 100 µg/mL P4. Panel I: green channel, panel II, red channel, panel III: superimposed green/red channels, panel IV: phase contrast. The white bar spans 20 µm. (**B**) Visualization of RAW 264.7 murine leukemia cells measured in the same conditions as cells in panel (**A**). (**C**) Visualization of MDA-MB-468 human breast carcinoma cells measured in the same conditions as cells in panel (**A**). (**D**) Visualization of HeLa human cervical carcinoma cells measured in the same conditions as cells in panel (A).

2.4.2. Cytosolic Calcium Rise and Reactive Oxygen Species (ROS) Production in Challenged Cells

Two main signalling stress mediators, and eventual inducers of cell death and apoptosis, are represented by a sustained cytosolic Ca^{2+} rise and reactive oxygen species (ROS) production [24]. The duration and intensity of these well-known stress signals are the key factors for an adequate cell response to dangers the cells are facing or, if too prolonged in time and/or too severe in its intensity, are the means to induce cell death, indicating the inability of the cells to overcome the challenge they are facing. Due to the similarity shown by the new identified protein chondrosin to the ryanodine receptor/channel (see Figure 2D,E), we decided to investigate the effect of chondrosin on the intracellular Ca^{2+} concentration rise by using a calcium-sensitive dye (Fluo3-AM) and fluorometric analysis (Figure 7A–D). Both fluo3-AM-loaded L929 and RAW 264.7 cells (panels A,B and C,D, respectively) were challenged with different P4 and DE concentrations (50 and 100 μg/mL and 100 μg/mL, respectively) and intracellular fluorescence was then monitored for 1 h total acquisition. Panels A and C show representative intracellular Ca^{2+} rise curves in single wells challenged with the two different P4 concentrations in the two cell lines (L929 and RAW 264.7, respectively) in the presence or absence of extracellular Ca^{2+} in the cell culture medium; conversely panels B and D show the slope/min ± SD for each stimulus calculated from the curves shown in panels A and B, respectively. In the presence of extracellular Ca^{2+} in the culture medium, both P4 and DE were able to induce a slow but unrelenting cytosolic Ca^{2+} rise in L929 and RAW 264.7 cells with respect to unchallenged control cells ("w Ca" lines in panels A and C, and black bars in panels B and D, respectively, ANOVA $p < 0.000001$ for both cell lines). Conversely, in the absence of extracellular Ca^{2+}, the intracellular rise of this important mediator was completely abolished over time after stimulation with both P4 and DE in both L929 and RAW 264.7 cell lines ("wo Ca" lines in A and C, and white bars in B and D, respectively). These data clearly indicate that chondrosin, in the P4 enriched fraction, is able to induce a significant intracellular Ca^{2+} rise by extracellular Ca^{2+} entry into the cytoplasm from the cell membrane probably by activating a plasma membrane Ca^{2+}-receptor/channel. Our hypothesis is focused on the possible activation, by direct interaction with chondrosin, of Cav 1.3 calcium channel, a L-type voltage-dependent ion channel, also recently described on the plasma membrane of RAW 264.7 cells [25]. The opening of this channel allows the extracellular Ca^{2+} entrance. Recently, in hippocampus neurons it has been indeed demonstrated the activation of this channel via physical interaction with the ryanodine receptor, which chondrosin closely resembles, with the consequent entrance of Ca^{2+} from the synaptic area [26].

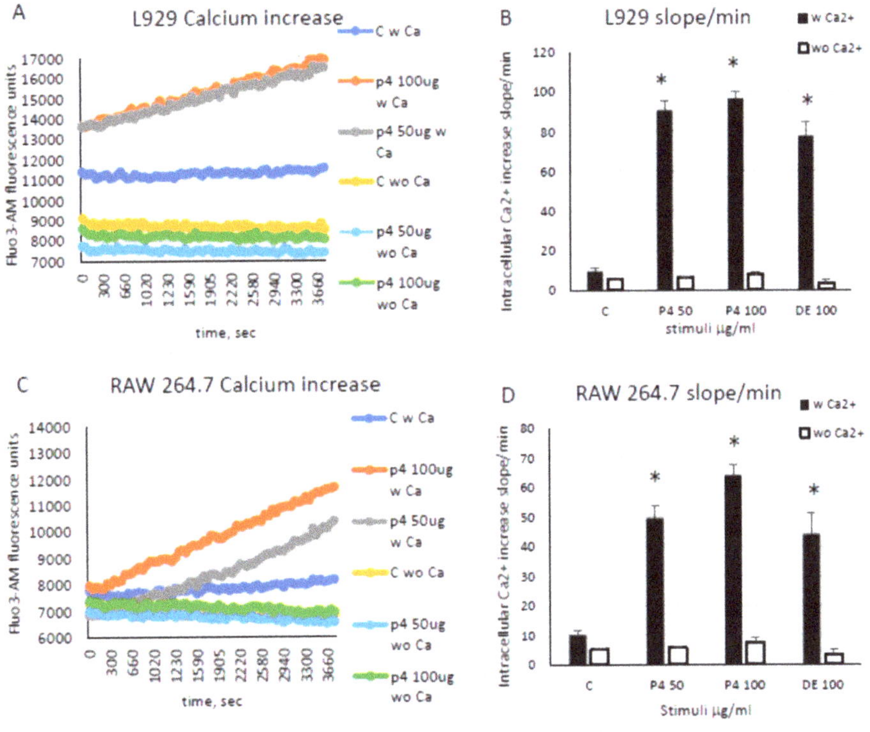

Figure 7. *Cont.*

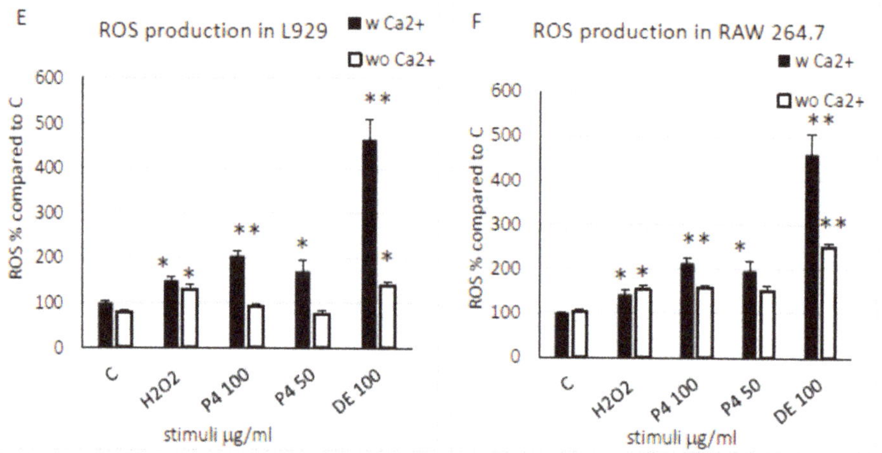

Figure 7. Intracellular Ca^{2+} and ROS quantification by fluorometric analysis. (**A**) Intracellular Ca^{2+} concentration increase evaluation over time in Fluo3-AM-loaded L929 murine tumorigenic fibroblasts challenged without (C w Ca) or with P4 at 100 and 50 µg/mL immediately before starting the fluorometric acquisition at 480/520 ex/em. The experiments were performed in the presence (w Ca) or absence (wo Ca) of Ca^{2+} in the extracellular medium. Each coloured line represents the recording at every minute of a single well of a 96-well plate for 1 h. Every line is representative of two experiments performed in triplicate. (**B**) Calculated slope/min of each intracellular Ca^{2+} increase in 1 h time interval (from experiment in **A**) for each condition of analysis performed in triplicate (control: C, P4 50 and 100 µg/mL, DE 100 µg/mL) in L929 murine tumorigenic fibroblasts. Slope/min was calculated from acquisitions either in the presence (black bars) or absence (white bars) of Ca^{2+} in the extracellular medium. Asterisks indicate significance in Tukey test (ANOVA for black bars $p < 0.000001$; Tukey vs. C, * $p < 0.0001$). (**C**) Intracellular Ca^{2+} concentration increase evaluation over time in RAW 264.7 murine leukemia cells measured under the same conditions as cells in panel (**A**). (**D**) Calculated slope/min of intracellular Ca^{2+} increase in RAW 264.7 murine leukemia cells was measured under the same conditions as cells in panel (**B**). Asterisks indicate significance in Tukey test (ANOVA for black bars $p < 0.000001$; Tukey vs. C, * $p < 0.0001$). (**E**) Intracellular ROS production measured by DCF fluorometric analysis in L929 murine tumorigenic fibroblasts incubated for 2 h with 200 µM H_2O_2 (positive control) or with 50 or 100 µg/mL P4 or 100 µg/mL DE, in the presence (black bars) or absence (white bars) of Ca^{2+} in the extracellular medium. Results are expressed as percentages of ROS production respect to the control (**C**) and are the mean ± SD of three experiments performed in quadruplicate. Asterisks indicate significance in Tukey test (ANOVA for black bars $p < 0.000001$; Tukey vs. C, ** $p < 0.0001$, * $p < 0.01$, respectively; ANOVA for white bars $p < 0.000001$, Tukey vs. C, * $p < 0.01$). (**F**) Intracellular ROS production measured by DCF fluorometric analysis in RAW 264.7 murine leukemia cells measured in the same conditions as cells in panel (**E**). Asterisks indicate significance in the Tukey test (ANOVA for black bars $p < 0.000001$; Tukey vs. C, ** $p < 0.0001$, * $p < 0.01$, respectively; ANOVA for white bars $p < 0.00005$, Tukey vs. C, ** $p < 0.0001$, * $p < 0.01$, respectively).

Since another important stress signal activating cell death pathways is intracellular ROS production, directly or indirectly stimulated by the extracellular stimulus/danger or by the Ca^{2+} second messenger rise, respectively [24,27], also this parameter was investigated in L929 and RAW 264.7 cells by using the ROS sensitive dye 2′,7′-dichlorodihydrofluorescein diacetate (DCF) and fluorometric analysis (Figure 7E,F). The analysis was performed either in the presence or absence of extracellular Ca^{2+} in the cell medium. In both cell lines (L929 panel E and RAW 264.7 panel F, respectively) it was possible to observe a significant intracellular ROS production compared to the control, in the presence of extracellular Ca^{2+} (black bars, ANOVA $p < 0.000001$ for both cell lines), after 2 h incubation with

P4 (50 and 100 μg/mL) and DE (100 μg/mL), similar to (P4) or significantly higher than (DE) the 200 μM H_2O_2 positive control stimulus. Conversely, in the absence of extracellular Ca^{2+} (white bars), a significant inhibition of ROS production after P4 and DE challenge was observed in both cell lines. In contrast, the positive H_2O_2 control remained essentially unaffected by the absence of the extracellular Ca^{2+}. These data indicate that while cytosolic ROS production in H_2O_2-challenged L929 and RAW 264.7 cells is not influenced by the extracellular Ca^{2+} concentration, in the case of P4 and DE challenged cells and, thus, in the presence of chondrosin, extracellular Ca^{2+} entry in the cells is totally (L929, panel E) or partially, but significantly (RAW 264.7, panel F), responsible for the consequent ROS production, depending on the cell line. This also indicates that cell type-specific responses and a different sensitivity to the stimulus can be observed in chondrosin-challenged cells. From these data we can fairly conclude that extracellular Ca^{2+} entry is a triggering signal for ROS production in chondrosin-challenged cells and that the significant cytosolic rise of these two important mediators is likely the main reason for the subsequent cytotoxic-apoptotic outcome in the tumour cells. Furthermore, from the analysis of Ca^{2+} and ROS data in DE-challenged cells, some other conclusions can be drawn on the cytotoxic activity of the *C. reniformis* protein-containing fractions. In particular it is to note that, in terms of signal intensity: (i) the intracellular Ca^{2+} rise in DE-challenged cells is of the same order of magnitude as the P4 stimulus (Figure 7 panels A–D), an effect likely due in both fractions to the chondrosin; and (ii) in the case of ROS intracellular production DE-challenged cells showed more than a two-fold increase compared to the P4 stimulus. This last result suggests the presence of a multifactorial component in the DE fraction, where the ROS increase is generated by the sum of a protein component causing the extracellular Ca^{2+} entry (very likely chondrosin) and of the action of another protein component probably directly stimulating a ROS production independent from extracellular Ca^{2+} entry. This is especially visible in the RAW 264.7 cell line (panel F). This significant difference in ROS production observed in the DE fraction compared to the P4 fraction, could also help to explain the higher rate of necrosis observed in DE-treated cells with respect to P4 (Figure 4), probably due to a more direct cytotoxic effect of the ROS overproduction in the first case relative to the second. The DE component responsible for the ROS overproduction and the higher rate of necrosis is lost in the P4 purified fraction enriched in chondrosin, where the ROS production is significantly lower and probably mainly due to the chondrosin action, through the stimulation of the extracellular Ca^{2+} entry. This allows to infer that, in the P4-treated cells, chondrosin exerts its action mainly by promoting apoptosis and in lesser extent, by a direct cytotoxic effect, contrary to what likely happens in the cells treated with the less purified DE fraction.

3. Conclusions

In this work we identified a new type of cytotoxic protein from the marine sponge *C. reniformis*, with unique features. Chondrosin is likely secreted to the surrounding environment when the sponge is subjected to a strong stress or after wounding. The structure of this toxin shows a domain with intriguing structural homology with the *N*-terminal region of the ryanodine receptor/Ca^{2+} channel. Furthermore, in this toxin, a short domain with high homology to defensins is also present. The presence of defensins regions and domains is known in many toxins of protein origin from arthropods to reptiles, while the toxic action of the N-terminal region of the ryanodine receptor/channel domain is observed for the first time. We demonstrated that the toxic action is mediated by an extracellular calcium intake followed by a cytoplasmic ROS overproduction, occurring mainly in some tumour cell lines (i.e., RAW 264.7 and L929). We suggest that this selective action could be related to the expression of Cav 1.3 ion voltage-dependent channel on the cell membranes of the affected cells. Recent publications have shown a physical interaction of the ryanodine receptor with the Cav 1.3 membrane receptor, with consequent extracellular calcium entrance. Due to the high similarity of chondrosin to the ryanodine receptor, this could also be the mechanism of action of the newly identified toxic protein from the marine sponge *C. reniformis*.

4. Materials and Methods

Chemicals: All reagents were acquired from Sigma-Aldrich (Milan, Italy), unless otherwise stated.

4.1. Preparation of Crude Extracts (CE) of *C. reniformis*

Specimens of *C. reniformis* were collected in the area of the Portofino Promontory (Liguria, Italy) at depths of 10–20 m and transferred to the laboratory in a thermic bag. During the transport, the temperature was maintained at 14–15 °C. A short-term animal housing, of no more than 24–48 h, was performed as described previously [28]. In particular, the sponges were stored at 14 °C in 200-L aquaria containing natural sea water collected in the same area of the Portofino Promontory with a salinity of 3.7% and equipped with an aeration system.

The sponge samples (20–40 g wet weight) were washed with sterile artificial sea water (ASW) and then were cut into very small pieces using a sterile scalpel and kept in a small volume of sterile TRIS-HCl 50 mM pH 8.0 containing an anti-protease mix (pepstatin and leupeptin 1mM) to protect the proteins from the action of eventual proteases released during squeezing. The fragments were vigorously squeezed with both a sterile gauze and a garlic squeezer in order to collect the liquid constituting a crude extract (CE). The procedure was performed at 0 °C on ice, to avoid the possible degradation of the CE components. The CE, with a final volume in the range of 30–50 mL depending on the dimensions of the sponge, was then centrifuged at 8000× *g* for 10 min at 4 °C to eliminate sponge debris and to obtain a clear CE.

4.1.1. Chemical Nature Assessment of CE Cytotoxic Activity

In order to investigate the chemical nature of the sponge cytotoxic activity, the CE was subjected to various treatments to assess the thermal stability, the molecular weight range and the sensitivity to trypsin digestion of the unknown compound(s). Following these steps, the cytotoxic activity was evaluated on the L929 cell line via the MTT test as described in Section 4.3.1. To assess the thermal stability of the cytotoxic component of the clear CE, the extract was heated for 10 min in a heat block at 100 °C and its activity was compared with an untreated sample. To establish the molecular range of the compound(s) involved in the cytotoxic activity, the clear CE was subjected to a dialysis step for 24 h, at 4 °C, against 100 volumes of 50 mM Tris-HCl buffer at pH 8.0, the cut-off of the dialysis membrane was 10,000 kDa to get rid of low-molecular weight sponge metabolites and mainly retaining the protein fraction obtaining a dialysed extract (DE). After that, in order to confirm the protein nature of the sponge cytotoxic activity, the DE was digested with porcine trypsin (Sigma-Aldrich, Milan) at 1:20 (*w:w*) or 1:50 (*w:w*) for 24 h at 37 °C. To confirm the trypsin digestion activity 20 μg of the undigested DE sample and 20 μg of the digested, samples were subjected to SDS-Page analysis on a 12% acrylamide gel. At the end of the run the gel was fixed in 40% ethanol, 10% acetic acid for 60 min and finally stained with colloidal Coomassie blue [29]. The cytotoxic activity of the trypsin-digested and undigested DE was then assessed by MTT test on the L929 cell line as described in Section 4.3.1.

4.1.2. Salting out of DE Proteins

The dialysed extract (DE) was concentrated to a final volume of 10–15 mL by centrifugation at 3500× *g*, at 4 °C, on "Macrosep®Advance Centrifugal Devices With Omega™ Membrane 10K" (PALL Corporation, NY, USA) with a 10,000 kDa cut-off. Protein concentration was then quantified by the Bradford method [30].

The following purification step was based on the salting out method by ammonium sulphate (AS) precipitation of protein fractions. In particular, a solution of 70% saturated AS was used to separate two protein fractions: a precipitated fraction (ASP) and a soluble fraction (ASS). The DE was diluted to a final protein concentration of 5 mg/mL in TRIS-HCl 50 mM pH 8.0, and was precipitated by putting the tube containing the solution in ice and slowly adding (drop by drop) a solution of concentrated ice-cold AS to finally reach a 70% of salt saturation of the entire solution. The slow addition was completed in 1 h and, afterwards, the 70% AS saturated solution was left to slowly stir maintaining the tube containing the solution in ice for further 2 h to let proteins precipitate. The suspension was then centrifuged at 5000× *g*, at 4 °C, for 30 min to recover a soluble protein fraction from the supernatant (ASS) and a precipitated protein fraction from the pellet (ASP). The ASS was again concentrated to a few mL by centrifugation at 4 °C as already described (Macrosep®Advance Centrifugal Devices cut-off 10,000 kDa), while the ASP was resuspended in a small volume (2 mL for each 5 mg of initial protein used for the salting out) of TRIS-HCl 50 mM, pH 8.0, and both ASS and ASP were dialysed against 100 volumes of TRIS-HCl 50 mM, pH 8.0, at 4 °C, to get rid of AS salt excess (cut-off 10,000 kDa). The protein quantification by Bradford assay was again performed on both fractions to calculate protein recovery.

4.1.3. HPLC Protein Purification

The protein separation by molecular weight gel filtration of the ASP purification step was carried out in a HPLC Agilent 1260 system (Agilent Technologies, Palo Alto, CA, USA). The separation was performed on an Agilent SEC-5 column (30 cm × 7.8 mm I.D., 5 μm) equipped with an Agilent SEC-5 guard column (5 cm × 7.8 mm I.D.) at 1 mL/min for 25 min in isocratic mode. Absorbance of the eluted fractions was monitored at 220 nm. The eluent was 0.1 M phosphate buffer, pH 6.0, with 0.1 M sodium sulphate buffer. Five fractions were collected from the column elution corresponded to five main peaks:

P1: from min 6 to min 8;
P2: 8 to 9.5 min;
P3: 9.5 to 10.5 min;
P4: 10.5 to 11.5 min; and
P5: 11.5 to 13.5 min.

Multiple runs were performed, and the five fractions collected were again concentrated by amicon filter centrifugation at 4 °C (cut-off 10,000 kDa, as already described in the previous paragraph) and the protein concentration of each purified fraction (P1 to P5) was then estimated by Bradford assay.

4.2. *Proteomic Analysis*

4.2.1. Protein Precipitation

A total of 50 μg of proteins were transferred into a Slide-A-Lyzer mini dialysis device (ThermoFischer Scientific, Milan, Italy) at 3500 kDa molecular weight cut-off (MWCO) and dialysed against 1L of deionized water at 4 °C, overnight. Proteins were then precipitated with five volumes of ice-cold acetone (80%) and centrifuged at 14,000× *g* for 30 min. The pellets were washed twice with ice-cold acetone (80%) and resuspended in 5 M urea, 2 M thiourea, 4% 3-[(3-Cholamidopropyl)dimethylammonio]-1-propanesulfonate,(CHAPS), 1% immobilized pH gradient (IPG) buffer, 20 mM 1,4-dithiothreitol (DTT), and traces of Bromophenol blue (BPB).

4.2.2. D Gel Electrophoresis

For the first dimension, 7-cm IPG strips (Bio-Rad Laboratories S.r.l., Segrate, MI, Italy), pH 3–10, were pre-hydrated at 50 V for 12 h in 5 M urea, 2 M thiourea, 4% CHAPS, 1% IPG buffer, 20 mM DTT, and traces of BBF. Isoelectric focusing (IEF) was performed at 300 V for 4 h, followed by a gradient of 300–1000 V in 30 min, 1000–5000 V in 90 min, and then kept at 5000 V for 4h.

The proteins in the strips were reduced for 10 min in 1% DTT in equilibration buffer (50 mM Tris–HCl with pH 8.8; 5 M urea; 2 M thiourea; 30% glycerol; 2% Sodium dodecyl sulfate (SDS); traces of BPB), and then alkylated for 10 min in 2.5% iodoacetamide in the same buffer. The proteins were then separated in a second dimension according to their apparent molecular mass on a 12% acrylamide gel, pH 8.8. After electrophoresis, the gels were fixed in 40% ethanol, 10% acetic acid for 60 min and stained with colloidal Coomassie blue [29].

4.2.3. In-Gel Digestion

The gel protein bands were excised and trypsin digested at 37 °C, overnight according to Shevchenko et al. [31]. Briefly, the gel pieces were de-stained in acetonitrile, reduced using 10 mM DTT in 100 mM ammonium bicarbonate for 30 min at room temperature (RT), and alkylated with 100 mM iodoacetamide in 100 mM ammonium bicarbonate for 30 min at RT in the dark. The tryptic peptide samples were extracted after digestion by sonicating for 10 min at RT, then vacuum dried and stored at −20 °C until MS/MS analysis.

4.2.4. Nano-LC Mass Spectrometry

Tryptic peptides were analysed by nano-HPLC-MS/MS using an Ultimate 3000 nano-HPLC system (managed by CHROMELEON software connected to a Hybrid Quadrupole-Orbitrap mass spectrometer (Q Exactive, Thermo Scientific, Waltham, MA, USA).

The pellets containing the tryptic peptides were resuspended immediately before analysis. The obtained solutions were firstly loaded from the sample loop onto a trapping column (Acclaim PepMap C18; 2 cm × 100 μm × 5 μm, 100 Å-ThermoScientific, Waltham, MA, USA) using the loading eluent (95–5% ACN/H_2O + 0.05% trifluoroacetic acid) at a flow rate of 5 μL/min for 5 min. The trapping column was then switched in-line with the separation column and the peptides were eluted increasing the organic solvent percentage at a flow rate of 300 nL/min. The separations were carried out at 35 °C using an Easy spray column (15 cm × 75 μm PepMap C18 3 μm Thermo Scientific) and applying a linear gradient from 4% to 95% of solution B (95–5% ACN/H_2O + 0.08% formic acid) for 55 min.

All the analyses were carried out in the 395–2000 *m/z* range, using a maximal ion injection time of 100 milliseconds. The resolution was set to 70,000 and the automatic gain control was set to 3×10^6 ions. The experiments were performed in data-dependent acquisition mode with alternating MS and MS/MS experiments. The minimum MS signal to obtain MS/MS was set to 500 ions and the most prominent ion signal was selected for MS/MS using an isolation window of 2 Da. The *m/z* values of signals already selected for MS/MS were put on an exclusion list for 5 s using dynamic exclusion. In all cases, one micro-scan was recorded. Collision-induced dissociation (CID) was done with a target value of 5000 ions, a maximal ion injection time of 50 ms, normalized collision energy of 35%. A maximum of 10 MS/MS experiments/MS scans were performed. Raw MS files were processed with the Thermo Scientific Proteome Discoverer software, version 1.4. Peak list files were obtained by the SEQUEST search engine against the *C. reniformis* protein database.

The deduced amino acid sequences database was obtained as described in [4] from *C. reniformis* transcriptome sequencing. This analysis allowed to obtain a series of putative proteins named isotig# (isotigs: contig combinations representing the full mRNAs) where # is a five-digit unique numeric identifier).

The resulting peptide hits were filtered for a maximum 1% FDR (false discovery rate) using the percolator tool. The peptide mass deviation was set to 10 ppm, and a minimum of six amino acids to identify peptides was required. The database search parameters were: mass tolerance precursor 20 ppm, mass tolerance fragment CID 0.8 Da, dynamic modification of deamidation (N, Q), oxidation (M) and static modification of alkylation with 2-Iodoacetamide (IAM) (C). In any case, the option "trypsin with two missed cleavages" was selected.

4.2.5. Protein Sequence Analysis and 3D Modelling

The amino acid sequences of identified proteins were first analysed using the Basic local alignment search tool (BLAST) algorithm at the National Centre for Biotechnology Information (http://blast.ncbi.nlm.nih.gov/Blast.cgi) in order to find identity with previously described proteins. Successively the sequences were analysed using the simple Modular Architecture Research Tool (SMART) program (http://smart.embl-heidelberg.de/) for the identification of conserved domains. The presence of signal peptides was detected using SignalP 4.1 server (http://www.cbs.dtu.dk/services/SignalP/), whereas the theoretical molecular weight and isoelectric point value of the mature protein were obtained using the Expasy tool: https://web.expasy.org/compute_pi/.

Finally, an in silico 3D-structure reconstruction of *C. reniformis* condrosin was performed with Phyre^2 free software http://www.sbg.bio.ic.ac.uk/phyre2/html/page.cgi?id=index using the normal modelling mode. [32].

4.3. Cell Cultures

The mouse macrophage leukemia cell line RAW 264.7, the mouse fibroblast tumorigenic L929, the MDA-MB-468 human breast carcinoma, the HeLa human cervical carcinoma and normal human primary dermal fibroblasts from adult foreskin (NHDF) were obtained from the American Type Culture Collection (LGC Standards srl, Milan, Italy) and cultured as described in the manufacturer's instructions. All cell lines, except NHDF cells, were cultured in high glucose Dulbecco's modified Eagle's medium (D-MEM) with glutamine (Microtech srl, Naples, Italy), supplemented with 10% foetal bovine serum (Microtech) with penicillin/streptomycin as antibiotics. NHDF primary cells were cultured in D-MEM supplemented with 15% FBS and penicillin/streptomycin. All cells were cultured at 37 °C in a humidified, 5% CO_2 atmosphere. Experiments were performed in quadruplicate on 96-well plates.

4.3.1. Cell Toxicity by MTT and LDH Tests

Experiments were performed in quadruplicate on 96-well plates as already described [33]. Briefly, RAW 264.7 macrophages were seeded at 25,000 cells/well, while all other cell lines were seeded at 10,000 cells/well and allowed to adhere overnight. Then the various dilutions of the different purification steps of the RE (final dilutions from 1 to 100 μg/mL of protein concentration) were added to each well and the plates incubated for 24 h at 37 °C. At the end of the experiments cell viability was assayed by MTT test (0.5 mg/mL final concentration) as already reported [34]. For the LDH test, cells were seeded and treated in the same manner as described above in 96-well plates in triplicate and after 24 h incubation the LDH release in the cell media was quantified in each well by the Cytotoxicity LDH Assay Kit-WST (Dojindo EU GmbH, Munich, Germany) following the manufacturer's instructions. Data are the means ± S.D. of three independent experiments performed in quadruplicate.

4.3.2. Apoptosis Detection by FACS Analysis and Confocal Microscopy

To measure the level of apoptosis in the four tumor cell lines (RAW 264.7, L929, MDA-MB-468 and HeLa) annexin-positive cell membrane staining and propidium iodide nuclear staining were measured in cells treated with DE and P4 dilutions after 6 and/or 24 h by both FACS analysis and confocal microscopy imaging.

To perform the FACS analysis the four cell lines were all seeded in 6-well tissue culture plates, in complete medium, at a density of 400,000 cells/well, except for RAW 264.7 cells that were seeded at a density of 800,000 cells/well. The day after cells were incubated in the presence or absence of different dilutions of DE and P4 (100 and 10 μg/mL) for 6 h or 24 h. At the end of the incubation, the cell media were removed from each wells and cells washed once with phosphate buffer saline (PBS) and treated with a trypsin- Ethylenediaminetetraacetic acid (EDTA) solution in PBS to detach cells still adherent to the plate and then centrifuged at 600× *g* for 5 min at RT. The pelleted cells were then stained using the Annexin V, Fluorescein isothiocyanate (FITC) Apoptosis Detection Kit (Dojindo EU, GmbH) following the manufacturer's instructions. FACS analysis was then performed on BD FACS Canto II flow cytometer (Becton Dickinson BD Italia spa, Milan, Italy) by FACS DIVA software 6.1.3 version with acquisition criteria of 10,000 events for each tube. The analysis strategy included the following plots and gates for untreated and treated samples: (a) FSC-A vs. SSC-A with a gate for live cells by light scatter properties; (b) FSC-A vs. FSC-H to exclude doublets; and (c) Annexin V FITC-A vs. Propidium Iodide-A (PI-A) to evaluate annexin V-/PI- live cells, annexin V+/PI− early apoptotic cells, annexin V+/PI+ dead cells or apoptotic. The results were expressed as the percentage of apoptotic cells in the live population.

Confocal microscopy images were obtained using a Leica TCS SL confocal microscope equipped with argon/He-Ne laser sources and a HCX PL APO CS 63.0 × 1.40 oil objective (Leica Microsystems, Wetzlar, Germany). For imaging cell apoptosis, the four tumor cell lines (RAW 264.7, L929, MDA-MB-468 and HeLa) were seeded in eight-well Lab-Teck chambered slides (Nalge Nunc Int., Naperville, IL, USA) at 50,000 cells/well, the day after cells were treated with 100 μg/mL P4 for 6 h. Subsequently, live cells were stained using the Annexin V, FITC Apoptosis Detection Kit (Dojindo EU, GmbH) following the manufacturer's instructions. Images of living cells (2 × digital zoom) were then acquired, in single stacks, both in the phase contrast mode as well as in fluorescence mode by applying a laser energy of 50% to the 488 nm line and acquiring in the emission range of 500–550 nm for the green fluorescence of annexin-positive cells and in the emission range of 600–670 nm for the red fluorescence of propidium iodide-positive cells.

4.3.3. Intracellular Calcium Detection

Experiments were performed in 96-well plates as already described [35]. Briefly, RAW 264.7 cells were plated at a density of 25,000 cells/well, while L929 cells were plated at a density of 10,000 cells/well and allowed to adhere overnight. Cells were then incubated for 45 min at 37 °C with 10 μM Fluo3-AM calcium sensitive dye in complete medium (Life Technologies, Milan, Italy). Subsequently, the wells were washed twice with Hank's Balanced Salt Solution (HBSS) to remove excess of dye from the medium and afterwards the experiment of intracellular calcium rise detection was performed in extracellular HBSS medium with or without Ca^{2+}, the latter also in the presence of 50 μM EDTA calcium chelator. Cells were treated or untreated with 50 or 100 μg/mL of P4 or 50 μg/mL of DE in the presence or absence of Ca^{2+} in the extracellular medium and the plates were immediately read on a Fluostar Optima BMG using 485/520 excitation/emission wavelengths for an interval of 1 h, recording each well fluorescence value every 15 s. Data are the means ± S.D. of two independent experiments performed in triplicate.

4.3.4. Intracellular ROS Detection

Experiments were performed in 96-well plates as already described [36]. Briefly, RAW 264.7 cells were plated at a density of 25,000 cells/well, while L929 cells were plated at a density of 10,000 cells/well and allowed to adhere overnight. Cells were then washed once with HBSS and incubated for 45 min at 37 °C with 10 μM 2′,7′-dichlorodihydrofluorescein diacetate dye in HBSS (Life Technologies, Milan, Italy). Subsequently, cells were washed with HBSS to remove excess of dye from the medium and then stimulation of ROS production was performed in extracellular HBSS medium with or without Ca^{2+}, the latter also in the presence of 50 μM EDTA calcium chelator. ROS production was evaluated after 2 h incubation at 37 °C either with 200 μM H_2O_2 (positive control), or with 50 or 100 μg/mL of P4 or 50 μg/mL of DE in the presence or absence of Ca^{2+} in the extracellular medium. The plates were finally read on a FLUOstar®Omega multi-mode microplate reader (BMG Labtech, Ortenberg, Germany) using 485/520 excitation/emission wavelengths. Data are the means ± S.D. of two independent experiments performed in which each condition was tested eight times.

4.4. Statistical Analysis

Statistical analysis was performed using one-way ANOVA plus Tukey's post-test (GraphPad Software, Inc., San Diego, CA, USA). p values < 0.05 were considered significant.

Supplementary Materials: The following are available online at http://www.mdpi.com/1660-3397/18/8/409/s1, Supplementary File S1. Chondrosin alignment using Phyre2 (see methods). Particularly relevant the high confidence with ryanodine receptor and the short identity with a region of beta chain of defensins.

Author Contributions: Conceptualization: M.P., S.S. and M.G.; methodology: M.P., S.S., C.O., G.D., A.S., D.F., T.A., M.G.; investigation: M.P., S.S., A.S., S.M., C.O., D.F., T.A., M.B.; writing: M.P., S.S., C.O., M.G.; review and editing: S.S., M.G., M.I.; supervision: S.S., M.G.; funding acquisition: M.G., M.I., M.P., G.D. and S.S. All authors have read and agreed to the published version of the manuscript.

Funding: This research was funded to M.G. and M.I. by MAECI - Ministry of Foreign Affairs and International Cooperation of Italian Republic and by the Ministry of Science and Technology of the State of Israel (Italian-Israeli Scientific track, project SMARTEX). This research was also partially funded by University of Genova funding to S.S. and by MIUR funding to M.P.

Acknowledgments: We are indebted to Jörn Piel for the critical reading of this manuscript and the stimulating discussions on protein structure

Conflicts of Interest: The authors declare no conflict of interest.

References

1. Parma, L.; Fassini, D.; Bavastrello, G.; Wilkie, I.C.; Bonasoro, F.; Carnevali, D.C. Ecology and physiology of mesohyl creep in *Chondrosia reniformis*. *J. Exp. Mar. Biol. Ecol.* **2012**, *428*, 24–31. [CrossRef]
2. Fassini, D.; Parma, L.; Lembo, F.; Candia Carnevali, M.D.; Wilkie, I.C.; Bonasoro, F. The reaction of the sponge *Chondrosia reniformis* to mechanical stimulation is mediated by the outer epithelium and the release of stiffening factor(s). *Zoology (Jena)* **2014**, *117*, 282–291. [CrossRef]
3. Pozzolini, M.; Bruzzone, F.; Berilli, V.; Mussino, F.; Cerrano, C.; Benatti, U.; Giovine, M. Molecular characterization of a nonfibrillar collagen from the marine sponge *Chondrosia reniformis* Nardo 1847 and positive effects of soluble silicates on its expression. *Mar. Biotechnol.* **2012**, *14*, 281–293. [CrossRef]
4. Pozzolini, M.; Scarfì, S.; Ghignone, S.; Mussino, F.; Vezzulli, L.; Cerrano, C.; Giovine, M. Molecular characterization and expression analysis of the first Porifera tumor necrosis factor superfamily member and of its putative receptor in the marine sponge *Chondrosia reniformis*. *Dev. Comp. Immunol.* **2016**, *57*, 88–98. [CrossRef]
5. Pozzolini, M.; Scarfì, S.; Gallus, L.; Ferrando, S.; Cerrano, C.; Giovine, M. Silica-induced fibrosis: An ancient response from the early metazoans. *J. Exp. Biol.* **2017**, *220*, 4007–4015. [CrossRef] [PubMed]
6. Nickel, M.; Brümmer, F. In vitro sponge fragment culture of *Chondrosia reniformis* (Nardo, 1847). *J. Biotechnol.* **2003**, *100*, 147–159. [CrossRef]
7. Pozzolini, M.; Gallus, L.; Ghignone, S.; Ferrando, S.; Candiani, S.; Bozzo, M.; Bertolino, M.; Costa, G.; Bavestrello, G.; Scarfì, S. Insights into the evolution of metazoan regenerative mechanisms: Roles of TGF superfamily members in tissue regeneration of the marine sponge *Chondrosia reniformis*. *J. Exp. Biol.* **2019**, *222*, jeb207894. [CrossRef] [PubMed]
8. Swatschek, D.; Schatton, W.; Kellermann, J.; Müller, W.E.G.; Kreuter, J. Marine sponge collagen: Isolation, characterization and effects on the skin parameters surface-pH, moisture and sebum. *Eur. J. Pharm. Biopharm.* **2002**, *53*, 107–113. [CrossRef]
9. Nicklas, M.; Schatton, W.; Heinemann, S.; Hanke, T.; Kreuter, J. Enteric coating derived from marine sponge collagen. *Drug Dev. Ind. Pharm.* **2009**, *35*, 1384–1388. [CrossRef]
10. Nicklas, M.; Schatton, W.; Heinemann, S.; Hanke, T.; Kreuter, J. Preparation and characterization of marine sponge collagen nanoparticles and employment for the transdermal delivery of 17β-estradiol-hemihydrate. *Drug Dev. Ind. Pharm* **2009**, *35*, 1035–1042. [CrossRef]
11. Pozzolini, M.; Scarfì, S.; Gallus, L.; Castellano, M.; Vicini, S.; Cortese, K.; Gagliani, M.; Bertolino, M.; Costa, G.; Giovine, M. Production, characterization and biocompatibility evaluation of collagen membranes derived from marine sponge *Chondrosia reniformis* Nardo, 1847. *Mar. Drugs* **2018**, *16*, 111. [CrossRef]
12. Pozzolini, M.; Millo, E.; Oliveri, C.; Mirata, S.; Salis, A.; Damonte, G.; Arkel, M.; Scarfì, S. Elicited ROS scavenging activity, photoprotective, and wound-healing properties of collagen-derived peptides from the marine sponge *Chondrosia reniformis*. *Mar. Drugs* **2018**, *16*, 465. [CrossRef] [PubMed]
13. Pozzolini, M.; Scarfì, S.; Mussino, F.; Salis, A.; Damonte, G.; Benatti, U.; Giovine, M. *Pichia pastoris* production of a prolyl 4-hydroxylase derived from *Chondrosia reniformis* sponge: A new biotechnological tool for the recombinant production of marine collagen. *J. Biotechnol.* **2015**, *208*, 28–36. [CrossRef] [PubMed]

14. Pozzolini, M.; Scarfì, S.; Mussino, F.; Ferrando, S.; Gallus, L.; Giovine, M. Molecular cloning, characterization, and expression analysis of a prolyl 4-hydroxylase from the marine sponge *Chondrosia reniformis*. *Mar. Biotechnol. (Ny)* **2015**, *17*, 393–407. [CrossRef] [PubMed]
15. Gökalp, M.; Wijgerde, T.; Sarà, A.; De Goeij, J.M.; Osinga, R. Development of an integrated mariculture for the collagen-rich sponge *Chondrosia reniformis*. *Mar. Drugs* **2019**, *17*, 29. [CrossRef]
16. Pronzato, R.; Manconi, R. Mediterranean commercial sponges: Over 5000 years of natural history and cultural heritage. *Mar. Ecol.* **2008**, *29*, 146–166. [CrossRef]
17. Mebs, D.; Weiler, I.; Heinke, H.F. Bioactive proteins from marine sponges: Screening of sponge extracts for hemagglutinating, hemolytic, ichthyotoxic and lethal properties and isolation and characterization of hemagglutinins. *Toxicon* **1985**, *23*, 955–962. [CrossRef]
18. Cheung, R.C.F.; Wong, J.H.; Pan, W.; Chan, Y.S.; Yin, C.; Dan, X.; Ng, T.B. Marine lectins and their medicinal applications. *Appl. Microbiol. Biotechnol* **2015**, *99*, 3755–3773. [CrossRef]
19. Lazcano-Perez, F.; A. Roman-Gonzalez, S.; Sanchez-Puig, N.; Arreguin-Espinosa, R. Bioactive peptides from marine organisms: A short overview. *Protein Pept. Lett.* **2012**, *19*, 700–707. [CrossRef]
20. Görg, A.; Weiss, W.; Dunn, M.J. Current two-dimensional electrophoresis technology for proteomics. *Proteomics* **2004**, *4*, 3665–3685. [CrossRef]
21. Deng, Z.; Bu, S.; Wang, Z.-Y. Quantitative analysis of protein phosphorylation using two-dimensional difference gel electrophoresis. *Methods Mol. Biol.* **2012**, *876*, 47–66. [CrossRef] [PubMed]
22. Wang, X.; Gao, B.; Zhu, S. Exon shuffling and origin of scorpion venom biodiversity. *Toxins* **2016**, *9*, 10. [CrossRef]
23. Fry, B.G.; Roelants, K.; Winter, K.; Hodgson, W.C.; Griesman, L.; Kwok, H.F.; Scanlon, D.; Karas, J.; Shaw, C.; Wong, L.; et al. Novel venom proteins produced by differential domain-expression strategies in beaded lizards and Gila Monsters (genus *Heloderma*). *Mol. Biol. Evol.* **2010**, *27*, 395–407. [CrossRef] [PubMed]
24. Zhou, D.R.; Eid, R.; Miller, K.A.; Boucher, E.; Mandato, C.A.; Greenwood, M.T. Intracellular second messengers mediate stress inducible hormesis and programmed cell death: A review. *Biochim. Biophys. Acta Mol. Cell Res.* **2019**, *1866*, 773–792. [CrossRef] [PubMed]
25. Fan, P.; Hu, N.; Feng, X.; Sun, Y.; Pu, D.; Lv, X.; Hao, Z.; Li, Y.; Xue, W.; He, L. Cav1.3 is upregulated in osteoporosis rat model and promotes osteoclast differentiation from preosteoclast cell line RAW264.7. *J. Cell. Physiol.* **2019**, *234*, 12821–12827. [CrossRef]
26. Kim, S.; Yun, H.-M.; Baik, J.-H.; Chung, K.C.; Nah, S.-Y.; Rhim, H. Functional interaction of neuronal Cav 1.3 L-type Calcium channel with ryanodine receptor type 2 in the rat hippocampus. *J. Biol. Chem.* **2007**, *282*, 32877–32889. [CrossRef]
27. Starkov, A.A.; Chinopoulos, C.; Fiskum, G. Mitochondrial calcium and oxidative stress as mediators of ischemic brain injury. *Cell Calcium* **2004**, *36*, 257–264. [CrossRef]
28. Pozzolini, M.; Mussino, F.; Cerrano, C.; Scarfì, S.; Giovine, M. Sponge cell cultivation: Optimization of the model *Petrosia ficiformis* (Poiret 1789). *J. Exp. Mar. Biol. Ecol.* **2014**, *454*, 70–77. [CrossRef]
29. Neuhoff, V.; Arold, N.; Taube, D.; Ehrhardt, W. Improved staining of proteins in polyacrylamide gels including isoelectric focusing gels with clear background at nanogram sensitivity using Coomassie Brilliant Blue G-250 and R-250. *Electrophoresis* **1988**, *9*, 255–262. [CrossRef] [PubMed]
30. Bradford, M.M. A rapid and sensitive method for the quantitation of microgram quantities of protein utilizing the principle of protein-dye binding. *Anal. Biochem.* **1976**, *72*, 248–254. [CrossRef]
31. Shevchenko, A.; Tomas, H.; Havlis, J.; Olsen, J.V.; Mann, M. In-gel digestion for mass spectrometric characterization of proteins and proteomes. *Nat. Protoc.* **2006**, *1*, 2856–2860. [CrossRef] [PubMed]
32. Kelley, L.A.; Mezulis, S.; Yates, C.M.; Wass, M.N.; Sternberg, M.J.E. The Phyre2 web portal for protein modeling, prediction and analysis. *Nat. Protoc.* **2015**, *10*, 845–858. [CrossRef] [PubMed]
33. Pozzolini, M.; Vergani, L.; Ragazzoni, M.; Delpiano, L.; Grasselli, E.; Voci, A.; Giovine, M.; Scarfì, S. Different reactivity of primary fibroblasts and endothelial cells towards crystalline silica: A surface radical matter. *Toxicology* **2016**, *361–362*, 12–23. [CrossRef] [PubMed]
34. Pozzolini, M.; Scarfì, S.; Benatti, U.; Giovine, M. Interference in MTT cell viability assay in activated macrophage cell line. *Anal. Biochem.* **2003**, *313*, 338–341. [CrossRef]

35. Magnone, M.; Bauer, I.; Poggi, A.; Mannino, E.; Sturla, L.; Brini, M.; Zocchi, E.; De Flora, A.; Nencioni, A.; Bruzzone, S. NAD^+ levels control Ca^{2+} store replenishment and mitogen-induced increase of cytosolic Ca^{2+} by Cyclic ADP-ribose-dependent TRPM2 channel gating in human T lymphocytes. *J. Biol. Chem.* **2012**, *287*, 21067–21081. [CrossRef] [PubMed]
36. Scarfi, S.; Magnone, M.; Ferraris, C.; Pozzolini, M.; Benvenuto, F.; Benatti, U.; Giovine, M. Ascorbic acid pre-treated quartz stimulates TNF-alpha release in RAW 264.7 murine macrophages through ROS production and membrane lipid peroxidation. *Respir. Res.* **2009**, *10*, 25. [CrossRef]

© 2020 by the authors. Licensee MDPI, Basel, Switzerland. This article is an open access article distributed under the terms and conditions of the Creative Commons Attribution (CC BY) license (http://creativecommons.org/licenses/by/4.0/).

marine drugs

MDPI

Article

The Protective Effect of Echinochrome A on Extracellular Matrix of Vocal Folds in Ovariectomized Rats

Ji Min Kim [1], Jeong Hun Kim [2], Sung-Chan Shin [3], Gi Cheol Park [4], Hyung Sik Kim [5,6], Keunyoung Kim [7], Hyoung Kyu Kim [8], Jin Han [8], Natalia P. Mishchenko [9], Elena A. Vasileva [9], Sergey A. Fedoreyev [9], Valentin A. Stonik [9] and Byung-Joo Lee [1,3,*]

1 Pusan National University School of Medicine and Medical Research Institute, Pusan National University, Yangsan 50612, Korea; ny5thav@hanmail.net
2 Biomedical Research Institute, Pusan National University Hospital, Busan 49241, Korea; kmky82@naver.com
3 Department of Otorhinolaryngology-Head and Neck Surgery and Biomedical Research Institute, Pusan National University Hospital, Busan 49241, Korea; cha-nwi@daum.net
4 Department of Otolaryngology-Head and Neck Surgery, Samsung Changwon Hospital, Sungkyunkwan University School of Medicine, Changwon 51353, Korea; uuhent@gmail.com
5 Department of Life Science in Dentistry, School of Dentistry, Pusan National University, Yangsan 50612, Korea; hskimcell@pusan.ac.kr
6 Institute for Translational Dental Science, Pusan National University, Yangsan 50612, Korea
7 Department of Nuclear Medicine and Biomedical Research Institute, Pusan National University Hospital, Busan 49241, Korea; buisket@naver.com
8 National Research Laboratory for Mitochondrial Signaling, Department of Physiology, College of Medicine, Cardiovascular and Metabolic Disease Center (CMDC), Inje University, Busan 47391, Korea; estrus74@gmail.com (H.K.K.); phyhanj@inje.ac.kr (J.H.)
9 G.B. Elyakov Pacific Institute of Bioorganic Chemistry, Far-Eastern Branch of the Russian Academy of Science, 690022 Vladivostok, Russia; mischenkonp@mail.ru (N.P.M.); vasilieva_el_an@mail.ru (E.A.V.); fedoreev-s@mail.ru (S.A.F.); stonik@piboc.dvo.ru (V.A.S.)
* Correspondence: voiceleebj@gmail.com; Tel.: +82-51-240-7528; Fax: +82-51-240-2162

Received: 2 December 2019; Accepted: 21 January 2020; Published: 24 January 2020

Abstract: Here, we investigated the effects of sex hormones on extracellular matrix (ECM)-related gene expression in the vocal fold lamina propria of ovariectomized (after ovary removal) rats and verified whether echinochrome A (ECH) exerts any therapeutic effects on ECM reconstitution after estrogen deficiency in ovariectomized rats. Sprague–Dawley female rats (9 weeks old) were acclimatized for a week and randomly divided into three groups ($n = 15$ each group) as follows: group I (sham-operated rats, SHAM), group II (ovariectomized rats, OVX), group III (ovariectomized rats treated with ECH, OVX + ECH). Rats from the OVX + ECH group were intraperitoneally injected with ECH at 10 mg/kg thrice a week after surgery for 6 weeks. And rats were sacrificed 6 weeks after ovariectomy. Estradiol levels decreased in OVX group compared with the SHAM group. ECH treatment had no effect on the levels of estradiol and expression of estrogen receptor β (ERβ). The evaluation of ECM components showed no significant changes in elastin and hyaluronic acid levels between the different groups. Collagen I and III levels were lower in OVX group than in SHAM group but increased in OVX + ECH group. The mRNA levels of matrix metalloproteinase (MMP)-1, -2, -8, and -9 were significantly higher in the OVX group than in the SHAM group, but decreased in the OVX + ECH group. Thus, changes were observed in ECM-related genes in the OVX group upon estradiol deficiency that were ameliorated by ECH administration. Thus, the vocal fold is an estradiol-sensitive target organ and ECH may have protective effects on the ECM of vocal folds in ovariectomized rats.

Keywords: echinochrome A; estradiol; extracellular matrix; vocal fold; ovariectomy

---

1. Introduction

Sex hormones are major factors that influence the activity of the vocal fold and voice production. Voice, a secondary sex characteristic, varies between males and females and changes with sexual maturation. Female voice is closely related to changes in female sex hormones. Laryngeal changes are evident and systematically fluctuate during the reproductive years with the menstrual cycle and affect voice changes throughout life [1,2].

In general, voice production relies on the extracellular matrix (ECM) of the connective tissue in the vocal fold. The ECM of the vocal fold lamina propria comprises interstitial proteins, such as collagen, elastin, and fibronectin, and glycosaminoglycans, such as hyaluronic acid. These ECM components have important biochemical functions and contribute to vocal fold function. These molecules play an important role in determining vocal fold viscoelasticity and affect clinical voice functions, such as phonation threshold pressure and vocal fundamental frequency [3–5].

During menopause, the decrease in the amount of estrogen causes dysfunctions of the connective tissues via ECM degradation. Previous studies have shown that the vocal fold is an estradiol-sensitive target organ and any decrease in estradiol levels may affect the expression of several ECM-related molecules in the vocal fold [6]. Hormone therapy is commonly used for the treatment of several menopausal symptoms and for the alleviation of menopausal voice complaints, but adverse-effects of hormone therapy have been reported [7–9]. Thus, here we investigated the mechanism underlying improvement in voice quality after menopause using a natural component of marine products.

Echinochrome A (ECH, 6-ethyl-2,3,5,7,8-pentahydroxy-1,4-naphthoquinone) is extracted from sea urchins (*Saphechinus mirabilis*) (Figure 1). Its chemical structure is appropriate for free-radical scavenging and includes 2,3,7-hydroxl groups, which are known for their antioxidant properties via regulation of mitochondrial biosynthesis [10]. Studies have shown that antioxidants improve ECM composition, suppress vocal fold wounds, and prevent inflammatory responses [11,12]. Thus, the antioxidant effects of ECH may be expected to play a role in improving the function of vocal fold ECM. Moreover, ECH also contains a 1,4-naphthoquinone ring, which is similar to that observed in vitamin K [13]. In postmenopausal women, vitamin K is reported to reduce menopausal symptoms; however, these studies are limited to bone metabolism or cardiovascular dysfunction [14]. Therefore, ECH may possibly alleviate menopausal symptoms owing to its structural similarity with vitamin K.

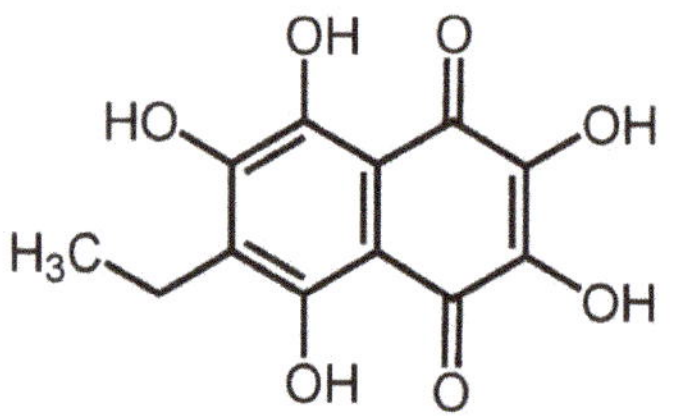

Figure 1. Chemical structure of echinochrome A.

To date, studies on vocal folds have focused on vocal fold aging and mechanisms of wound healing. However, reports on sex hormone-specific female vocal aging are scarce. Moreover, the existing reports on female vocal fold aging are mainly morphological studies of the vocal fold of elderly women and the underlying cellular mechanisms of sex hormone-induced vocal fold changes are yet unknown. Thus, the purpose of the present study was to investigate the effects of sex hormones on the alteration of the expression of ECM-related genes in the vocal fold lamina propria of ovariectomized female rats (after surgical ovary removal) and to verify whether ECH exerts any preventive effects on ECM reconstitution following estradiol deficiency in ovariectomized female rats.

2. Results

2.1. *Effect of ECH on Serum Estradiol Level and Expression of Estrogen Receptor β*

Figure 2A shows the changes in the serum level of estradiol. The level of serum estradiol decreased in the OVX group (10.82 ± 4.35 ng/mL, $p < 0.001$ vs. SHAM) compared with that reported in the SHAM group (10.82 ± 4.25 ng/mL); however, estradiol concentration in the OVX group was similar to that reported in the OVX + ECH group (11.34 ± 5.56 ng/mL). To evaluate the effect of sex hormone on sex hormone receptors, we performed immunohistochemistry and quantitative polymerase chain reaction (qPCR) analyses to determine the expression levels of two isoforms, *Esr2a* and *Esr2b*, in vocal fold lamina propria. ERβ expression was similar between all groups (Figure 2B). According to our previous research, *Esr1* expression was undetected on the lamina propria of female vocal fold with qPCR [6]. Hence, we evaluated the expression levels of *Esr2a* and *Esr2b* using qPCR. The expression level of *Esr2a* and *Esr2b* showed no significant differences between all groups (Figure 2C). Ovariectomy led to a significant decrease in the amount of estradiol and ECH had no effect on both serum estradiol level and ERβ expression.

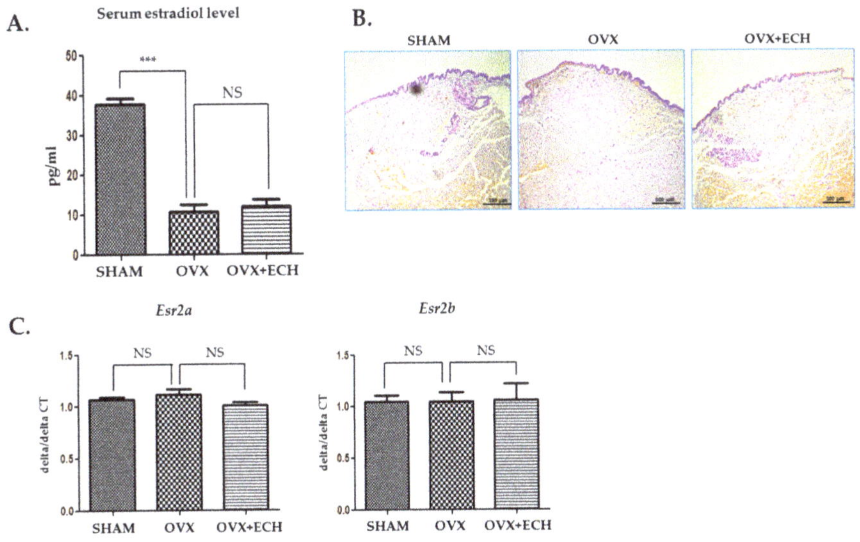

Figure 2. Serum estradiol levels and expression of estrogen receptor β. The level of serum estradiol decreased in the ovariectomized rat, OVX group compared with the SHAM group. ECH treatment did not affect serum estradiol level (**A**). Immunohistochemistry (IHC) staining analyses of representative estrogen receptor β (ERβ) in the lamina propria of vocal folds. The immune-positive area for ERβ was not changed between groups (**B**). Quantitative polymerase chain reaction (qPCR) analyses of genes encoding representative *Esr2a* and *Esr2b* in the lamina propria of vocal folds. The expression of *Esr2a* and *Esr2b* was not changed between groups. The scale bar in each panel is equal to 100 μm (40× magnification). One-way ANOVA test; NS not significant and *** $p < 0.001$ vs. SHAM.

2.2. *Effect of ECH on Hyaluronic Acid and Hyaluronic Acid Synthase (Has1, Has2, Has3)*

We determined the concentration of hyaluronic acid with Alcian blue staining. The blue stain was decolorized following hyaluronidase digestion. Hyaluronic acid appeared to be evenly distributed throughout the vocal fold and no significant difference was observed between all groups (Figure 3A,B). The OVX and OVX + ECH groups showed no significant changes in the expression levels of the hyaluronic acid synthase 1 (*Has1*) gene in qPCR. Hyaluronic acid synthase 2 (*Has2*) and 3 (*Has3*) gene levels decreased in the OVX group but failed to change in the OVX + ECH group (Figure 3C).

The results confirmed no statistical difference in the total density of hyaluronic acid between different groups. Six weeks after ovariectomy, the expression levels of *Has2* and *Has3* were affected; however, no significant difference was observed in the expression level of *Has1*. ECH treatment had no effect on hyaluronic acid level at 6 weeks after ovariectomy.

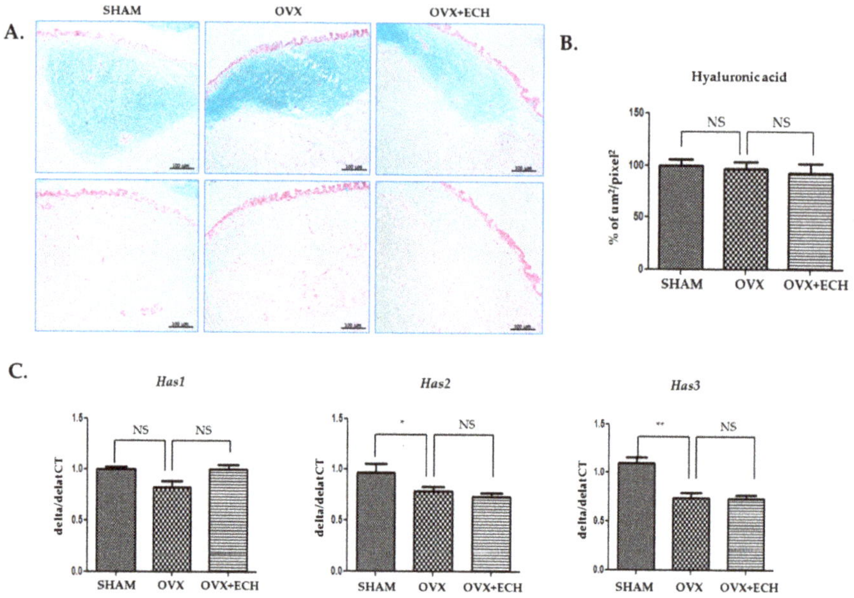

Figure 3. Hyaluronic acid of vocal fold lamina propria. (**A**) Alcian blue stained staining analyses and (**B**) the densities of hyaluronic acid in the lamina propria of vocal folds. The concentration of hyaluronic acid was not changed between groups. Quantitative polymerase chain reaction (qPCR) analyses of genes encoding representative hyaluronic acid synthase (*Has*) 1, 2, and 3 in the lamina propria of vocal folds. The expression of *Has1* was not changed between groups. The expression of *Has2* and *Has3* decreased significantly in the OVX group compare with the SHAM group, but ECH treatment had no effect. The scale bar in each panel is equal to 100 μm (40× magnification). One-way ANOVA test; NS not significant and * $p < 0.05$, ** $p < 0.01$ vs. SHAM.

2.3. *Effect of ECH on Collagen and Procollagen (Col1a1, Col1a2, Col3a1)*

Collagen I and III are the major types of collagen in the vocal fold lamina propria of rats. The density of collagen I, as evident from immunohistochemical staining, was lower in the OVX group (27.6%, $p < 0.05$ vs. SHAM) than in SHAM group (Figure 4A,B). The decrease in collagen I expression in the OVX group was restored to the level detected in the SHAM group after ECH treatment. The mRNA expression level of procollagen was confirmed with qPCR and no significant difference was observed in the expression levels of *Col1a1* and *Col1a2* between the OVX and SHAM groups. However, the expression levels of *Col1a1* and *Col1a2* increased in the OVX + ECH treatment group compared with those in the OVX group, which were higher than the levels observed in SHAM group (Figure 4C). Collagen III deposition showed a pattern similar to that of collagen I. The density of collagen III in the stained areas from the OVX group was lower than that in the stained areas of the SHAM group. The expression of collagen III in the OVX + ECH group increased compared with that in the OVX group (Figure 4D,E). The expression level of *Col3a1* was confirmed with qPCR. *Col3a1* gene expression was significantly upregulated in the OVX group compared to that in SHAM group, but its expression in the OVX + ECH group was similar to that reported in the OVX group (Figure 4F). These results reveal that ECH treatment increases the protein expression of collagen I via upregulation in the expression levels of *Col1a1* and *Col1a2*. However, mRNA and protein levels of collagen I and III in the OVX group were partially inconsistent. Hence, we confirmed the expression of matrix metalloproteinases (MMPs).

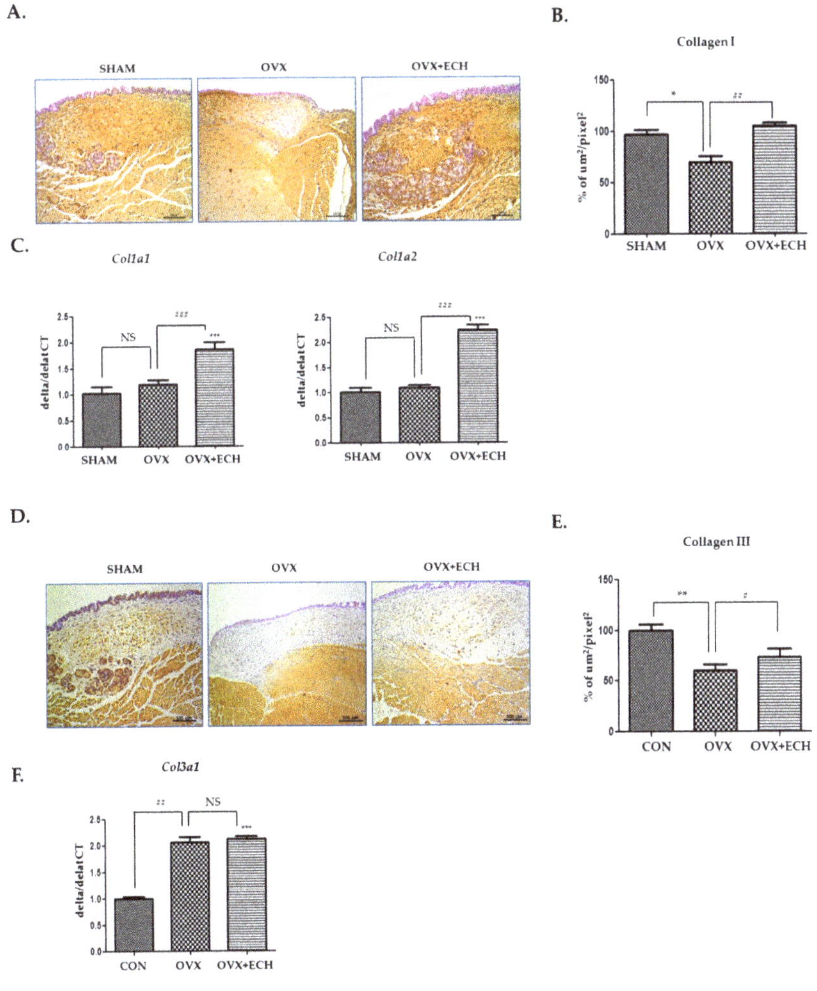

Figure 4. Collagens I and III of the vocal fold lamina propria. Immunohistochemistry (IHC) staining analyses of representative (**A**) collagen I and (**B**) the densities of collagen I in the lamina propria of vocal folds. The immune-positive area for collagen I was decreased in the OVX group and increased in the OVX + ECH group. (**C**) Quantitative polymerase chain reaction (qPCR) analyses of genes encoding representative procollagen *Col1a1* and *Col1a2* in the lamina propria of vocal folds. The expression of *Col1a1* and *Col1a2* did not change in the OVX group compared with the SHAM group, but was significantly elevated in the OVX + ECH group. IHC staining analyses of representative (**D**) collagen III and (**E**) the densities of collagen III in the lamina propria of vocal folds. The immune-positive area for *Col3a1* was decreased in the OVX group and increased in the OVX + ECH group. (**F**) qPCR analyses of genes encoding representative procollagen *Col3a1* in the lamina propria of vocal folds. The expression of *Col3a1* increased in the OVX group compared with the SHAM group, but there was no change in the OVX + ECH group. The scale bar in each panel is equal to 100 μm (40× magnification). One-way ANOVA test; NS not significant, * $p < 0.05$, ** $p < 0.01$ and *** $p < 0.001$ vs. SHAM; # $p < 0.05$, ## $p < 0.01$ and ### $p < 0.001$ vs. OVX.

2.4. *Effect of ECH on Two Elastin Genes (*Eln *and* Cela1*)*

To investigate the expression level of elastin, Verhoeff's elastin staining technique was used. Immunohistochemical staining revealed slightly lower elastin intensity for the OVX group than for the SHAM group, but no statistical significance was reported. The OVX + ECH group showed no change in elastin expression (Figure 5A,B). We examined the expression levels of *Eln* and *Cela1* with qPCR. *Eln* tropoelastin is a precursor of elastin and assembles into elastic fibers. The expression of *Eln* decreased in the OVX group compared with that in the SHAM group, but increased with ECH treatment to the level reported in the SHAM group. The expression level of *Cela1* elastase, an elastin-degrading enzyme, also slightly increased in the OVX group without any statistical significance; ECH treatment had no effect on *Ela* expression level (Figure 5C) but affected the expression level of *Cela1*; however, no significant difference was observed in the expression levels of elastase and immunohistochemical elasatin proteins in elastic fibers.

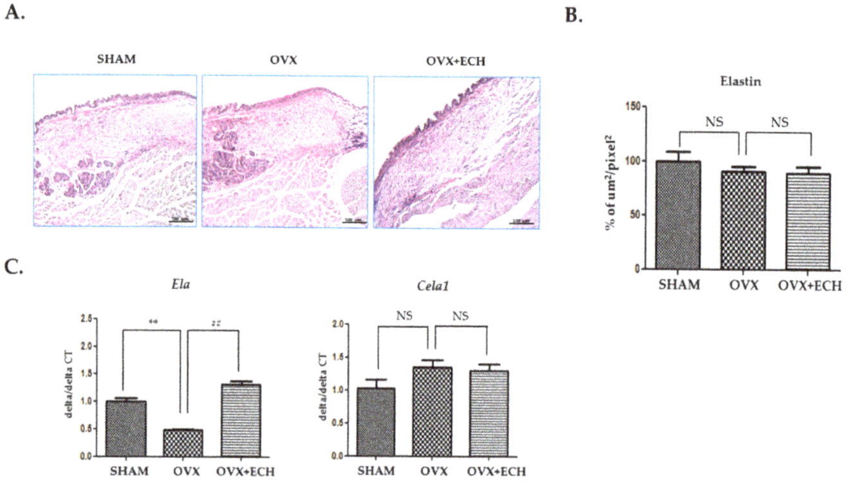

Figure 5. Elastin of vocal fold lamina propria. (**A**) Van Gieson stained staining analyses and (**B**) the densities of elastin fibers in the lamina propria of vocal folds. The expression of elastin was not changed in each group. Quantitative polymerase chain reaction (qPCR) analyses of genes encoding representative *Eln* and *Cela1* in the lamina propria of vocal folds (**C**). The expression of *Eln* decreased significantly in the OVX group compared with the SHAM group, but ECH treatment increased *Eln* level. The expression of *Cela1* was not changed in each group. The scale bar in each panel is equal to 100 μm (40× magnification). One-way ANOVA test; NS not significant; ** $p < 0.01$ vs. SHAM and ## $p < 0.01$ vs. OVX.

2.5. *Effect of ECH on Matrix Metalloproteinases (MMPs)*

We tested the expression levels of *Mmp1*, *Mmp2*, *Mmp8*, and *Mmp9* to determine any inconsistencies between the protein and mRNA levels of collagen (Figure 4). Some MMPs act as collagenase and are involved in the pathological remodeling of tissues. We screened the expression of the genes encoding interstitial MMPs (*Mmp1*, *Mmp8*) and gelatinase MMPs (*Mmp2*, *Mmp9*) in each group with qPCR. The expression level of *Mmp1* and *Mmp8* significantly increased in the OVX group compared with that in the SHAM group, but ECH treatment resulted in a decrease in *Mmp1* and *Mmp8* expression levels (Figure 6). Moreover, the expression level of *Mmp2* and *Mmp9* was significantly higher in the OVX group than in the SHAM group and ECH treatment ameliorated this effect (Figure 6). The expression of MMPs in the OVX group was significantly higher than that in the SHAM group, but ECH treatment reduced these upregulated levels. Thus, *Mmp1*, *Mmp2*, *Mmp8*, and *Mmp9* expression levels increased at 6 weeks after ovariectomy, which resulted in collagen degradation and consequently decreased the expression of collagen, while ECH treatment suppressed collagen degradation by reducing the levels of MMPs.

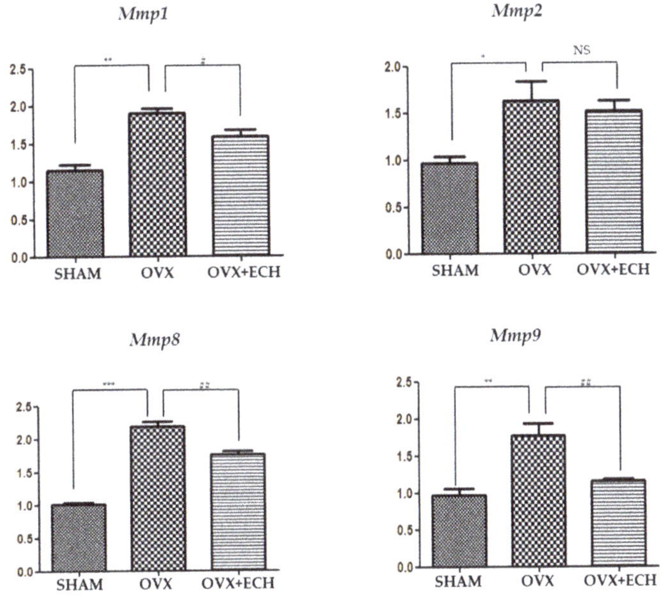

Figure 6. Matrix metalloproteinases in vocal fold lamina propria. Quantitative polymerase chain reaction (qPCR) analyses of genes encoding representative matrix metalloproteinases (*Mmp1*, *Mmp2*, *Mmp8*, *Mmp9*) in the lamina propria of vocal folds. The expression of the matrix metalloproteinases MMPs increased significantly in the OVX group compare with the SHAM group, but ECH treatment decreased MMP levels. One-way ANOVA test; NS not significant; * $p < 0.05$, ** $p < 0.01$ and *** $p < 0.001$ vs. SHAM; # $p < 0.05$ and ## $p < 0.01$ vs. OVX.

3. Discussion

Changes in sex hormones with menopause affect the female voice. Female sex hormones affect the larynx and vocal folds, thereby influencing voice production. The most drastic change in female voice occurs during menopause. After menopause, women show restricted vocal frequency perturbation range and lower habitual fundamental frequency [15]. These changes may affect social life, especially for professional singers. According to previous reports, the decrease in estradiol levels may cause changes in the connective layers of the vocal fold in postmenopausal women [16]. In addition, estradiol deficiency may cause atrophy of laryngeal muscles and stiffening of laryngeal cartilage. Our previous study evaluated voice changes induced by sex hormones [17]. We have previously reported the effects of ECM production and degradation on vocal fold lamina propria in ovariectomized rats [6]. Population surveys show that many women report voice deepening after menopause, but this observation was not common among men of similar age [18]. This result is also consistent with our previous study. We investigated the changes in the expression of ECM-related genes in orchiectomized (after testis removal) male rats and detected no significant changes. These results suggest that the lamina propria of the vocal fold is an estradiol-sensitive target organ.

Loss of ovarian function after menopause decreases the biological functions of several organs, usually owing to estrogen deficiency. Physical changes caused by menopause include abdominal fat accumulation, osteoporosis, cardiovascular disease, and dry mouth. Thus, estrogen replacement therapy, designed to alleviate menopausal symptoms, may be helpful for menopausal voice therapy [19,20]. Hormone therapy has long been used for the treatment of several menopause-related complaints. Estrogen replacement therapy may alleviate menopause-related voice complaints [21,22]. Vocal quality changes are common in women after estrogen replacement therapy in response to the management of menopause-related conditions. Estrogen replacement therapy has been used to forestall menopause-associated voice changes, especially among professional singers. Cruso et al. showed that the larynx possesses receptors for ovarian sex hormones and that estrogen plays an important role in laryngeal tropism [3]. These previous evidences suggest that estrogen replacement therapy may provide prevention, and possibly treatment, of pathophysiologies, such as vocal cord dystrophy, which are common among postmenopausal women. However, the safety of estrogen replacement therapy is still controversial. Therefore, non-hormonal alternatives, including mineral and vitamin supplements, phytoestrogens, natural hormones, and phytochemicals, are being investigated [23]. In particular, the pharmacological mechanism underlying the effects of isoflavones, the most studied flavonoids, is known. Isoflavones exert antioxidant effects and alleviate menopause-related complications [24–26]. Therefore, ECH, a natural marine substance with strong antioxidant properties, may be potentially useful to improve menopausal symptoms. In this direction, we used ECH to verify any changes in vocal cord and voice caused by menopause.

Oxidative stress is related to voice changes caused by vocal scar and aging [27–29]. Antioxidants have been used to prevent vocal fold scars by improving vocal fold wound healing [11,12]. A study was conducted to improve voice after aging [30,31]. However, no studies have been directed to improve voice quality and the cellular mechanisms underlying the effect of these antioxidants on vocal fold lamina propria in menopause are unknown. Therefore, to better understand this menopause-related vocal fold change, we analyzed the preventive effects of ECH on the distribution and production of ECM within the lamina propria of the vocal fold in ovariectomized rats.

ECH is one of the several spinochromes in sea urchins. It has a naphthazarin fragment, which makes it suitable for metal ion chelation. The chemical structure of ECH is appropriate for free-radical scavenging, owing to the presence of 2,3,7-hydroxyl groups. Hence, the antioxidant properties of ECH are related to the regulation of mitochondrial biosynthesis [32,33]. ECH exerts several biological effects. In animal experimental models, ECH reduced glucose concentration, lipid peroxidation, and activities of arginases, such as alanine aminotransferase (ALT), aspartate aminotransferase (AST), alkaline phosphatase (ALP), and gammaglutamyl transpeptidase (γ-GT). Moreover, ECH increased levels of insulin, nitric oxide, and endogenous antioxidant enzymes in the rat liver [34]. In addition, ECH exhibited protective effects and reduced infarct size by up to 45% in a myocardial ischemia/reperfusion injury model by enhancing mitochondrial functions [35]. It is effective against peptic ulcer-induced oxidative stress in rats and this effect is mediated via alleviation of gastric acidity [36]. However, so far, no study has explored the effects of strong antioxidant properties and biological activities of ECH on the vocal fold. Thus, here we investigated the effects of sex hormones on the alteration in the expression of ECM-related genes of vocal fold lamina propria in ovariectomized rats and verified whether ECH exerts any preventive effects on ECM reconstitution following estradiol deficiency in ovariectomized rats. Ovariectomized rats are widely used for the study of prevention and treatment strategies for postmenopausal women because the rat ovariectomized state closely mimics the hormonal conditions of postmenopausal women [37,38].

Analysis of ECM components at 6 weeks after ovariectomy revealed no changes in hyaluronic acid concentration and elastin levels. Hyaluronic acid is one of important components of the ECM and contributes to the viscoelastic properties of the vocal fold lamina propria [39]. Elastic fibers serve as scaffolds for structural maintenance and provide tensile strength and resilience [40]. The expression levels of *Has 2, 3* and *Eln* were slightly different, but the changes in hyaluronic acid and elastin in vocal fold lamina propria were insignificant. These findings differed in part from our previous findings at 12 weeks after ovariectomy [6]. The change in ECM owing to the reduction in estradiol seems to be somewhat different over time.

Collagen level decreased in the OVX group, but the down-regulated collagen level was increased by ECH treatment. Decreased collagen level in the lamina propria correlated with stiffness that disturbed the pliable mucosal wave. Collagen I is ubiquitous and mainly appears as fibrillary bundles. It provides high-tensile strength [39,40]. Collagen III is present in most tissues that require flexibility and elasticity [40,41]. The OVX group showed downregulated collagen I and III levels, which were restored after ECH treatment. Contrary to the results of the histological analysis, the expression levels of *Col1a1, Col1a2,* and *Col3a1* increased in the OVX + ECH group; however, the downregulation in the expression of these procollagen molecules was not observed in the OVX group.

To address these discrepancies, we evaluated MMP expression. MMPs belong to a family of enzymes involved in the turnover of the ECM. The expression of MMPs is stable in normal resting tissues but gets up-regulated during physiological and pathological stress and tissue repair. The expression of MMPs is reflective of the amount of collagenase and was found to be increased in the OVX group and suppressed in the OVX + ECH group. These findings may be related to the lower deposition of collagen I and III in the vocal fold lamina propria, as higher levels of collagenase in the OVX group resulted in the degradation of collagen. The results revealed that the most significant ECM component among the SHAM, OVX, and OVX + ECH groups was collagen. Thus, the ECM component that exerted maximum effects on the vocal fold in the OVX group was collagen and that ECH treatment modulated collagen expression and remodeled the lamina propria of the vocal fold by increasing collagen synthesis and decreasing collagen degradation. In contrast, hyaluronic acid concentration and elastin levels were not significantly different in all groups and ECH treatment had no influence on the expression level of hyaluronic acid and elastin until 6 weeks after ovariectomy. According to our previous study, hyaluronic acid concentration and elastin levels significantly decreased at 12 weeks after ovariectomy [6]. Thus, collagen synthesis and degradation seem to be the most important factors controlling early voice change caused by menopause.

Thus, the expression levels of hyaluronic acid and elastin were unchanged in the lamina propria of the vocal fold from the OVX group. Collagen I and III levels were significantly decreased in the lamina propria of the vocal fold in ovariectomized rats. However, ECH treatment increased the synthesis of collagen and decreased its degradation. We observed changes in several ECM-related genes in the OVX group after estradiol deficiency and ECH was shown to improve the altered expression of these genes in the OVX group (Figure 7). Thus, the vocal fold is an estradiol-sensitive target organ and ECH may have protective effects on ECM of vocal folds in ovariectomized rats.

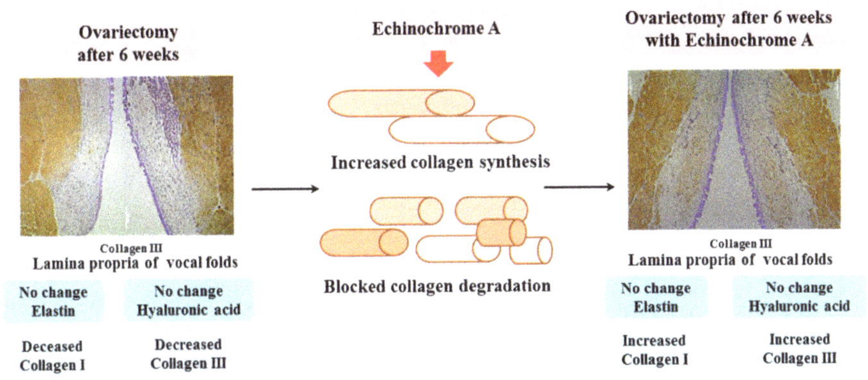

Figure 7. Summary of the current study. To summarize, hyaluronic acid and elastin were unchanged in the lamina propria of the vocal fold from the OVX group. Collagen I and III levels were significantly decreased in the lamina propria of the vocal fold in ovariectomized rats. However, ECH treatment increased the synthesis of collagen and decreased its degradation. We observed changes in several ECM-related genes in the OVX group after estradiol deficiency and ECH was shown to improve the altered expression of ECM components in the OVX group. Thus, the vocal fold is an estradiol-sensitive target organ and ECH may have protective effects on the ECM of vocal folds in ovariectomized rats.

4. Material and Methods

4.1. Animals

Forty-five female Sprague–Dawley rats, aged nine weeks, were used in this study (Samtako, Osan, Korea). Each group was weight-matched at the beginning of the study. After a week for acclimatization, rats were randomly divided into three groups. Group I (n = 15, sham-operated rats, called\SHAM), group II (n = 15, ovariectomized surgery rats, called OVX), and group III (n = 15, ovariectomized surgery rats treated with ECH, called OVX + ECH). Rats were sacrificed 6 weeks after ovariectomy. Six rats were used for histological study and nine rats were used for qPCR. All rats were maintained on a light/dark cycle of 12 h and provided rat chow with water ad libitum in a pathogen-free room. Animal care and research protocols were based on the principles and guidelines adopted by Guide for the Care and Use of Laboratory Animals (National Institutes of Health publication). This study was approved by the Review Board of Pusan National Hospital (IRB No.2018-04-017) and informed consent was waived.

4.2. Echinochrome A

Echinochrome A is insoluble in water and, therefore, it is used for medical purposes in the form of injection, registered in Russia as the drug Histochrome (P N002363/02). Histochrome, trade name soluble echinochrome A sodium salt, does not contain other components. We used Histochrome, containing 0.2 mg/mL echinochrome A, produced by Pacific Institute of Bioorganic Chemistry, Far East Branch of the Russian Academy of Sciences.

4.3. Establishment of the Ovariectomized Rat Model

The rats were anesthetized using isoflurane inhalation (3% dissolved in oxygen). The ovariectomy (OVX) was as follows: rats were anesthetized and an incision made at the midline of the abdomen with the bilateral ovaries being revealed. In the OVX group, the ovaries were ligated and cut off bilaterally followed by the closure of the abdominal cavity. In the Sham operations group (SHAM), OVX surgery was performed by exposing the ovaries without the excision of ovaries. After ovariectomized surgery, rats were intraperitoneally injected with ECH at 10 mg/kg three times a week during 6 weeks (OVX + ECH).

4.4. Plasma Estradiol Analysis

Concentrations of estradiol in serum were measured by rat-specific estradiol enzyme-linked immunosorbent (ELISA) assay plates coated with a biotin-conjugated binding protein kit purchased from Calbiotech (Spring Valley, CA, USA). A cardiac puncture was performed and the blood spun at 3000 rpm for 30 min. Plasma was separated from the blood collected during exsanguination, immediately frozen in liquid nitrogen, and then stored at −80 °C.

4.5. Histology and Morphometric Analysis

The larynx was isolated from each rat and prepared for fixation overnight in 4% formalin. We used an automatic tissue processor for paraffin embedding (Leica, Wetzlar, Germany), TP1020, semi-enclosed benchtop tissue processor) and dispensing (Leica, Wetzlar, Germany) EG1150H, heated paraffin embedding module). Cross-sections (8 μm thick) were placed on glass slides and sections were prepared for immunohistochemistry, Verhoeff–Van Gieson elastin staining and Alcian blue staining. For staining analyses, slides were de-paraffinized with xylene and then hydrated through a series of washes in 100%, 85%, 75%, and 50% ethanol and finally water. We selected proper middle portions of lamina propria tissue for representative figures use undertaken at 200X pictures by light microscope (Leica, Wetzlar, Germany) DM4000/600M, versatile upright microscope for materials analysis). For quantitative analyses of collagen I, collagen III, elastin, and hyaluronic acid expression, we measured positively stained areas through image analysis using a system composed of a light microscope. Morphometric determination was undertaken at 40X pictures from the whole part of the lamina propria using the morphometric method, that used an image analysis system program composed of a light microscope (Leica, Wetzlar, Germany) Basic LAS V3.8 software). For the immunohistochemical analysis of vocal fold lamina propria, three non-overlapping areas were analyzed at 400X and a total of nine areas were analyzed in each section. Results were expressed as stained area per total area in micrometers squared. Data were expressed as medians and ranges.

4.6. Verhoeff–Van Gieson Elastin Staining

The Verhoeff–Van Gieson elastin staining method was performed to identify atrophy of elastic tissues. The sections were first placed in an iron hematoxylin solution for 10 min and then rinsed in distilled water and differentiated in 2% ferric chloride. After rinsing in distilled water and placing in 95% alcohol, the samples were counterstained with Van Gieson solution (Sigma Aldrich; St. Louis, MO, USA) for 5 min. The samples were then dehydrated in graded alcohol and then cleared in xylene and mounted.

4.7. Alcian Blue Staining

Alcian blue staining and a hyaluronidase digestion technique were performed to identify hyaluronic acid. Duplicate sections of the control samples were incubated in hyaluronidase (Sigma Aldrich, St. Louis, MO, USA) at 37 °C for one hour. After the wash, sections with and without hyaluronidase digestion were stained with Alcian blue stain (pH 2.5) for 30 min. Sections were washed and counterstained with nuclear fast red stain. Areas containing hyaluronic acid remained unstained in digested slides and stained blue in undigested slides.

4.8. Immunohistochemistry

De-paraffinized sections were washed with phosphate-buffered saline (PBS) and blocked for 1 h at room temperature with 2% bovine serum albumin (BSA) containing 0.3% Triton X-100 in PBS. They were then incubated for 24 h at 4 °C with the following primary antibodies: anti-estrogen receptor β (200 ug/mL) (Santa Cruz Biotechnology, Dallas, TA, USA), anti-collagen I, and anti-collagen III (1:400) (Abcam, Cambridge, UK). After the primary antibody was removed by rinsing, sections were incubated with secondary antibodies for 1 h at room temperature. The following goat-anti rabbit secondary antibodies (1:1000) (ENZO Biochem, NY, USA) were used for double-staining with DAB (3,3-diaminobenzidine) staining. Incubation with phosphate-buffered saline supplemented with 1% bovine serum albumin instead of the primary antibody served as a negative control.

4.9. Quantitative PCR

To confirm mRNA expression, we isolated whole lamina propria of the vocal fold with a syringe needle under microscope and used the real time PCR method. Tissue RNA was extracted using the TRIzol system (Life Technologies, Rockville, MD, USA). A reverse transcription kit (Applied Biosystems, Foster City, CA, USA) was used to perform reverse transcription according to the manufacturer's protocol. Quantitative PCR was performed according to the SYBR ®Green PCR protocol (Applied Biosystems, Foster city, CA, USA). Each sample was tested in quintuplicate. Reaction conditions were: 10 min at 95 °C (one cycle); 10 s at 95 °C; and 30 s at 60 °C (40 cycles). Final primer concentration was 0.1 μM and sequences can be found in Table 1. Gene-specific PCR products were continuously measured by an ABI PRISM 7900 HT Sequence Detection System (PE Applied Biosystems, Waltham, CT, USA). All the primers used for qPCR analysis had been designated using Primer Express software 1.5 (Applied Biosystems, Foster city, CA, USA) and synthesized by Invitrogen. (Invitrogen Life Technologies, Carlsbad, CA, USA). Normalization consisted of using the differences between the cycle thresholds (delta CT) and the expression level for *Rn18s* to calculate the delta CT/target gene delta CT ratio. Delta/delta CT corresponds to the differences between the delta CT the internal control gene.

Table 1. Sequence of primers.

Esr2a (estrogen receptor βI)	Forward	GCTTCGTGGAGCTCAGCCTG
	Reverse	AGGATCATGGCCTTGACACAGA
Esr2b (estrogen receptor βII)	Forward	GAAGCTGAACCACCCAATGT
	Reverse	CAGTCCCACCATTAGCACCT
Has1 (hyaluronic acid synthase 1)	Forward	CCACTGCACATTTGGGGATG
	Reverse	GAATAGCATCTGGAGCGCGA
Has2 (hyaluronic acid synthase 2)	Forward	ACTGGGCAGAAGCGTGGATTATGT
	Reverse	AACACCTCCAACCATCGGGTCTTCTT
Has3 (hyaluronic acid synthase 3)	Forward	GCACCATTGAGATGCTTCGG
	Reverse	TACCTCACGCTGCTCAGGAA
Eln (tropoelastin)	Forward	TTCTGGGAGCGTTTGGAG
	Reverse	CCTTGAAGCATAGGAGAGACCT
Cela1 (chymotrypsin-like elastase family member 1)	Forward	TCCTAGGAGCCAGGCCATT
	Reverse	GGGTAGATAGGAGAAAGTCCAAACC
Col1a1 (collagen, type I, alpha 1)	Forward	AGTCCATCTTTGCCAGGAGAACCA
	Reverse	CGGCAGGACCAGGAAGACC
Col1a2 (collagen, type I, alpha 2)	Forward	CCGAGGCAGAGATGGTGTT
	Reverse	GCAGCAAAGTTCCCAGTAAGA
Col3a1 (collagen, type III, alpha 1)	Forward	ACTGACCAAGGTAGTTGCATCCCA
	Reverse	CCAGGGTCACCATTTCTCC
Mmp1 (matrix metallopeptidase 1)	Forward	ATGAGACGTGGACCGACAAC
	Reverse	TGAGTGAGTCCAAGGGAGTG
Mmp2 (matrix metallopeptidase 2)	Forward	GTC ACT CCG CTG CGC TTT TCT CG
	Reverse	GAC ACA TGG GGC ACC TTC TGA
Mmp8 (matrix metallopeptidase 8)	Forward	CAGACAACCCTGTCCAACCT
	Reverse	GGATGCCGTCTCCAGAAGTA
Mmp9 (matrix metallopeptidase 9)	Forward	CGGAGCACGGGGACGGGTATC
	Reverse	AAGACGAAGGGGAAGACGCACATC
Rn18s (18s RNA)	Forward	AACCCGTTGAACCCCATT
	Reverse	GGGCAGGGACTTAATCAACG

4.10. Statistical Analysis

Unless otherwise noted, all quantitative data were reported as the mean standard error of the mean from at least three parallel repeats. One-way analysis of variance was used to determine significant differences between groups in which $p < 0.05$ was considered statistically significant.

5. Conclusions

We observed changes in genes expression associated with ECM production and degradation in the lamina propria of the vocal fold after the induction of menopause by ovariectomy in a rat experimental model. The changes in the genes related to the generation and degradation of ECM were observed after the administration of ECH. This study suggests that the antioxidant properties of ECH may have protective effects on the vocal fold caused by lamina propria ECM deposition. These results indicate that the vocal fold is an estradiol-sensitive target organ and that ECH may have protective effects on the ECM of vocal folds in ovariectomized rats.

Author Contributions: J.M.K. performed the research, analyzed the data, and drafted the manuscript. J.H.K. and S.-C.S. carried out the animal surgeries. G.C.P., H.S.K., K.K., H.K.K., and J.H. participated in the experimental studies. N.P.M., E.A.V., S.A.F., and V.A.S. purified the Echinochrome A. B.-J.L. corresponded our study and alignment experiment. All authors have read and agreed to the published version of the manuscript.

Funding: This work was supported by the National Research Foundation of Korea (NRF) grant funded by the Korean government (No. 2016R1D1A3B01015539, NRF-2017R1E1A1A01074316).

Acknowledgments: This work was supported by the National Research Foundation of Korea (NRF) grant funded by the Korean government (2017K1A3A1A49070056). The study was carried out under support of the Ministry of Education and Science of the Russian Federation (RFMEFI61317 × 0076) using the equipment of the Collective Facilities Center (The Far Eastern Center for Structural Molecular Research (NMR/MS) PIBOC FEB RAS).

Conflicts of Interest: The authors declare no conflict of interest.

References

1. Huber, J.E.; Stathopoulos, E.T.; Curione, G.M.; Ash, T.A.; Johnson, K. Formants of children, women, and men: The effects of vocal intensity variation. *J. Acoust. Soc. Am.* **1999**, *106*, 15–32.
2. Meurer, E.M.; Osório Wender, M.C.; Von Eye Corleta, H.; Capp, E. Female suprasegmental speech parameters in reproductive age and postmenopause. *Maturitas* **2004**, *48*, 71–77. [CrossRef] [PubMed]
3. Caruso, S.; Roccasalva, L.; Sapienza, G.; Zappalá, M.; Nuciforo, G.; Biondi, S. Laryngeal cytological aspects in women with surgically induced menopause who were treated with transdermal estrogen replacement therapy. *Fertil. Steril.* **2000**, *74*, 1073–1079. [PubMed]
4. Firat, Y.; Engin-Ustun, Y.; Kizilay, A.; Ustun, Y.; Akarcay, M.; Selimoglu, E.; Kafkasli, A. Effect of intranasal estrogen on vocal quality. *J. Voice* **2009**, *23*, 716–720. [CrossRef] [PubMed]
5. Mendes-Laureano, J.; Sá, M.F.S.; Ferriani, R.A.; Reis, R.M.; Aguiar-Ricz, L.N.; Valera, F.C.P.; Küpper, D.S.; Romão, G.S. Comparison of fundamental voice frequency between menopausal woman and woman at menacme. *Maturitas* **2006**, *55*, 195–199. [PubMed]
6. Kim, J.M.; Shin, S.C.; Park, G.C.; Lee, J.C.; Jeon, Y.K.; Ahn, S.J.; Thibeault, S.; Lee, B.J. Effect of sex hormones on extracellular matrix of lamina propria in rat vocal fold. *Laryngoscope* **2019**. [CrossRef]
7. Raj, A.; Gupta, B.; Chowdhury, A.; Chadha, S. A Study of Voice Changes in Various Phases of Menstrual Cycle and in Postmenopausal Women. *J. Voice* **2010**, *24*, 363–368.
8. Kahwati, L.C.; Haigler, L.; Rideout, S. What is the best way to diagnose menopause? *J. Fam. Pract.* **2005**, *54*, 1000–1002.
9. D'Haeseleer, E.; Depypere, H.; Claeys, S.; Wuyts, F.L.; De Ley, S.; Van Lierde, K.M. The impact of menopause on vocal quality. *Menopause* **2011**, *18*, 267–272. [CrossRef]
10. Jeong, S.H.; Kim, H.K.; Song, I.S.; Noh, S.J.; Marquez, J.; Ko, K.S.; Rhee, B.D.; Kim, N.; Mishchenko, N.P.; Fedoreyev, S.A.; et al. Echinochrome a increases mitochondrial mass and function by modulating mitochondrial biogenesis regulatory genes. *Mar. Drugs* **2014**, *21*, 4602–4615. [CrossRef]
11. Mizuta, M.; Hirano, S.; Hiwatashi, N.; Kobayashi, T.; Tateya, I.; Kanemaru, S.I.; Nakamura, T.; Ito, J. Effect of AST on age-associated changes of vocal folds in a rat model. *Laryngoscope* **2014**, *124*, E411–E417. [CrossRef] [PubMed]
12. Mizuta, M.; Hirano, S.; Hiwatashi, N.; Tateya, I.; Kanemaru, S.I.; Nakamura, T.; Ito, J. Effect of astaxanthin on vocal fold wound healing. *Laryngoscope* **2014**, *124*, E1–E7. [CrossRef] [PubMed]
13. Lennikov, A.; Kitaichi, N.; Noda, K.; Mizuuchi, K.; Ando, R.; Dong, Z.; Fukuhara, J.; Kinoshita, S.; Namba, K.; Ohno, S.; et al. Amelioration of endotoxin-induced uveitis treated with the sea urchin pigment echinochrome in rats. *Mol. Vis.* **2014**, *7*, 171–177.
14. Borrelli, F.; Ernst, E. Alternative and complementary therapies for the menopause. *Maturitas* **2010**, *66*, 333–343. [CrossRef]
15. Wuyts, F.L.; De Bodt, M.S.; Molenberghs, G.; Remacle, M.; Heylen, L.; Millet, B.; Van Lierde, K.; Raes, J.; Van De Heyning, P.H. The Dysphonia Severity Index: An Objective Measure of Vocal Quality Based on a Multiparameter Approach. *J. Speech Lang. Hear. Res.* **2000**, *43*, 796–809. [CrossRef]

16. Pattie, M.A.; Murdoch, B.E.; Theodoros, D.; Forbes, K. Voice changes in women treated for endometriosis and related conditions: The need for comprehensive vocal assessment. *J. Voice* **1998**, *12*, 366–371. [CrossRef]
17. Kuhn, M.A. Histological changes in vocal fold growth and aging. *Curr. Opin. Otolaryngol. Head Neck Surg.* **2014**, *22*, 460–465. [CrossRef]
18. Lindholm, P.; Vilkman, E.; Raudaskoski, T.; Suvanto-Luukkonen, E.; Kauppila, A. The effect of postmenopause and postmenopausal HRT on measured voice values and vocal symptoms. *Maturitas* **1997**, *28*, 47–53. [CrossRef]
19. Baker, J. A report on alterations to the speaking and singing voices of four women following hormonal therapy with virilizing agents. *J. Voice* **1999**, *13*, 496–507. [CrossRef]
20. Silverman, E.M.; Zimmer, C.H. Effect of the Menstrual Cycle on Voice Quality. *Arch. Otolaryngol.* **1978**, *104*, 7–10. [CrossRef]
21. Chernobelsky, S.I. A study of menses-related changes to the larynx in singers with voice abuse. *Folia Phoniatr. Logop.* **2002**, *54*, 2–7. [CrossRef] [PubMed]
22. Samsioe, G. The role of ERT/HRT. *Best Pract. Res. Clin. Obstet. Gynaecol.* **2002**, *16*, 371–381. [CrossRef] [PubMed]
23. Morán, J.; Garrido, P.; Alonso, A.; Cabello, E.; González, C. 17β-Estradiol and genistein acute treatments improve some cerebral cortex homeostasis aspects deteriorated by aging in female rats. *Exp. Gerontol.* **2013**, *48*, 414–421. [CrossRef]
24. Maskarinec, G.; Takata, Y.; Franke, A.A.; Williams, A.E.; Murphy, S.P. A 2-Year Soy Intervention in Premenopausal Women Does Not Change Mammographic Densities. *J. Nutr.* **2004**, *134*, 3089–3094. [CrossRef] [PubMed]
25. Koebnick, C.; Reimann, M.; Carlsohn, A.; Korzen-Bohr, S.; Bügel, S.; Hallund, J.; Rossi, L.; Branca, F.; Hall, W.; Williams, C.; et al. The acceptability of isoflavones as a treatment of menopausal symptoms: A European survey among postmenopausal women. *Climacteric* **2005**, *8*, 230–242. [CrossRef] [PubMed]
26. Cianci, A.; Cicero, A.F.G.; Colacurci, N.; Matarazzo, M.G.; De Leo, V. Activity of isoflavones and berberine on vasomotor symptoms and lipid profile in menopausal women. *Gynecol. Endocrinol.* **2012**, *28*, 699–702. [CrossRef] [PubMed]
27. Fitzpatrick, A.M.; Teague, W.G.; Holguin, F.; Yeh, M.; Brown, L.A.S. Airway glutathione homeostasis is altered in children with severe asthma: Evidence for oxidant stress. *J. Allergy Clin. Immunol.* **2009**, *123*, 146–152. [CrossRef]
28. Karbiener, M.; Darnhofer, B.; Frisch, M.T.; Rinner, B.; Birner-Gruenberger, R.; Gugatschka, M. Comparative proteomics of paired vocal fold and oral mucosa fibroblasts. *J. Proteom.* **2017**, *23*, 11–21. [CrossRef]
29. Lin, T.C.; Chen, J.C.; Liu, C.H.; Lee, C.Y.; Tsou, Y.A.; Chuang, C.C. A feasibility study on non-invasive oxidative metabolism detection and acoustic assessment of human vocal cords by using optical technique. *Sci. Rep.* **2017**, *5*, 17002. [CrossRef]
30. Tellis, C.M.; Rosen, C.; Close, J.M.; Horton, M.; Yaruss, J.S.; Verdolini-Abbott, K.; Sciote, J.J. Cytochrome C oxidase deficiency in human posterior cricoarytenoid muscle. *J. Voice* **2011**, *25*, 387–394. [CrossRef]
31. Diamond, J.; Skaggs, J.; Manaligod, J.M. Free-radical damage: A possible mechanism of laryngeal aging. *Ear Nose Throat J.* **2002**, *81*, 531–533. [CrossRef] [PubMed]
32. Lebedev, A.V.; Levitskaya, E.L.; Tikhonova, E.V.; Ivanova, M.V. Antioxidant properties, autooxidation, and mutagenic activity of echinochrome a compared with its etherified derivative. *Biochemistry (Moscow)* **2001**, *8*, 885–893. [CrossRef] [PubMed]
33. Lebedev, A.V.; Ivanova, M.V.; Krasnovid, N.I.; Kol'tsova, E.A. Acidity and interaction with superoxide anion radical of echinochrome and its structural analogs. *Vopr. Med. Khim.* **1999**, *45*, 123–130.
34. Mohamed, A.S.; Soliman, A.M.; Marie, M.A.S. Mechanisms of echinochrome potency in modulating diabetic complications in liver. *Life Sci.* **2016**, *15*, 41–49. [CrossRef]
35. Boulet, M.J.; Oddens, B.J. Female voice changes around and after the menopause—An initial investigation. *Maturitas* **1996**, *23*, 15–21. [CrossRef]
36. Abitbol, J.; Abitbol, P.; Abitbol, B. Sex hormones and the female voice. *J. Voice* **1999**, *13*, 424–446. [CrossRef]
37. Ward, P.D.; Thibeault, S.L.; Gray, S.D. Hyaluronic acid: Its role in voice. *J. Voice* **2002**, *16*, 303–309. [CrossRef]
38. Hirano, S. Current treatment of vocal fold scarring. *Curr. Opin. Otolaryngol. Head Neck Surg.* **2005**, *13*, 143–147. [CrossRef]

39. Hansen, J.K.; Thibeault, S.L. Current understanding and review of the literature: Vocal fold scarring. *J. Voice* **2006**, *20*, 110–120. [CrossRef]
40. Thibeault, S.L. Advances in our understanding of the Reinke space. *Curr. Opin. Otolaryngol. Head Neck Surg.* **2005**, *13*, 148–151. [CrossRef]
41. Hirschi, S.D.; Gray, S.D.; Thibeault, S.L. Fibronectin: An interesting vocal fold protein. *J. Voice* **2002**, *16*, 310–316. [CrossRef]

© 2020 by the authors. Licensee MDPI, Basel, Switzerland. This article is an open access article distributed under the terms and conditions of the Creative Commons Attribution (CC BY) license (http://creativecommons.org/licenses/by/4.0/).

marine drugs

MDPI

Article

Neurotrophic Effect of Fish-Lecithin Based Nanoliposomes on Cortical Neurons

Catherine Malaplate [1,†], Aurelia Poerio [1,2,†], Marion Huguet [1], Claire Soligot [1], Elodie Passeri [1,2], Cyril J. F. Kahn [2], Michel Linder [2], Elmira Arab-Tehrany [2,*] and Frances T. Yen [1,*]

1 Research Unit Animal and Functionality of Animal Products, Quality of Diet and Aging Team (UR AFPA) Laboratory, Qualivie Team, University of Lorraine, 54505 Vandoeuvre-lès-Nancy, France
2 LIBio Laboratory, University of Lorraine, 54505 Vandoeuvre-lès-Nancy, France
* Correspondence: elmira.arab-tehrany@univ-lorraine.fr (E.A.-T.); frances.yen-potin@univ-lorraine.fr (F.T.Y.); Tel.: +33-3-72-74-41-05 (E.A.T.); +33-3-72-74-41-50 (F.T.Y.)
† Co-first authors.

Received: 16 May 2019; Accepted: 1 July 2019; Published: 9 July 2019

Abstract: Lipids play multiple roles in preserving neuronal function and synaptic plasticity, and polyunsaturated fatty acids (PUFAs) have been of particular interest in optimizing synaptic membrane organization and function. We developed a green-based methodology to prepare nanoliposomes (NL) from lecithin that was extracted from fish head by-products. These NL range between 100–120 nm in diameter, with an n-3/n-6 fatty acid ratio of 8.88. The high content of n-3 PUFA (46.3% of total fatty acid content) and docosahexanoic acid (26%) in these NL represented a means for enrichment of neuronal membranes that are potentially beneficial for neuronal growth and synaptogenesis. To test this, the primary cultures of rat embryo cortical neurons were incubated with NL on day 3 post-culture for 24 h, followed by immunoblots or immunofluorescence to evaluate the NL effects on synaptogenesis, axonal growth, and dendrite formation. The results revealed that NL-treated cells displayed a level of neurite outgrowth and arborization on day 4 that was similar to those of untreated cells on day 5 and 6, suggesting accelerated synapse formation and neuronal development in the presence of NL. We propose that fish-derived NL, by virtue of their n-3 PUFA profile and neurotrophic effects, represent a new innovative bioactive vector for developing preventive or curative treatments for neurodegenerative diseases.

Keywords: n-3 fatty acids; nanoparticles; brain

1. Introduction

Polyunsaturated fatty acids (PUFA) have been extensively studied for their effects in neuronal development and growth, where investigations have particularly focused on n-3 PUFA for their therapeutic effects on neurodegenerative diseases, such as Alzheimer's disease. Both n-3 and n-6 PUFA have significant roles in membrane structure and function and in cell signaling. They also play important roles as substrates for the synthesis of lipid mediators that are involved in inflammation. Indeed, the consumption of n-3 PUFA docosahexanoic (DHA) and eicosapentaenoic (EPA) acids has been shown to decrease the amounts of n-6 arachidonic acid (AA), which is a precursor of the production of eicosanoids that are involved in inflammation [1]. DHA and EPA are precursors of the anti-inflammatory resolvins, and they may also exert an anti-oxidative role by modulating the activity of proteins that are involved in oxidative stress in the central nervous system [2]. PUFAs are also known to be directly involved in the regulation of gene expression in the brain [3].

Numerous studies have focused particularly on n-3 PUFA's role on membrane structure and function. Indeed, DHA represents 60% of PUFA in neuronal membranes. Lipid rafts are needed for axon guidance, allowing for cone growth and cell polarization of neurons for the formation of new synaptic connections [4]. The growth-associated protein 43 (GAP43) is an abundant raft-protein that is involved in the development of axons and nerve growth, and its expression can be induced by fatty acids, such as DHA and oleic acid, in immunofluorescence studies [5,6]. Both cell and animal studies have also demonstrated increased neuronal differentiation and neurite outgrowth in the presence of PUFA [7,8].

It is clear that n-3 PUFA provide beneficial effects in neuronal development and growth by increasing membrane fluidity [9–11], or as activators of cell signaling functions [3,12]. Furthermore, by improving synaptic plasticity and the formation of new synaptic connections, they are key in the prevention of neuronal damage that can be associated with aging or neurodegenerative diseases, such as Alzheimer's disease.

These fatty acids must be obtained either directly from the diet, or are produced by synthesis in the liver from precursors linoleic and α-linoleic acid before transport and delivery to the brain, since neurons lack the enzymes for the *de novo* synthesis of DHA and arachidonic acid. Providing the means for the efficient delivery of PUFA to the brain would thus be of interest towards maintaining brain membrane integrity and synaptic function in the aging process for preventive purposes and also as adjuvant for better response to therapeutics [13].

We have developed a green extraction technique to prepare nanoliposomes from natural resources (patent n° FR 2.835.703, [14]). These soft nanoparticles contain multiple bilayers that are composed of natural lecithin surrounding an aqueous compartment. Its unique physicochemical characteristics allows the incorporation of hydrophilic, amphiphilic, or hydrophobic molecules, and, by virtue of the lipid bilayer, these nanoliposomes can fuse with cell membranes, thereby delivering the liposome contents to the target tissue. Nanoliposomes the offer advantages of low toxicity, of being modifiable with respect to size and surface, biocompatibility, and biodegradability [15]. Nanoliposomes that are prepared using lecithin derived from fish by-products, which represent a major source of n-3 PUFA, show positive effects on cell proliferation with a stimulation of cell activity in mesenchymal stem cells [16], as well as in neuronal cells [17]. Here, we report the further characterization of these nanoliposomes. Increased metabolic mitochondrial activity and neural network formation was observed in the presence of nanoliposomes [17], suggesting the potential effects on synapse formation and neurogenesis. It remained to be determined whether the nanoliposome-induced effects were neuron-specific, since the cells used were shown to express the glial fibrillary acidic protein GFAP which is found only in glial cells. Here, we investigate this further by examining the effect of nanoliposomes on specific synaptic and neurogenesis markers in purified primary culture preparations of rat embryo cortical neurons.

2. Results and Discussion

2.1. Lipid Classes

In salmon lecithin, phosphatidylcholine was the major class of phospholipids and it represented 42% of this fraction (Table 1). The triacylglycerol (TAG) content in lecithin was 31.20 ± 0.4% and the amount of polar fraction was 67.65 ± 0.9%. A small amount of cholesterol was detected in the fraction, at a level of 1.15 ± 0.1%.

2.2. Fatty Acid Analyses

Analyses by gas chromatography revealed that fatty acid composition of salmon lecithin consists of a variety of polyunsaturated fatty acids (PUFA) (Table 2). A number of PUFAs of omega 3 and omega 6 were identified in salmon lecithin, of which C22:6 n-3 (26.26%) and C20:5 n-3 (11.03%) were the most significant. C18:1 n-9 (13.87%) and C16:0 (20.67%) were the two major monounsaturated and saturated fatty acids, respectively. The n-3/n-6 ratio was 8.88 with a ratio of DHA/EPA of 2.38.

Table 1. Lipid classes and fraction of polar lipids composition of salmon lecithin.

Name	Salmon Lecithin
Total phospholipids (%)	67.7 ± 1.1
Phosphatidylcholine, PC (%)	42.4 ± 0.5
Phosphatidylethanolamine, PE (%)	7.7 ± 0.1
Phosphatidylserine, PS (%)	9.1 ± 0.1
Phosphatidylinositol, PI (%)	13.0 ± 0.3
Sphingomyelin, SPM (%)	1.5 ± 0.1
Lysophosphosphatidylcholine, LPC (%)	2.8 ± 0.1
Other phospholipids (%)	23.5 ± 0.2
Triglycerides, TAGs (%)	31.2 ± 0.8
Cholesterol, CHOL (%)	1.2 ± 0.1
Free fatty acids, FFA (%)	ND

Table 2. Fatty acid composition of salmon lecithin.

Saturated Fatty Acids (SFA)		Monounsaturated Fatty Acids (MUFA)		Polyunsaturated Fatty Acids (PUFA)	
Fatty acid	% (SD) *	Fatty acid	% (SD)	Fatty acid	% (SD)
C14:0	2.72 (0.04)	C14:1n9	0.33 (0.02)	C18:2n6	1.20 (0.04)
C15:0	1.13 (0.01)	C16:1n7	3.23 (0.07)	C18:3n3	0.35 (0.01)
C16:0	20.67 (0.15)	C18:1n9	13.87 (0.13)	C20:4n6	3.52 (0.02)
C17:0	0.88 (0.05)	C20:1n9	2.11 (0.06)	C20:5n3 [1]	11.03 (0.13)
C18:0	6.10 (0.05)	C22:1n9	0.79 (0.08)	C22:5n3	3.93 (0.33)
C20:0	0.35 (0.03)			C22:6n3 [2]	26.26 (0.09)
C22:0	1.55 (0.06)				
SFA	33.40	MUFA	20.32	PUFA	46.28

* Mean (SD) % of total fatty acid composition of nanoliposomes (mean and standard deviation of triplicate determinations).
[1] EPA, [2] DHA.

2.3. Liposome Size and Electrophoretic Mobility Measurements and Morphological Properties

The particle sizes of different nanoliposome preparations were immediately measured after sonication. The liposome size depends on the viscosity of the material and agitation parameters, including sonication amplitude and time. The size of the nanoliposome also depends on fatty acid composition (the presence of LC-PUFA), lipid profile, and the surface-active properties of the lecithin, like as the percentage and type of polar head [16,18]. The hydrodynamic diameter of nanoliposomes for salmon lecithin was 110 ± 0.32 nm, and the polydispersity index was 0.29 ± 0.00. The polar fraction of lecithin (phosphate residues) has a negative charge. The electrophoretic mobility of nanoliposomes from salmon lecithin was −3.5 ± 0.09 μmcm/Vs with a relatively high stability, According to the electrophoretic light scattering (ELS) results, according to the electrophoretic light scattering (ELS) results. Different types of phospholipids, such as phosphatidylserine (PS), phosphatidic acid (PA), phosphatidylglycerol (PG), phosphatidylinositol (PI), phosphatidylethanolamine (PE), and phosphatidylcholine (PC) were present in salmon lecithin. Their charge is negative, except for PC and PE, which does not exhibit a net charge at physiological pH. Therefore, these anionic fractions most likely account for the negative electrophoretic mobility [19]. Nanoliposome stability measured by particle size at 4 °C and 37 °C over a one-month period showed no significant variation between day 0 and day 30.

The images that were obtained by Transmission Electron Microscopy (TEM) showed that prepared nanoliposomes were in the form of multilamellar vesicles (MLV). The bilayer nature of the vesicles was visible in these micrographs (Figure 1). We also observed some droplets in each formulation, because of the presence of small quantities of oil (10%). We used Atomic Force Microscopy (AFM) in order to observe the morphological property in nanometric scale. The results showed that, despite the variety of fatty acids in salmon lecithin, we did not observe phase segregation.

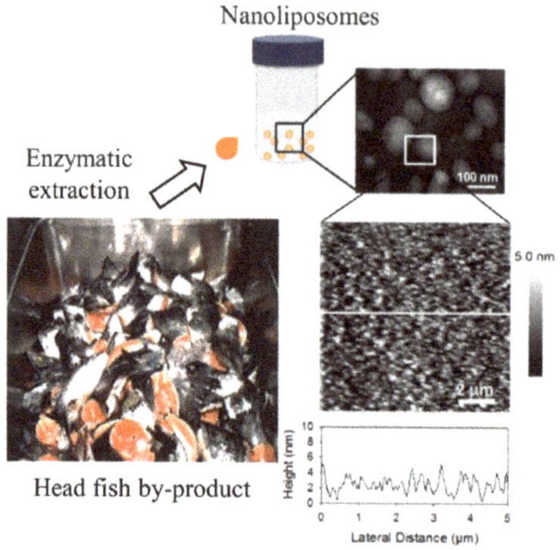

Figure 1. Formation and characterization of nanoliposomes from natural lecithin. Schematic diagram of the study, demonstrating the extraction of lecithin from marine source followed by generation of nanoliposomes; the inset shows a representative Transmission Electron Microscopy (TEM) image of the fabricated nanoliposomes and Atomic Force Microscopy (AFM) images of supported lipid bilayers made of phospholipids from salmon lecithin.

2.4. Membrane Fluidity

Membrane fluidity of nanoliposome is one of the important parameters that affect the release of active molecules and drugs from nanoliposomes, which reflects the order and dynamics of phospholipid alkyl chains [20]. Membrane fluidity depends on the lipid composition of nanoliposomes. By increasing the percentage of unsaturated FAs, the packing between the phospholipids decreases and keeps the level of hydration, thus maintaining membrane fluidity [21].

Nanoliposomes that were prepared from salmon lecithin had a membrane fluidity of 3.20 ± 0.03 when they contained higher proportions of PUFA. The lipid fluidity was expected to increase the permeant diffusion rate and partitioning tendency, which yields a possible squaring effect on the enhancement factor.

2.5. Treatment of Primary Cultured Neurons with Nanoliposomes

We investigated the effect of these lipid particles on the maturation of primary cultures of rat cortical neurons in view of the high amounts of n-3 fatty acids. Neurons were prepared and plated on day 0 in vitro (D0). To assess potential cytotoxic effects of NL, a set of cultured cells were treated with increasing concentrations of NL on D3, and incubated 24 h. MTT assay on D4 revealed a small decrease in cell viability at 50 µg/mL NL, which became statistically significant at NL concentrations $\geq$ 100 µg/mL (Figure 2). Cell viability was not significantly changed in the presence of 10 µg/mL NL, which was therefore selected as the concentration to be used for the study.

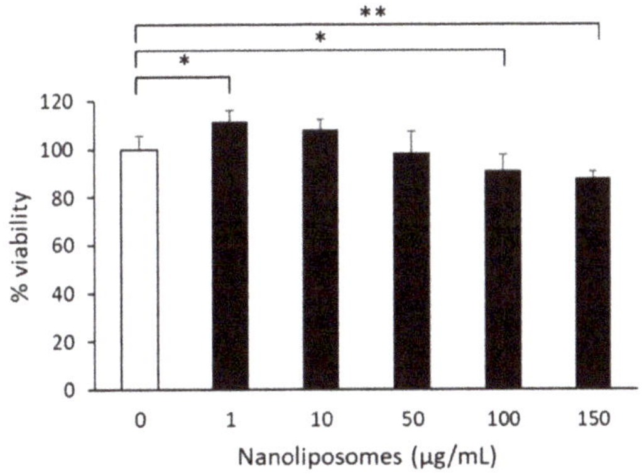

Figure 2. Cytotoxicity of nanoliposomes. Primary cultures of rat embryo cortical neurons were incubated in medium containing the indicated concentrations of nanoliposomes on day 3 in vitro. After 24 h, MTT assay was performed to assess cell viability. Mean and SD are shown for quadruplicate determinations. Statistical significance is shown as compared to that obtained for cells incubated in absence of nanoliposomes (* $p < 0.05$, ** $p < 0.01$).

The primary cultures of neurons were prepared and then incubated in the absence or presence of NL. Since significant changes in the maturation process of the neuronal network are observed after D3, cell culture media was replaced with the same media supplemented with 10 μg/mL NL on D3. The cell lysates were then prepared on D4 for immunoblotting studies to assess the changes in protein levels of different markers of neuronal functions. A similar set of cells that were treated in an identical manner, but cultured in the absence of NL, were used as controls that allowed us to establish the baseline; cell lysates were prepared on D4, D5, and D6. The results in Figure 3 revealed that there was a general tendency of higher protein levels of markers of neuronal and cone growth (β-tubulin and GAP43) in control cells without NL, as well as synaptic proteins (SNAP25, PSD95, synaptophysin), when comparing the protein levels on lysates from D5 or D6 to those of D4, with the exception of the post-synaptic PSD95 marker on D6. The two structural markers, β-tubulin and GAP43 protein levels, also showed similar profiles when compared with D5 or D6 to D4. The latter protein is indicative of cytoskeletal development that is conducive with axonal and dendritic growth. Interestingly, in cells that were incubated in the presence of NL on D3, the protein profiles appeared to be similar to that of D5 or D6, rather than D4 control cells in the absence of NL, with the exception of synaptophysin, which suggests the accelerated maturation of these cells in the presence of the NL. Unfortunately, data analysis did not reveal any statistically significant differences, with the exception of synaptophysin levels between D4 and D5. This could be due, in part, to the variation of protein levels between the different culture preparations, despite a similar trend in three separate cultures, as shown in the representative immunoblot (Figure 3A). Immunofluorescence studies were performed on cells that were labeled with the different markers to evaluate the morphology of the neurons during culture since the maturation of a neuron involves several stages including growth cone, axon, and synaptic button formation.

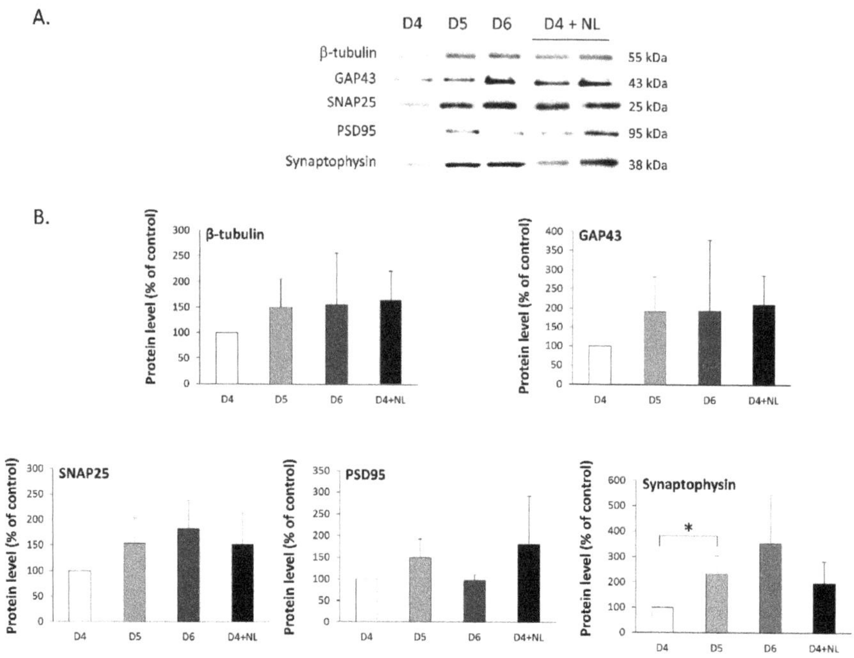

Figure 3. Immunoblots of pre- and post-synaptic markers in primary cultures of cortical neurons treated with fish nanoliposomes (NL). (**A**) Representative immunoblots of cell lysates prepared from primary cultures of rat embryo cortical neurons at different times following preparation (D = days in vitro) to detect GAP43, SNAP25, PSD95, synaptophysin, and β-tubulin, as indicated; D4 + NL are cells incubated 24 h with 10 μg/mL NL between D3 and D4; D4, D5, and D6 are control cells incubated in the absence of NL and recovered on D4, D5 and D6. (**B**) Protein levels following densitometric analysis of immunoblots. Results are expressed as % of control (D4) (mean ± SD of 3 experiments using three different NL preparations on three different cell culture preparations. (* $p < 0.05$).

Image analysis (Figure 4A) showed that GAP43 expression increased with neuronal extensions and could be seen as being granular with spots in control cells on D5 as compared to those on D4. This protein is transported along neurons from the cellular body to cone growth and therefore is a maker for neuronal growth. On D6, GAP43 was present primarily as granular fluorescent spots that were localized at growth cones and axons, most likely participating in the formation of new extensions. Cells that were incubated with NL exhibited a GAP43 profile on D4 that was similar to that of control cells on D5, with staining in both neuronal extensions and as granular with spots, indicating the accelerated state of outgrowth in the presence of NL as compared to untreated cells.

With neuronal growth, the formation of synapses should be observed. Co-labeling of the pre- and post-synaptic markers PSD95 (green) and SNAP25 (red) would normally indicate the formation of a functional synapse with both pre- and post-synaptic button formations, which immunoblots could not detect. Image analyses to count spots on ImageJ revealed a higher number of SNAP25 (granular red puncta) as compared to that of PSD95 (granular green puncta) in untreated cells on D4 (Figure 4B). The merging of images revealed as orange spots were indicative of colocalization of both markers, and they were also detected in untreated cells on D4 and increased when compared to values that were obtained for D5 and D6 combined. In cells that were treated with NL, statistically significant increases in SNAP25 and PSD95 individually, as well as SNAP25 + PSD95 orange spots were observed, as compared to untreated cells (D4), which is indicative of a higher number of synapse formations in the presence of these lipid particles.

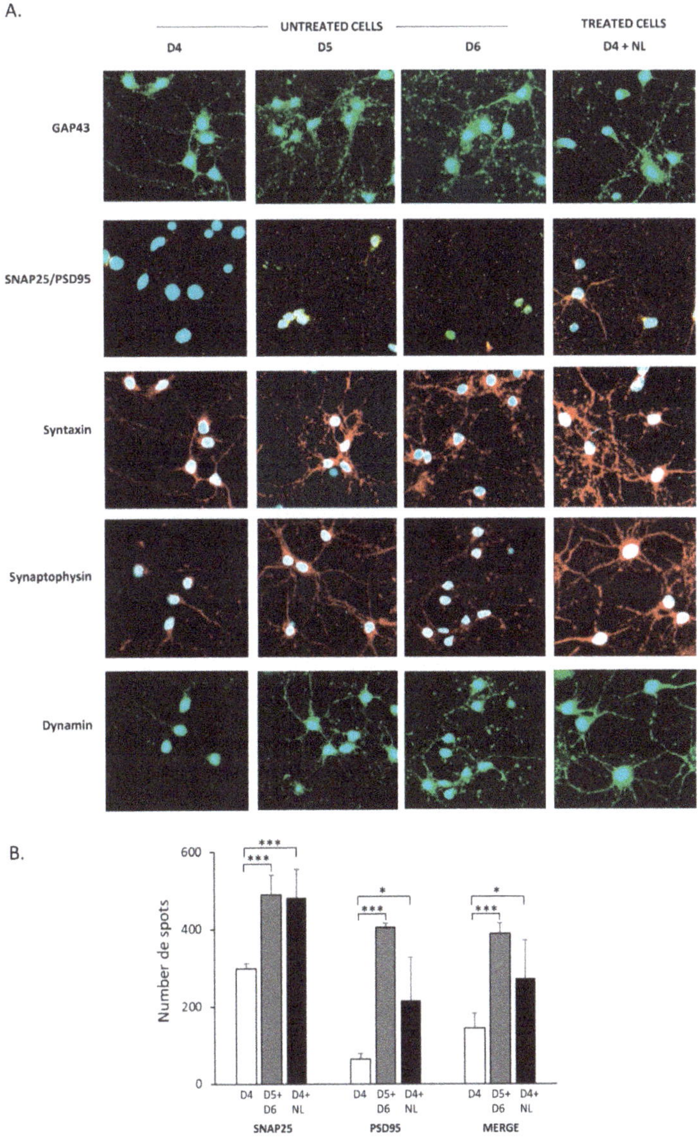

Figure 4. Cell localization of synaptic markers in primary cultures of cortical neurons treated with fish nanoliposomes (NL). (**A**). Immunofluorescence was used to detect different synaptic markers in primary cultures of rat embryo cortical neurons at the indicated times (D = days in vitro); D4 + NL are cells incubated 24 h with 10 µg/mL NL between D3 and D4; D4, D5, and D6 are control cells incubated in the absence of NL and recovered on D4, D5, and D6. Representative images are shown here obtained using the confocal microscope (120× magnification, Fluoview Fv10i, Olympus). (**B**). Image analysis of SNAP24/PSD95 labeling. The number of labeled spots of SNAP25 (red), PSD95 (green) and SNAP25 + PSD95 together (merge, orange), indicating colocalization are indicated for untreated cells on D4 (open bar, n = 4), on D5 and D6 (combined data shown as gray bar, n = 3), and for NL-treated cells on D4 (solid bar, n = 8). Statistically significant differences are shown as compared to the untreated cells (D4) for the corresponding label measured (* $p < 0.05$, *** $p < 0.001$).

The presence of syntaxin, as part of the SNARE complex located at cell membrane synaptic terminals, was detected in neurons, appearing to be transported along the neuronal extensions. Synaptophysin, which is part of a complex with synaptobrevin and is important in neuronal development, is localized around the cellular body and along the axons on D4. While syntaxin labeling was already granular on D5, that of synaptophysin remained detectable along the axons, which may be due to the different roles and functional localizations. On D6, syntaxin labeling was found around the cellular body, which could indicate the continuous synthesis of this protein. Labeling of dynamin I, a GTPase that is involved in synaptic vesicle recycling, was very similar to that of synaptophysin. In NL-treated cells, syntaxin, synaptophysin and dynamin labeling profiles were very similar to those of D5 and D6, detected on both axons and around the cellular bodies.

Embryonic cortical neuron development in vitro proceeds through several stages that are identified by morphological changes that occur during maturation. Neurons establish distinct compartments that initially form as neuritis as they grow and differentiate, which become axons, and finally lead to the formation of synaptic contacts through dendritic spines and axon terminals to establish the neural network [22]. Image analysis of labeled cells by immunofluorescence revealed the different structural and morphological changes that occur between D4 and D6 of culture consistent with neuronal development and differentiation, including neurite outgrowth and synaptogenesis, as suggested by the tendencies that were observed in the immunoblots. Preliminary data indicate that the presence of NL may also activate cell survival pathways (Poerio et al, unpublished data), which suggests the potential neuroprotective properties of these NL. In summary, these results indicate that the presence of NL accelerates the maturation processes of embryonic rat cortical neurons in primary culture.

3. Materials and Methods

Salmon lecithin was obtained by enzymatic hydrolysis in our laboratory, as described before [23]. Lipidic fractions were extracted by a low temperature enzymatic process that is solvent-free. The following materials were used in the present study: acetonitrile and diethyl ether (Sigma-Aldrich, Lyon, France), boron trifluoride-methanol (BF3) (Supelco, Bellfonte, PA, USA), chloroform (VWR-Prolabo, Milan, Italy), hexane, methanol, and formic acid (Carlo-Erba, Peypin, France), and ammoniac (Merck KGaA, Darmstadt, Germany). All of the organic solvents used were analytical grade reagents.

3.1. Fatty Acids Composition

Fatty acid methyl esters (FAMEs) from salmon lecithin were prepared as described by Ackman (1998) [24]. Subsequently, FAMEs were analyzed while using a Shimadzu 2010 gas chromatography (Shimadzu, Marne-la-Vallée, France) system that was equipped with a flame-ionization detector. FAME was injected into a fused silica capillary column (60 m, 0.25 mm i.d. × 0.20 μm film thicknesses, SPTM2380 Supelco, Bellfonte, PA, USA). Injector and detector temperatures were settled at 250 °C. The column temperature was fixed initially at 120 °C for 3 min., then raised to 180 °C at a rate of 2 °C $min.^{-1}$, and maintained at 220 °C for 25 min. Individual fatty acids were identified while using standard mixtures (PUFA1 from a marine source and PUFA2 from a vegetable source; Supelco, Sigma-Aldrich, Bellefonte, PA, USA). The results are shown as mean ± SD of triplicate analyses.

3.2. Lipid Classes

The lipid classes of different lipid fractions from salmon lecithin were determined while using the Iatroscan MK-5 TLC-FID (Iatron Laboratories Inc., Tokyo, Japan). The measurement was performed according to the protocol that is described in detail in our previous paper [25]. Two migrations were done to determine the proportion of neutral and polar lipid fractions. All of the standards were purchased from Sigma (Sigma– Aldrich Chemie GmbH, Munich, Germany). Area percentages of each pic are presented as the mean ± SD of three repetitions.

3.3. Preparation of Nanoliposomes

Salmon lecithin was extracted by a controlled enzymatic procedure, according to the Linder et al. Patent [14] that was slightly modified. The use of a protease, namely Alcalase 2.4L (Novo Nordisk, Bagsvaerd, Denmark), lead to recovering most of the lipid fraction after a controlled hydrolysis degree by the pH-stat method [26]. The protease was inactivated by heating at 90 °C during 15 min. before a centrifugation step (85 °C, 15 min. 4000× *g*). A freeze-dried step of the substrate, containing the lipid and protein fractions, was done, and acetone at −18 °C was added to separate the lecithin and neutral lipids, according to Hasan et al. [27].

One gram of lecithin was dissolved in ethanol, and then a thin lipid film was formed on the wall of the flask by means of a Rotavapor (Laborita 4000 Heidolph, UK) and by completely evaporating the organic solvent under vacuum, followed by hydration with 49 mL of distilled water, and the suspension was agitated for 5 h under nitrogen. The samples were then sonicated (sonicator probe, Sonics & Materials Inc., CT, USA) at 40 KHz and 40% of full power for 360 s (1 s on, 1 s off) to obtain a homogeneous solution. The liposome samples were stored in glass bottles in the dark at 4 °C.

3.4. Liposome Size and Electrophoretic Mobility Measurements

The mean size and electrophoretic mobility of liposomes were measured by dynamic light scattering (DLS) while using a Malvern Zetasizer Nano ZS (Malvern Instruments Ltd, UK). The samples were diluted (1:200) with ultrapure distilled water prior to measuring size and electrophoretic mobility. The size distribution of particle as well as the dispersed particles electrophoretic mobility was measured to evaluate the surface net charge around droplets. Measurements were made at 25 °C with a fixed scattering angle of 173°, the refractive index (RI) at 1.471, and absorbance at 0.01. The presented sizes are the z-average mean (dz) for the liposomal hydrodynamic diameter (nm). The measurements of electrophoretic mobility were performed in standard capillary electrophoresis cells that were equipped with gold electrodes at the same temperature. At least three independent measurements were performed for each condition.

3.5. Stability of Nanoliposomes

The nanoliposomes were stored in a drying-cupboard at 37 °C for 30 days. Mean particle size, electrophoretic mobility, and polydispersity index of all formulations were analyzed every three days. The same protocol described previously was used for each analysis.

3.6. Transmission Electron Microscopy (TEM)

Nanoliposomes were negatively stained according to the protocol of Colas et al. (2007) [28] and then visualized on TEM. Briefly, the samples were diluted 25-fold with distilled water to reduce the concentration of the particles. The same volume of the diluted solution was mixed with an aqueous solution of ammonium molybdate (2%) as a negative staining agent. The samples were examined using a Philips CM20 Transmission Electron Microscope (Philips, Dresden, Germany) associated with an Olympus TEM CCD camera after 3 min. incubation at room temperature and 5 min. incubation on a copper mesh coated with carbon.

3.7. Atomic Force Microscopy Imaging

An Image of the supported lipid bilayers (SLBs) was acquired on a Bruker AFM Dimension FastScan (Bruker, Billerica, MA, USA) with NPG tips (Bruker, Billerica, MA, USA) with a spring constant of about 0.32 N/m (manufacturer data). An image was obtained at room temperature in Peak Force QNM mode, shortly after SLB formation. An image of 5 µm size was acquired at least for two different samples and two different areas per sample. Images were analyzed using Nanoscope Analysis (v140r2, Bruker, Billerica, MA, USA).

3.8. Membrane Fluidity of Nanoliposomes

The membrane fluidity of all samples was measured by fluorescence anisotropy. TMA–DPH was used as fluorescent probe, which is a compound that contains a cationic trimethylammonium (TMA) substitute that acts as a surface anchor to improve the localization of the fluorescent probe of membrane interiors, DPH. This measurement was carried out according to the method that was described by Maherani et al. [29]. Briefly, the solution of TMA–DPH (1 mM in ethanol) was added to the liposome suspension to reach a final concentration of 4 µM and 0.2 mg/mL for the probe and the lipid, respectively. The mixture was lightly stirred for at least 1 h at room temperature and protected from light. Subsequently, 180 µL of the solution was distributed into each well of a 96-well black microplate. The fluorescent probe was vertically and horizontally oriented in the lipid bilayer. The fluorescent intensity of the samples was measured with Tescan INFINITE 200R PRO that was equipped with fluorescent polarizers. The samples were excited at 360 nm and emission was recorded at 430 nm under constant stirring at 25 °C. The Magellan 7 software was used for data analysis. The polarization value (P) of TMA–DPH was calculated while using the following equation:

$$P = \frac{I_{||} - GI_{\perp}}{I_{||} + 2GI_{\perp}} \tag{1}$$

where $I_{||}$ is the fluorescent intensity parallel to the excitation plane, $I_{\perp}$ is the fluorescent intensity perpendicular to the excitation plane, and G is the factor that accounts for transmission efficiency. Membrane fluidity is defined as 1/P. The results were presented as mean ± SD of triplicate analyses.

3.9. Cell Culture

Cell culture studies were performed at the Bioavailability–Bioactivity (Bio-DA) platform. The primary cultures of cortical neurons from rat fetuses (embryonic day 16–17) were prepared, as described previously [30]. Cells were plated at 10×10^4 cells/cm^2 onto plates or slides pre-coated with poly-L-ornithine (15 µg/mL for plates, 150 µg/mL for slides, Sigma), and culture in neuronal culture medium M2 composed of DMEM-F12 (Invitrogen, Illkirch, France) medium containing 0.5 µM insulin, 60 µM putrescine, 30 nM sodium selenite, 100 µM transferrin, 10 nM progesterone, and 0.1% (*w*/*v*) ovalbumin (Sigma). The cell cultures were maintained at 35 °C in 6% CO_2. The absence of glial fibrillary acidic protein (GFAP) following immunoblotting of cell lysates verified the purity of the neurons (data not shown). Neurons were incubated for up to five days, where day (D) 0 is the day of the preparation of the primary culture. The cells were incubated in the presence of NL on Day 3 for 24 h. Cytotoxicity of NL on cells was determined while using the MTT assay, as described previously [30].

3.10. Immunoblotting

On D4, D5, and D6, the cells were washed with ice-cold PBS (Invitrogen). Cell lysates were prepared using RIPA buffer, as previously described [30]. Equal volumes of cell lysates were applied to SDS-PAGE, and transferred to PVDF for immunoblotting [30]. The following antibodies were used at 1/1000 dilution: anti-synaptophysin (Cell Signaling 4329S), anti-SNAP25 (Santa Cruz sc-7538), anti-PSD95 (Cell Signaling, 2507S), anti-GAP43 (Cell signaling, 8945S), and anti-β-tubulin (Sigma T5201). Secondary antibodies, anti-mouse HRP-linked, and anti-rabbit HRP linked from Cell Signaling and anti-goat HRP-linked from Santa Cruz were used to detect the bands with Supersignal chemiluminescence ECL kit (Millipore, Molsheim, France). Gel images were obtained while using the Fusion Imaging System (Fusion Fx5; Vilber Lourmat, France), and densitometric analysis was performed using the freeware ImageJ.

3.11. Immunofluorescence Analyses

Cortical neurons cultured on slides were fixed in PBS containing 4% (*w*/*v*) paraformaldehyde for 30 min. at room temperature, and then permeabilized by incubation with Dulbecco's PBS (DPBS,

Invitrogen) containing 30% Cas-Block and 0.2% (v/v) Triton X-100. The cells were incubated with the primary antibody diluted in the same solution for 2 h at room temperature. After washing with DPBS, the slides were incubated in the dark in the presence of secondary antibodies that were conjugated to a fluorophore in DBPS. Cell nuclei were stained using 4,6-diamidino-2-phenylindole (DAPI). Images were obtained while using a confocal microscope (Fluoview Fv10i, Olympus, Rungis, France); analysis of SNAP25 and PSD95 spots was performed using ImageJ (particle analysis after subtraction of background; spots counted were visually verified using the outline option).

3.12. Statistical Analyses

All of the results are shown as the mean ± SD, unless otherwise indicated. The values for each set of cells that were treated with NL were calculated as % of control cells incubated in the absence of NL from the same experiment before statistical analysis. Statistical analysis was performed while using ANOVA followed by a Scheffe's post hoc test; significance was considered as $p < 0.05$.

4. Conclusions

In conclusion, these results demonstrate that the supplementation of NL in the culture media accelerate the development of neural networks in primary cultures of rat cortical neurons. Treatment with NL appeared to accelerate neuronal development, neurite outgrowth, and synaptogenesis, thus demonstrating a beneficial role of these pure NL on neuronal development by virtue of their intrinsic properties, which may also include neuroprotective effects. We would propose that, as multilayer vesicles with improved fusogenic properties, these PUFA-rich NL could represent a means towards providing cells with PUFA in a synergistic and efficient way, rather than directly using PUFA as fatty acids. Indeed, PUFA supplementation may be a necessary adjuvant for the aging brain to be more responsive to the therapeutic treatment of age-related neurodegenerative diseases, such as Alzheimer's disease [13]. Furthermore, nanoliposomes can also serve as a carrier of active molecules, thus serving a dual role in not only in providing the necessary lipid components for optimal membrane organization, but also in the delivery of active molecules for preventive or curative treatments of neurodegenerative diseases.

Author Contributions: Conceptualization, validation, formal analysis: C.M., E.A.-T., F.T.Y.; investigation: A.P., C.M., M.H., C.S.-H., E.P., M.L., methodology: M.H., C.S.-H., M.L., writing, review and editing: A.P., C.M., C.J.F.K., E.A.-T., F.T.Y.; supervision: C.M., E.A.-T., F.T.Y.

Funding: This research received no external funding.

Acknowledgments: The author acknowledge support of *NanoLipoN* by the "Impact Biomolecules" project of the "Lorraine d'Excellence" (Investissement d'avenir-ANR) and French Ministry of Higher Education, Research and Innovation, the scientific research pole A2F (Agronomy, food sciences and forestry) of the Université de Lorraine.

Conflicts of Interest: The authors declare no conflict of interest. The funders had no role in the design of the study; in the collection, analyses, or interpretation of data; in the writing of the manuscript, or in the decision to publish the results.

References

1. Calder, P.C. Omega-3 Fatty Acids and Inflammatory Processes. *Nutrients* **2010**, *2*, 355–374. [CrossRef] [PubMed]
2. Serini, S.; Calviello, G. Long-chain omega-3 fatty acids and cancer: Any cause for concern? *Curr. Opin. Clin. Nutr. Metab. Care* **2018**, *21*, 83–89. [CrossRef] [PubMed]
3. Kitajka, K.; Sinclair, A.J.; Weisinger, R.S.; Weisinger, H.S.; Mathai, M.; Jayasooriya, A.P.; Halver, J.E.; Puskas, L.G. Effects of dietary omega-3 polyunsaturated fatty acids on brain gene expression. *Proc. Natl. Acad. Sci. USA* **2004**, *101*, 10931–10936. [CrossRef] [PubMed]
4. Guirland, C.; Zheng, J.Q. Membrane Lipid Rafts and Their Role in Axon Guidance. In *Axon Growth and Guidance*; Bagnard, D., Ed.; Springer: New York, NY, USA, 2007; Volume 621, pp. 144–154. ISBN 978-0-387-76714-7.

5. Cao, D.; Xue, R.; Xu, J.; Liu, Z. Effects of docosahexaenoic acid on the survival and neurite outgrowth of rat cortical neurons in primary cultures. *J. Nutr. Biochem.* **2005**, *16*, 538–546. [CrossRef] [PubMed]
6. Tabernero, A.; Lavado, E.M.; Granda, B.; Velasco, A.; Medina, J.M. Neuronal differentiation is triggered by oleic acid synthesized and released by astrocytes: Oleic acid induces neuronal differentiation. *J. Neurochem.* **2008**, *79*, 606–616. [CrossRef] [PubMed]
7. Kawakita, E.; Hashimoto, M.; Shido, O. Docosahexaenoic acid promotes neurogenesis in vitro and in vivo. *Neuroscience* **2006**, *139*, 991–997. [CrossRef] [PubMed]
8. Sakamoto, T.; Cansev, M.; Wurtman, R.J. Oral supplementation with docosahexaenoic acid and uridine-5′-monophosphate increases dendritic spine density in adult gerbil hippocampus. *Brain Res.* **2007**, *1182*, 50–59. [CrossRef] [PubMed]
9. Innis, S.M. Dietary (n-3) Fatty Acids and Brain Development. *J. Nutr.* **2007**, *137*, 855–859. [CrossRef]
10. Shindou, H.; Koso, H.; Sasaki, J.; Nakanishi, H.; Sagara, H.; Nakagawa, K.M.; Takahashi, Y.; Hishikawa, D.; Iizuka-Hishikawa, Y.; Tokumasu, F.; et al. Docosahexaenoic acid preserves visual function by maintaining correct disc morphology in retinal photoreceptor cells. *J. Biol. Chem.* **2017**, *292*, 12054–12064. [CrossRef]
11. Li, D.; Wahlqvist, M.L.; Sinclair, A.J. Advances in n-3 polyunsaturated fatty acid nutrition. *Asia Pac. J. Clin. Nutr.* **2019**, *28*, 1–5.
12. Hishikawa, D.; Valentine, W.J.; Iizuka-Hishikawa, Y.; Shindou, H.; Shimizu, T. Metabolism and functions of docosahexaenoic acid-containing membrane glycerophospholipids. *FEBS Lett.* **2017**, *591*, 2730–2744. [CrossRef] [PubMed]
13. Colin, J.; Thomas, M.H.; Gregory-Pauron, L.; Pinçon, A.; Lanhers, M.C.; Corbier, C.; Claudepierre, T.; Yen, F.T.; Oster, T.; Malaplate-Armand, C. Maintenance of membrane organization in the aging mouse brain as the determining factor for preventing receptor dysfunction and for improving response to anti-Alzheimer treatments. *Neurobiol. Aging* **2017**, *54*, 84–93. [CrossRef] [PubMed]
14. Linder, M.; Fanni, J.; Parmentier, M.; Regnault, P. Procédé d'extraction d'huile par voie enzymatique et obtention d'hydrolysats protéiques à fonctionnalités dirigées. *Brev. FR* **2002**, *2*, 703.
15. Maherani, B.; Arab-Tehrany, E.; Mozafari, M.R.; Gaiani, C.; Linder, M. Liposomes: A Review of Manufacturing Techniques and Targeting Strategies. *Curr. Nanosci.* **2011**, *7*, 436–452. [CrossRef]
16. Arab Tehrany, E.; Kahn, C.J.F.; Baravian, C.; Maherani, B.; Belhaj, N.; Wang, X.; Linder, M. Elaboration and characterization of nanoliposome made of soya; rapeseed and salmon lecithins: Application to cell culture. *Colloids Surf. B Biointerfaces* **2012**, *95*, 75–81. [CrossRef] [PubMed]
17. Latifi, S.; Tamayol, A.; Habibey, R.; Sabzevari, R.; Kahn, C.; Geny, D.; Eftekharpour, E.; Annabi, N.; Blau, A.; Linder, M.; et al. Natural lecithin promotes neural network complexity and activity. *Sci. Rep.* **2016**, *6*, 25777. [CrossRef] [PubMed]
18. Benedet, J.A.; Umeda, H.; Shibamoto, T. Antioxidant Activity of Flavonoids Isolated from Young Green Barley Leaves toward Biological Lipid Samples. *J. Agric. Food Chem.* **2007**, *55*, 5499–5504. [CrossRef]
19. Chansiri, G.; Lyons, R.T.; Patel, M.V.; Hem, S.L. Effect of surface charge on the stability of oil/water emulsions during steam sterilization. *J. Pharm. Sci.* **1999**, *88*, 454–458. [CrossRef]
20. Belhaj, N.; Arab-Tehrany, E.; Linder, M. Oxidative kinetics of salmon oil in bulk and in nanoemulsion stabilized by marine lecithin. *Process Biochem.* **2010**, *45*, 187–195. [CrossRef]
21. Leekumjorn, S.; Cho, H.J.; Wu, Y.; Wright, N.T.; Sum, A.K.; Chan, C. The role of fatty acid unsaturation in minimizing biophysical changes on the structure and local effects of bilayer membranes. *Biochim. Biophys. Acta (BBA) Biomembr.* **2009**, *1788*, 1508–1516. [CrossRef]
22. Arimura, N.; Kaibuchi, K. Neuronal polarity: From extracellular signals to intracellular mechanisms. *Nat. Rev. Neurosci.* **2007**, *8*, 194–205. [CrossRef] [PubMed]
23. Linder, M.; Matouba, E.; Fanni, J.; Parmentier, M. Enrichment of salmon oil with n-3 PUFA by lipolysis, filtration and enzymatic re-esterification. *Eur. J. Lipid Sci. Technol.* **2002**, *104*, 455–462. [CrossRef]
24. Ackman, R.G. Remarks on official methods employing boron trifluoride in the preparation of methyl esters of the fatty acids of fish oils. *J. Am. Oil Chem. Soc.* **1998**, *75*, 541–545. [CrossRef]
25. Hasan, M.; Belhaj, N.; Benachour, H.; Barberi-Heyob, M.; Kahn, C.J.F.; Jabbari, E.; Linder, M.; Arab-Tehrany, E. Liposome encapsulation of curcumin: Physico-chemical characterizations and effects on MCF7 cancer cell proliferation. *Int. J. Pharm.* **2014**, *461*, 519–528. [CrossRef] [PubMed]
26. Gbogouri, G.A.; Linder, M.; Fanni, J.; Parmentier, M. Analysis of lipids extracted from salmon (Salmo salar) heads by commercial proteolytic enzymes. *Eur. J. Lipid Sci. Technol.* **2006**, *108*, 766–775. [CrossRef]

27. Hasan, M.; Ben Messaoud, G.; Michaux, F.; Tamayol, A.; Kahn, C.J.F.; Belhaj, N.; Linder, M.; Arab-Tehrany, E. Chitosan-coated liposomes encapsulating curcumin: Study of lipid–polysaccharide interactions and nanovesicle behavior. *RSC Adv.* **2016**, *6*, 45290–45304. [CrossRef]
28. Colas, J.C.; Shi, W.; Rao, V.M.; Omri, A.; Mozafari, M.R.; Singh, H. Microscopical investigations of nisin-loaded nanoliposomes prepared by Mozafari method and their bacterial targeting. *Micron* **2007**, *38*, 841–847. [CrossRef]
29. Maherani, B.; Arab-tehrany, E.; Kheirolomoom, A.; Reshetov, V.; Stebe, M.J.; Linder, M. Optimization and characterization of liposome formulation by mixture design. *Analyst* **2012**, *137*, 773–786. [CrossRef]
30. Colin, J.; Allouche, A.; Chauveau, F.; Corbier, C.; Pauron-Gregory, L.; Lanhers, M.C.; Claudepierre, T.; Yen, F.T.; Oster, T.; Malaplate-Armand, C. Improved Neuroprotection Provided by Drug Combination in Neurons Exposed to Cell-Derived Soluble Amyloid-β Peptide. *J. Alzheimer's Dis.* **2016**, *52*, 975–987. [CrossRef]

© 2019 by the authors. Licensee MDPI, Basel, Switzerland. This article is an open access article distributed under the terms and conditions of the Creative Commons Attribution (CC BY) license (http://creativecommons.org/licenses/by/4.0/).

marine drugs

MDPI

Article

Fucoidan-Stabilized Gold Nanoparticle-Mediated Biofilm Inhibition, Attenuation of Virulence and Motility Properties in *Pseudomonas aeruginosa* PAO1

Fazlurrahman Khan [1,†], Panchanathan Manivasagan [1,†], Jang-Won Lee [2], Dung Thuy Nguyen Pham [2], Junghwan Oh [1,3] and Young-Mog Kim [1,2,*]

1 Marine-Integrated Bionics Research Center, Pukyong National University, Busan 48513, Korea; fkhan055@pknu.ac.kr (F.K.); manimaribtech@gmail.com (P.M.); jungoh@pknu.ac.kr (J.O.)
2 Department of Food Science and Technology, Pukyong National University, Busan 48513, Korea; ananias93@naver.com (J.-W.L.); dungpham0495@gmail.com (D.T.N.P.)
3 Department of Biomedical Engineering, Pukyong National University, Busan 48513, Korea
* Correspondence: ymkim@pknu.ac.kr; Tel.: +82-51-629-5832
† These authors contributed equally to this work.

Received: 28 February 2019; Accepted: 29 March 2019; Published: 3 April 2019

Abstract: The emergence of antibiotic resistance in *Pseudomonas aeruginosa* due to biofilm formation has transformed this opportunistic pathogen into a life-threatening one. Biosynthesized nanoparticles are increasingly being recognized as an effective anti-biofilm strategy to counter *P. aeruginosa* biofilms. In the present study, gold nanoparticles (AuNPs) were biologically synthesized and stabilized using fucoidan, which is an active compound sourced from brown seaweed. Biosynthesized fucoidan-stabilized AuNPs (F-AuNPs) were subjected to characterization using UV-visible spectroscopy, Fourier transform infrared spectroscopy (FTIR), field emission transmission electron microscopy (FE-TEM), dynamic light scattering (DLS), and energy dispersive X-ray diffraction (EDX). The biosynthesized F-AuNPs were then evaluated for their inhibitory effects on *P. aeruginosa* bacterial growth, biofilm formation, virulence factor production, and bacterial motility. Overall, the activities of F-AuNPs towards *P. aeruginosa* were varied depending on their concentration. At minimum inhibitory concentration (MIC) (512 μg/mL) and at concentrations above MIC, F-AuNPs exerted antibacterial activity. In contrast, the sub-inhibitory concentration (sub-MIC) levels of F-AuNPs inhibited biofilm formation without affecting bacterial growth, and eradicated matured biofilm. The minimum biofilm inhibition concentration (MBIC) and minimum biofilm eradication concentration (MBEC) were identified as 128 μg/mL. Furthermore, sub-MICs of F-AuNPs also attenuated the production of several important virulence factors and impaired bacterial swarming, swimming, and twitching motilities. Findings from the present study provide important insights into the potential of F-AuNPs as an effective new drug for controlling *P. aeruginosa*-biofilm-related infections.

Keywords: antibiofilm; fucoidan; motility; nanoparticles; *Pseudomonas aeruginosa*; virulence factors

---

1. Introduction

The formation of biofilm by *Pseudomonas aeruginosa* contributes to its survival in adverse environmental conditions, defense against the host immune system, and resistance to antimicrobial compounds such as conventional antibiotics, resulting in extreme complications in preventing and eradicating this opportunistic pathogen from infected patients and medical facilities [1–4]. Apart from the formation of the biofilm matrix, several virulence factors are also produced, which further aid the bacteria in causing chronic infections [2,5]. With the rapid pace of emergence and spread of

P. aeruginosa with biofilm-forming ability, current anti-biofilm and anti-virulence approaches have mainly targeted the following: (1) attachment of planktonic cells, (2) cell-to-cell communication networks and regulatory systems, and (3) eradication of pre-existing matured biofilm structures [6,7]. Furthermore, these modern anti-biofilm approaches highly favor treatments which are bioactive, cost-effective, and less toxic [8–11].

Recently, nanomaterials have become popular, owing to their various physiochemical advantages resulting from their nano-scale size, such as high surface area to volume ratio, low toxicity, and high stability [12,13]. The gold nanoparticle (AuNP) possesses these properties, and is one of the commonly-used nanoparticles, with several applications in catalysis, electronics, nonlinear optics, drug delivery, and disease diagnosis in medical fields [14–18]. In comparison with chemical methods, which employ surfactants in the synthesis of this nanoparticle (NP), biological methods employing 'green' materials such as biopolymers provide significant benefits in terms of reducing NP aggregation, production costs, simple isolation, and environmental friendliness [19–22]. The morphology regarding size, shape, and crystalline properties, as well as the biocompatibility and stability of biosynthesized AuNP, are also significantly improved [23]. Although several biological systems are currently used to synthesize NPs, edible marine algae are highly preferred due to their widespread availability and richness in bioactive compounds, which could act as active stabilizing and reducing agents [24]. The bioactive compound fucoidan used in the present study is a fucose-rich and sulfated polysaccharide present in diverse brown seaweed species. Fucoidan has been extensively utilized as an important antitumor, antibacterial, antiviral, anti-inflammatory, and antioxidant agent owing to its biodegradable, biocompatible, non-toxic, and water-soluble characteristics [25,26]. In efforts to overcome antibiotic resistance in bacteria, previous studies have shown that both biosynthesized AuNPs and fucoidan-synthesized-NPs exhibit high antibacterial activity towards a variety of bacteria [27–29]. Therefore, the present study aimed to synthesize and characterize fucoidan-stabilized gold nanoparticles (F-AuNPs), as well as to evaluate their application as a potential anti-biofilm and anti-virulence drug against *P. aeruginosa*.

2. Materials and Methods

2.1. Bacterial Strains, Culture Media, Chemicals, and Growth Conditions

The study was performed using *P. aeruginosa* PAO1 KCTC 1637 obtained from Korean Collection for Type Cultures, Daejeon, Korea as the reference strain. The liquid and solid media used for the growth and cultivation of *P. aeruginosa* were tryptic soya broth (TSB; Difco Laboratory Inc., Detroit, MI, USA) and tryptic soya agar (TSA) plate. The pH of the media was adjusted to 7.2. Fucoidan ($\geq$95%) sourced from *Fucus vesiculosus*) and hydrogen tetrachloroaurate (III) were obtained from Sigma-Aldrich Co. (St. Louis, MO, USA). All the reagents and chemicals used in the present study were of analytical grade. The growth condition of *P. aeruginosa* was aerobic and the growth temperature was maintained at 35 °C throughout the experiment.

2.2. Synthesis and Characterization of F-AuNPs

The chemical synthesis and instrumental characterization of F-AuNPs were carried out according to the procedure described previously [30]. The F-AuNPs were synthesized by mixing fucoidan (5.0 mg) into a solution of $HAuCl_4.3H_2O$ (1×10^{-4} M) at the temperature of 80 °C for 30 min under continuous stirring. The color change of the solution into dark ruby red was considered as an initial indicator of F-AuNP formation. Furthermore, F-AuNP formation was also monitored by measuring absorbance spectra using DU-530 spectrophotometer (Beckman Coulter, Fullerton, CA, USA). The resulting solution was centrifuged (12,000$\times$ g for 30 min), followed by washing with deionized water. The unreacted gold was dispersed into water and dialyzed using a 12,000 Da molecular weight cut-off dialysis tube for 24 h at room temperature in order to remove it from the mixture.

Different physiochemical properties, including size, morphology, stability and composition, of newly synthesized F-AuNPs were characterized using various instruments and methods. The morphology of F-AuNPs was determined using field emission transmission electron microscopy (FETEM) JEM-2100F (JEOL Ltd., Tokyo, Japan). The particle size of the F-AuNPs was measured using dynamic light scattering (DLS) with the help of an electrophoretic light scattering spectrophotometer (ELS-800, OTSUKA Electronic Co., Ltd., Osaka, Japan). The room temperature and fixed angle (90°) in the spectrophotometer were set for scattering and measuring the spectra. The elemental composition of F-AuNPs was determined using energy dispersive X-ray diffraction (EDX; Hitachi, S-2400, Tokyo, Japan). The functional groups of each component present in F-AuNPs were determined by Fourier transform infrared spectroscopy (FTIR). The FTIR of F-AuNPs was carried out in a diffuse reflectance mode with a range of wavelengths from 4000 to 400 cm^{-1}. Finally, the crystalline structure of the F-AuNPs was examined using X-ray diffraction (XRD; X'Pert-MPD system, Philips, Almelo, The Netherlands).

2.3. Determination of Minimum Inhibitory Concentrations of F-AuNPs and Growth of P. aeruginosa Cells in the Presence of F-AuNPs

Minimum inhibitory concentration (MIC) was defined as the complete inhibition of bacterial growth with no visible turbidity by the action of F-AuNPs at the lowest concentration. Determination of MIC of F-AuNPs against *P. aeruginosa* PAO1 followed the guidelines from the Clinical and Laboratory Standards Institute (CLSI), 2016 [31]. Briefly, the cell culture of *P. aeruginosa* was grown overnight and then added to a 96 well microtiter plate. Two-fold serial diluted concentrations of F-AuNPs (1024 to 32 μg/mL) (10 mg/mL stock prepared in sterilized distilled water) were added to the plate. The plate was then incubated at 35 °C for 24 h under orbital agitation (120 rpm) in the microtiter plate reader (BioTek, Winooski, VT, USA). After incubation, the optical density (OD) of the grown bacterial cells at 600 nm was measured. Similarly, the growth property of *P. aeruginosa* in the presence of different concentrations of F-AuNPs was also measured using a similar method to that discussed above. The only difference was the measurement of OD of the grown cells, which was monitored at time intervals of every 2 h in the microplate reader. Both MIC and growth assays were performed in triplicate.

2.4. Crystal Violet Staining Method for the Biofilm Assays

The crystal violet method was used for the quantitative estimation of biofilm formation in the presence and absence of the compound, following the procedure described earlier [8]. The minimum concentration of F-AuNP that inhibited *P. aeruginosa* biofilm formation (minimum biofilm inhibition concentration: MBIC) was also determined. Briefly, the *P. aeruginosa* cell culture (grown overnight in TSB) was diluted to a turbidity of 0.05 at 600 nm, and then treated with different concentrations of F-AuNPs (ranging from 16 to 256 μg/mL). After 24 h of incubation at 35 °C, the planktonic cells were discarded, while the attached cells were washed three times with water and then stained with crystal violet (0.1%). After 20 min of incubation, the crystal violet dye was discarded and the attached cells were again washed thrice with water. The adhered cells were re-suspended with 95% ethyl alcohol followed by the OD determination at the wavelength of 570 nm. Simultaneously, the *P. aeruginosa* growth property in the presence of F-AuNPs was also determined in static conditions by measuring the OD at 600 nm. For both biofilm and growth analysis, each concentration of F-AuNPs was repeated three times.

Crystal violet assay was also performed to investigate the eradication effect of F-AuNPs on pre-formed matured *P. aeruginosa* biofilm. The minimum concentration at which F-AuNPs exhibited eradication effect on pre-formed matured biofilm (minimum biofilm eradication concentration: MBEC) was also determined. The first step was to allow the formation of biofilm for 24 h by incubating *P. aeruginosa* in TSB without F-AuNPs in the 96 well microtiter plate, as discussed earlier [8]. Briefly, after incubation, the planktonic cells were removed and attached biofilm cells were washed thrice with fresh TSB media. The established biofilm cells were treated with different concentrations of F-AuNPs (16–256 μg/mL) in fresh TSB media. The microtiter plate was then incubated at 35 °C for 24 h, and quantified for biofilm cells after staining with 0.1% crystal violet following the procedure described in detail in the biofilm assay section. The experiment was performed in triplicate.

2.5. Microscopic Examination of the Biofilm Formed Cells

Visualization of the cell morphology and biofilm architecture was carried out by using microscopes such as the scanning electron microscopy (SEM) and fluorescence microscopy. The procedure used for the SEM sample preparation was adopted as discussed earlier [8,32]. Briefly, the cell culture was allowed to grow in TSB media on the surface of nylon membranes (0.5 × 0.5 cm) placed in a 24 well microtiter plate in the presence and absence of F-AuNPs (256 μg/mL). The 24 well microtiter plate was incubated for 24 h at 35 °C. The biofilm cells were directly fixed by formaldehyde and glutaraldehyde and kept at 4 °C temperature overnight. After removing the unattached cells, the fixed cells were washed three times with phosphate buffer saline (PBS; pH 7.4), followed by dehydration in increasing concentrations of ethyl alcohol at 50, 70, 80, 90, 95 and 100%. The adhered cells on the nylon membrane were freeze-dried using a freeze dryer machine (FD8518, ilShinBiobase Co., Ltd., Dongducheon, Korea), followed by fixation to SEM stubs. The affixed membrane was further coated with gold for 120 s with the help of an ion-sputter (E-1010, Hitachi, Tokyo, Japan). The prepared samples were visualized for the study of cell morphology using JSM-6490LV (JEOL, Tokyo, Japan) at the magnification of ×5000 and voltage of 15 kV. Similarly, the biofilm architecture was also observed using a Leica DMI300B fluorescence microscope at a magnification value of ×40, as described earlier [8]. However, for the fluorescence microscope, (Leica Microsystems, Wetzlar, Germany), the sample was prepared on the glass pieces and was placed in a 6 well microtiter plate. Before visualization of the cells, the biofilm cells on the surface of glass pieces were washed three times with PBS, followed by staining with 10 μg/mL working concentration of acridine orange dye. The stained cells were again washed with PBS and observed under a fluorescence microscope.

2.6. Determination of Hemolytic and Protease Activities

The hemolytic property of *P. aeruginosa* in the presence of F-AuNPs was determined using the red blood cells (RBCs) following the procedure described previously [8,33]. Briefly, the *P. aeruginosa* cell culture was grown overnight and was then supplemented with different concentrations of F-AuNPs (ranging from 32 to 256 μg/mL) in a 96 well microtiter plate, followed by incubation at 35 °C for 12 h in shaking condition (120 rpm). The treated and non-treated bacterial cell cultures (50 μL) were mixed with diluted RBCs. A negative control was prepared by mixing the F-AuNPs (256 μg/mL) with diluted RBCs. The bacterial cell culture mixed with RBCs was incubated at 35 °C for 1 h in shaking incubator (120 rpm). The mixture was centrifuged at 16,600× *g* for 10 min, and the OD of supernatant containing hemolyzed RBCs was determined by measuring at 543 nm. The experiment was performed in triplicate.

The production and activity of the protease enzyme from *P. aeruginosa* were tested in the presence and absence of F-AuNPs on casein agar plate, as described in the previous protocol [8,33]. The casein agar plate was prepared by mixing casein powder (10%) into autoclaved Bacto agar (2%) in 100 mL distilled water. The filtered supernatant (10 μL), which was obtained from the overnight grown *P. aeruginosa* cell culture (initial turbidity of 0.05 at 600 nm) in the presence of different concentrations of F-AuNPs (16–256 μg/mL), was loaded in the holes of a casein agar plate. After 24 h of incubation at 35 °C temperature, diameters (cm) of the clear zones around the holes were measured to determine the inhibition of F-AuNPs to bacterial protease activity. Analysis of protease activity was performed in two replicates using two independent cultures.

2.7. Quantitative Estimation of Virulence Factor Production

The impact of F-AuNPs on the production of several virulence factors from *P. aeruginosa*, such as pyocyanin, pyoverdine, and rhamnolipid, was examined in the present study. The methodology of the assays of each virulence factor production was adopted from the previous protocol [8,33]. For the estimation of virulence factors production such as rhamnolipid and pyocyanin, TSB media was used, whereas for the estimation of siderophore-like pyoverdine, iron-limited minimal salt media (MSM) along with 2% sodium succinate (SS) was used. The cell culture (5 mL) of *P. aeruginosa* (initial turbidity of 0.05 at 600 nm) grown overnight was incubated with various concentrations of F-AuNPs in test tubes containing either TSB (for pyocyanin and rhamnolipid assays) or MSM + 2% SS (for pyoverdine assays), and was incubated under shaking condition at 35 °C for 12 h. After 12 h of incubation, for the pyocyanin estimation, the cell-free supernatant was mixed with chloroform for the extraction of green-blue colored pigment, as described in detail in a previous study [34]. The collected blue-green colored sample turned a pink color when it was acidified with HCl (0.2N), and was then quantified by measuring the OD at 520 nm. The rhamnolipid from the supernatant was extracted using an organic solvent i.e., diethyl ether, and the quantification was carried out by orcinol colorimetric method following the detailed procedure described earlier [35]. The total content of rhamnolipid was quantified by measuring the OD at 421 nm. For the estimation of pyoverdine, the supernatant was directly quantified by the OD at 405 nm, as discussed earlier [36]. All experiments were performed in triplicate.

2.8. Assays of Motility Properties of P. aeruginosa

The effect of F-AuNPs at sub-MICs on different types of motility such as swarming, swimming, and twitching of *P. aeruginosa* was tested as described previously [33,37]. Two sub-MIC levels were selected for all motility assays (32 μg/mL and 256 μg/mL). To check the swarming motility, the Bacto agar (0.4%) plate prepared in Luria Britani (LB) broth containing casamino acid (0.5%) and glucose (0.5%) was used. For swimming motility, the Bacto agar (0.3%) was also used, however, it was prepared in distilled water along with 1% NaCl and 0.25% tryptone. Each plate was also supplemented with different concentrations of F-AuNPs. The *P. aeruginosa* cell culture (10 μL) was grown overnight and then placed on the center of swarming and swimming agar plates, followed by incubation at 35 °C for 24 h. The experiment was repeated two times. The two movements were demonstrated by the zone of cell travelling on the agar after incubation for 24 h. The assay for twitching motility was slightly different compared to the swarming and swimming motilities, and was performed following the protocol described previously. For the twitching motility assay, the overnight grown cell culture (10 μL) was firstly stubbed a thin layer in the center of Petri dishes, followed by pouring of Bacto agar (1.5%) prepared in LB supplemented with glucose (30 mM) and casamino acid (0.2%). After 24 h of incubation, the total agar content was discarded and the cells attached to the surface of the plate were stained with crystal violet (0.1%), then were washed with water and air dried. The crystal violet stained area of the cells is the indicator of twitching motility. The assay of twitching motilities was also performed in replicates.

2.9. Statistical Analysis

All graphs in the present study were constructed using GraphPad Prism 7.0 (GraphPad Software Inc., San Diego, CA, USA). All data in the present study were obtained from one-way ANOVA and are represented as mean ± standard deviation.

3. Results

3.1. Synthesis and Characterization of F-AuNPs

F-AuNPs were synthesized by the reduction of ionic gold (Au^{3+}) in a chloroauric acid solution with the help of fucoidan. Fucoidan, which is a negatively charged polymer derived mainly from marine seaweed, acts as a stabilizing and reducing agent. The initial indication and confirmation of F-AuNP synthesis were established by checking the appearance of ruby red color, as well as by measuring absorbance spectra using UV-visible spectrophotometry (Figure 1A). The maximum absorbance peak was found at 570 nm, which was almost coincident with the peak obtained (566 nm) during the synthesis of AuNPs by Manivasagan et al. [30].

The morphology of the synthesized F-AuNPs was characterized using field emission transmission electron microscopy (FE-TEM) (Figure 1B). The distribution of F-AuNP sizes was also determined using dynamic light scattering (DLS) (Figure 1C). The results of FE-TEM and DLS showed that F-AuNPs were spherical in shape and ranged in size from 15 to 119 nm; the average size of the particles was ~53 nm (Figure 1C). Furthermore, chemical interactions between different functional groups present in the polymeric fucoidan and AuNPs were determined by Fourier transform infrared spectroscopy (FTIR). The FTIR results (Figure 1D) demonstrated that fucoidan showed characteristic peaks at 845 cm^{-1} and 1159–1260 cm^{-1}, corresponding to the S=O asymmetric stretching and C–O–S stretching of sulfate groups, respectively. The bands in the spectra at 1633 cm^{-1} and 1637 cm^{-1} in both fucoidan and F-AuNPs correspond to the N–H bending of amines. Similarly, the bands at 3441 cm^{-1} and 3444 cm^{-1} in both fucoidan and F-AuNPs spectra correspond to the O–H stretching of alcohol, whereas the bands at 2932 cm^{-1} and 2933 cm^{-1} spectra correspond to the C–H stretching of alkanes. Figure 1E represents the UV-visible absorbance spectra of freshly prepared and one-month old F-AuNPs.

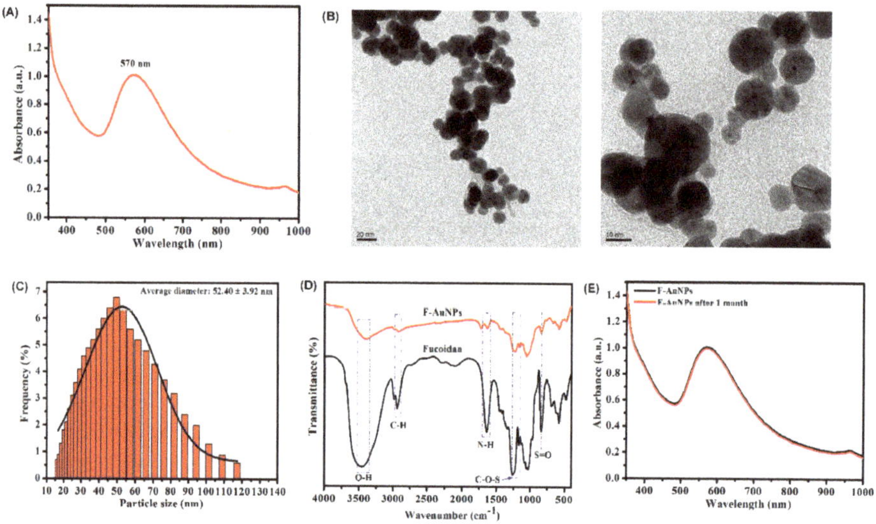

Figure 1. Synthesis and characterization of fucoidan-stabilized gold nanoparticles (F-AuNPs). (**A**) UV-visible-absorbance spectra of F-AuNPs, (**B**) field emission transmission electron microscopy (FE-TEM) image of F-AuNPs, (**C**) dynamic light scattering (DLS) histogram of particle size distribution, and (**D**) Fourier transform infrared spectroscopy (FTIR) spectrum of F-AuNPs, and (**E**) UV-visible absorbance spectra of the freshly synthesized and one-month old F-AuNPs.

Different diffraction peaks in Figure 2A as observed by X-ray diffraction (XRD) indicated the crystalline nature of the F-AuNPs. The value of each peak in the XRD patterns, as observed at 38.13°, 44.43°, 64.66°, and 77.66°, showed the reflection of a crystalline metallic gold particle with values of (111), (200), (220), and (311), respectively (Figure 2A). The above results concur with the XRD patterns of gold nanoparticles reported previously [30,38]. Finally, we also determined the presence of gold as a major constituent in the F-AuNPs by energy dispersive X-ray diffraction (EDX) (Figure 2B). Among the major peaks in the spectrum, the peak appearing at 2.2 keV is a characteristic peak of gold present in the F-AuNPs, whereas the peak at 8.2 keV is that of Cu available from the grid used. The elemental composition of F-AuNPs has also been analyzed previously using EDX with similar peak profiles [30].

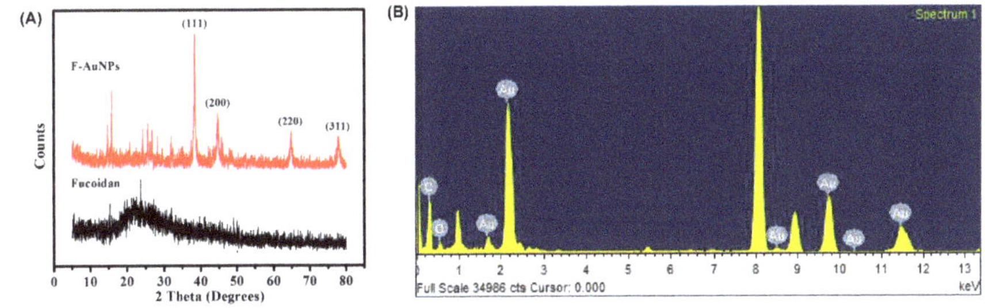

Figure 2. (**A**) The X-ray diffraction (XRD) pattern of F-AuNPs and (**B**) X-ray spectrum of the F-AuNPs.

3.2. *Determination of Minimum Inhibitory Concentration (MIC) of F-AuNPs and Growth Properties of P. aeruginosa in the Presence of F-AuNPs*

Before investigating the start of biofilm inhibition and the virulence attenuating properties of synthesized F-AuNPs, the MIC was determined using different concentrations (ranging from 16–1024 µg/mL) of F-AuNPs. The MIC was determined by measuring the OD of bacterial cell growth at 600 nm after 24 h of incubation under shaking conditions (120 rpm). Figure 3A clearly shows a significant inhibition of *P. aeruginosa* growth at 512 and 1024 µg/mL of F-AuNPs. Hence, based on the above results, the MIC value of F-AuNPs for *P. aeruginosa* was assigned as 512 µg/mL (Figure 3A). The growth profile of *P. aeruginosa* in the presence of different concentrations (ranging from 16–1024 µg/mL) of F-AuNPs was also determined by measuring the OD_{600} at 2 h time intervals up to 24 h during incubation under agitation (120 rpm). The growth pattern of *P. aeruginosa* in the presence of each subinhibitory concentration (sub-MIC) of F-AuNPs was found to be similar to the control (Figure 3B). Thus, based on the above results, it is evident that F-AuNPs at sub-MIC levels caused a bactericidal effect to bacterial cells throughout the experiment.

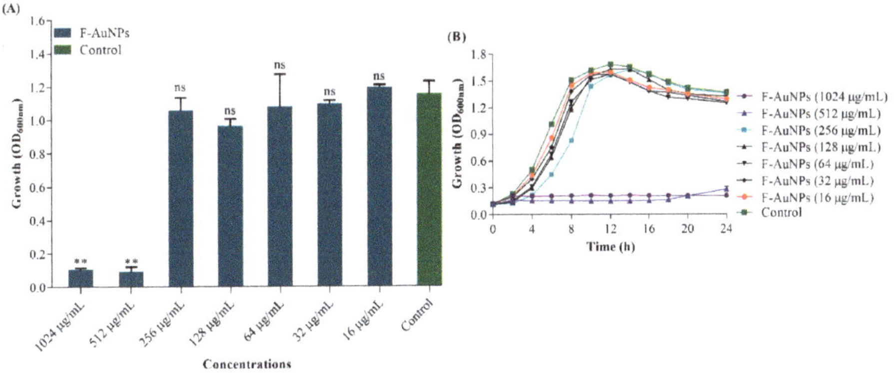

Figure 3. (**A**) Determination of minimum inhibitory concentration of F-AuNPs at 600 nm wavelength and (**B**) growth curve analysis of *P. aeruginosa* in the presence of different concentrations of F-AuNPs at every 2 h time interval the OD at 600 nm wavelength. The experiments were performed in triplicate with two independent cultures. ** $p < 0.01$ considered as significant and ns indicates non-significant as compared to the control (not treated by F-AuNPs).

3.3. *Biofilm Inhibition Properties of F-AuNPs*

The anti-biofilm activity of F-AuNPs against *P. aeruginosa* was determined by crystal violet staining assays and OD measurements at 570 nm. As shown in Figure 4A, the sub-MIC levels of F-AuNPs when incubated with *P. aeruginosa* cells cultured overnight (initial turbidity of 0.05 at 600 nm) exhibited concentration-dependent biofilm inhibition. In comparison to the non-treated control, F-AuNPs at

128 μg/mL and 256 μg/mL concentrations showed approximately 86% and 84% biofilm inhibition, respectively. The minimum biofilm inhibitory concentration (MBIC) of F-AuNPs for *P. aeruginosa* was therefore assigned as 128 μg/mL (Figure 4A). The growth property of *P. aeruginosa* in the presence of sub-MIC of F-AuNPs was also checked by measuring the OD at 600 nm (Figure 4B). The results showed that there were no bactericidal effects at each concentration of F-AuNPs when incubated under static conditions (without shaking).

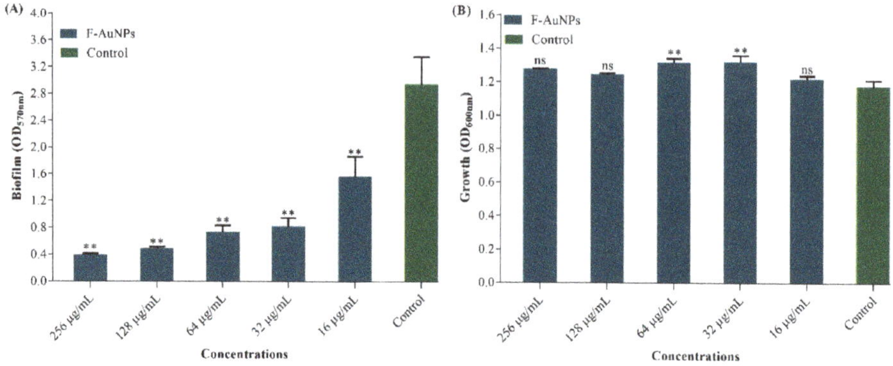

Figure 4. Biofilm inhibition properties of different concentration of F-AuNPs. (**A**) Biofilm assays and (**B**) growth analysis of *Pseudomonas aeruginosa*. The experiment was repeated three times for each concentration of F-AuNPs. ** $p < 0.01$ considered as significant and ns indicates non-significant as compared to the control (not treated by F-AuNPs).

Furthermore, the effects of F-AuNPs on cell morphology as well as biofilm architecture were examined using a scanning electron microscope (SEM) and fluorescence microscopy for the 24 h treated and non-treated cells (Figure 5). The results of SEM analysis of the cell culture incubated along with F-AuNPs (256 μg/mL) for 24 h showed a lack of cells attached to the nylon surface, whereas the cell culture not treated with F-AuNPs showed dense layers of sessile cells adhered to the nylon surface (Figure 5A). The results obtained from fluorescence microscopy using acridine orange dye (10 μg/mL) showed a significant reduction of green fluorescence in the presence of F-AuNPs (256 μg/mL), while non-treated cells (control) exhibited intense green fluorescence (Figure 5B). Fluorescence microscopy analysis also confirmed that F-AuNPs inhibited the attachment of cells to the glass surface as compared to the control. Thus, based on crystal violet assays, SEM, and fluorescence microscopy studies, it can be concluded that F-AuNPs disrupted the attachment of sessile cells to surfaces, which initiated the formation of biofilms.

Apart from the inhibition of biofilm formation at the initial stage by F-AuNPs, the dispersion of mature biofilm established by *P. aeruginosa* was also studied (Figure 6). The 24 h old established mature biofilm was treated with different concentrations (ranging from 16–256 μg/mL) of F-AuNPs. The results showed that higher concentration (from 128–256 μg/mL) exhibited stronger dispersion of established mature biofilm, as compared to the lower concentration (16–64 μg/mL). The minimum biofilm eradication concentration (MBEC) of F-AuNPs on pre-formed mature *P. aeruginosa* biofilm was therefore selected as 128 μg/mL.

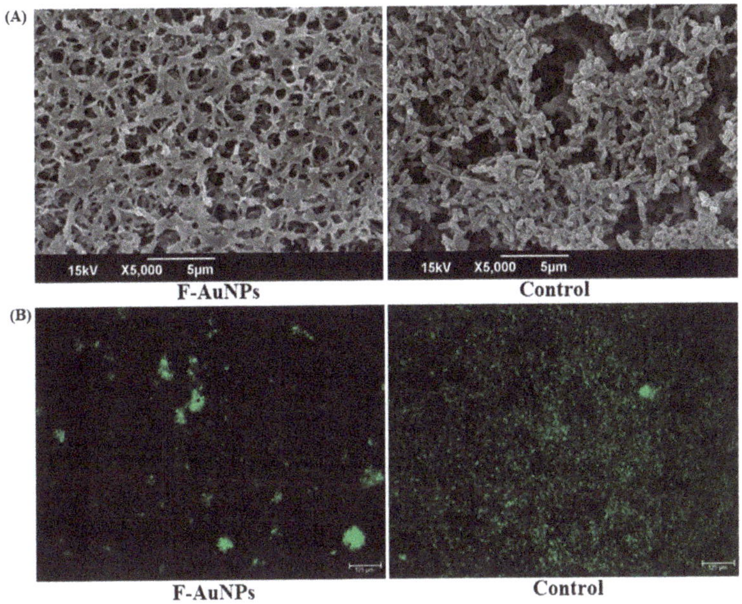

Figure 5. Microscopic examination of biofilm cells and biofilm architecture after 24 h of incubation with F-AuNPs (256 μg/mL). (**A**) SEM image and (**B**) fluorescence image of biofilm cells.

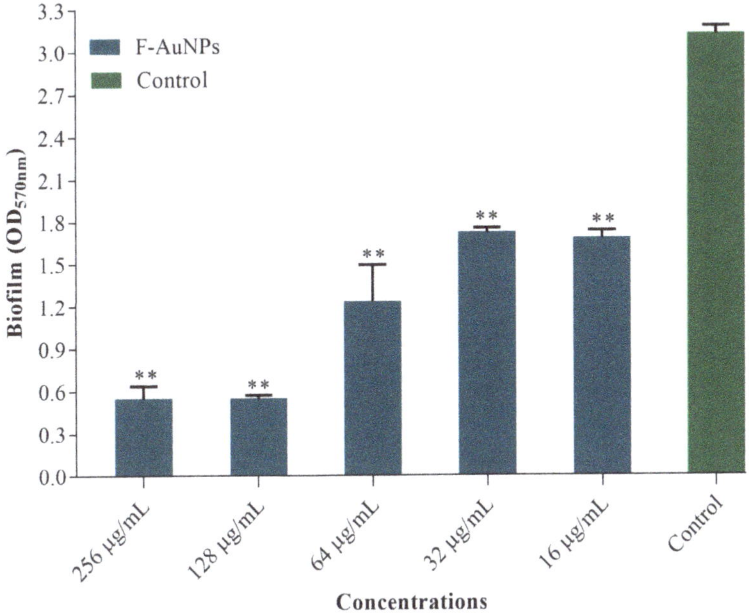

Figure 6. Dispersion of established mature biofilm of *P. aeruginosa* in the presence of F-AuNPs. The 24 h established matured biofilm was analyzed by crystal violet staining method and OD measurement at 570 nm. The experiment was repeated three times for each F-AuNP concentration. ** $p < 0.01$ versus the control (not treated by F-AuNPs).

3.4. Antivirulence, Antihemolytic and Protease Inhibitory Activity of F-AuNPs

The sub-MICs of F-AuNPs were also checked for inhibitory effects on the bacterial production of several virulence factors during biofilm formation that are essential for colonization and pathogenesis. Production of pyocyanin from *P. aeruginosa* in the presence of different concentrations of F-AuNPs was determined spectrophotometrically at 520 nm. The results showed a significant loss in the inhibition of pyocyanin, in which pyocyanin production at 32, 128, and 256 μg/mL concentrations of F-AuNPs were found to be approximately 79.4%, 81.9%, and 87.7%, respectively (Figure 7A). Similarly, the amount of rhamnolipid production was determined by using an orcinol colorimetric assay and OD measurements at 421 nm. Concentrations of 32, 128, and 256 μg/mL of F-AuNPs reduced rhamnolipid production by 54%, 50%, and 53%, respectively, which represents almost equal inhibition at all concentrations tested (Figure 7B). Production of another virulence factor, pyoverdine, which is one of the siderophores required for iron acquisition from the environment was also checked in the presence of different sub-MICs of F-AuNPs. Pyoverdine production was measured directly in the supernatant at a wavelength of 405 nm. The results showed that at 256 μg/mL, inhibition of pyoverdine production by *P. aeruginosa* was 91.6%, whereas, at 128 μg/mL and 32 μg/mL, bacterial pyoverdine generation was inhibited by almost 95% (Figure 7C).

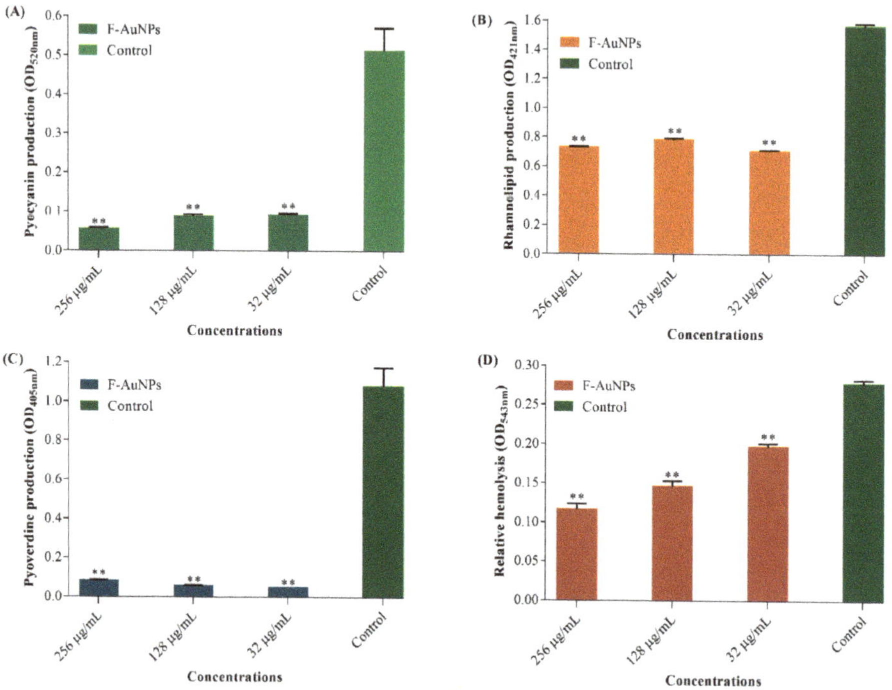

Figure 7. Effect of F-AuNPs on the production of virulence factors and hemolytic activity in *P. aeruginosa*. (**A**) Production of pyocyanin, (**B**) production of rhamnolipid, (**C**) production of pyoverdine, and (**D**) hemolytic activity. The determination of virulence factor production and hemolytic activity from the F-AuNPs treated sample were carried out as a relative value in comparison to the control. All the experiments were performed in triplicate. ** $p < 0.01$ versus the control (not treated by F-AuNPs).

In addition to the virulence factor production assays, we checked the hemolytic activity of *P. aeruginosa* in the presence of different sub-MICs of F-AuNPs. Bacterial cell cultures treated with F-AuNPs were mixed with diluted RBCs, followed by 1 h of incubation at 35 °C. The hemolyzed RBCs present in the supernatant were monitored at 543 nm. The results showed that with

F-AuNPs at concentrations of 32, 128, and 256 μg/mL, the inhibition of hemolytic activity was 29%, 47.5%, and 59%, respectively (Figure 7D). Previous reports identified the fact that synthesis and production of protease enzymes from the cells are also functionally important in the pathogenesis of *P. aeruginosa* [39,40]. Hence, the production of protease enzymes in the presence of sub-MICs of F-AuNPs on casein-containing agar plates was assayed, and the results were revealed by the diameter (cm) of clear zones appearing around the treatment-loaded agar holes. As shown in Figure 8A,B, the maximum inhibitory effect of F-AuNPs over the bacterial production of proteases was exhibited at high concentrations (128 and 256 μg/mL).

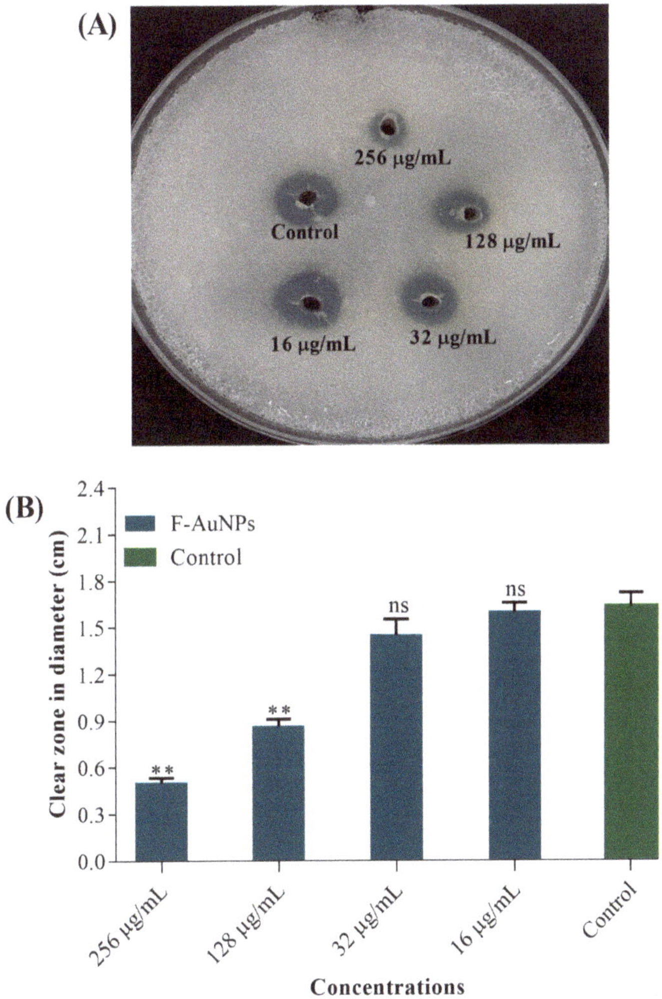

Figure 8. Protease inhibitory activity of F-AuNPs at sub-MICs in *P. aeruginosa*. (**A**) The image of the casein-containing agar plate showing protease activity, and (**B**) diameter (cm) of clear zones appearing around the holes. All the experiments were performed in triplicate. ** $p < 0.01$ considered as significant, ns indicates non-significant as compared to the control (not treated by F-AuNPs).

3.5. Motility Impairment Properties of F-AuNPs

Different types of motilities, such as swimming, swarming, and twitching, exhibited by *P. aeruginosa* have been well studied, and these motilities play a significant role in biofilm formation as well as infection of host cells [41–43]. The various types of motilities are due to the presence of surface appendages on *P. aeruginosa* such as flagellae and pili [42,43]. In the present study, the activity of F-AuNPs at sub-MIC levels (32 and 256 μg/mL) on various types of motilities of *P. aeruginosa* such as swimming, swarming, and twitching was studied on agar plates. Swimming motility was monitored in Bacto agar (0.3%) media containing NaCl (1%) and tryptone (0.25%). As shown in Figure 9A,B, flagellar-mediated swimming motility was completely inhibited in comparison to the control (absence of the drug).

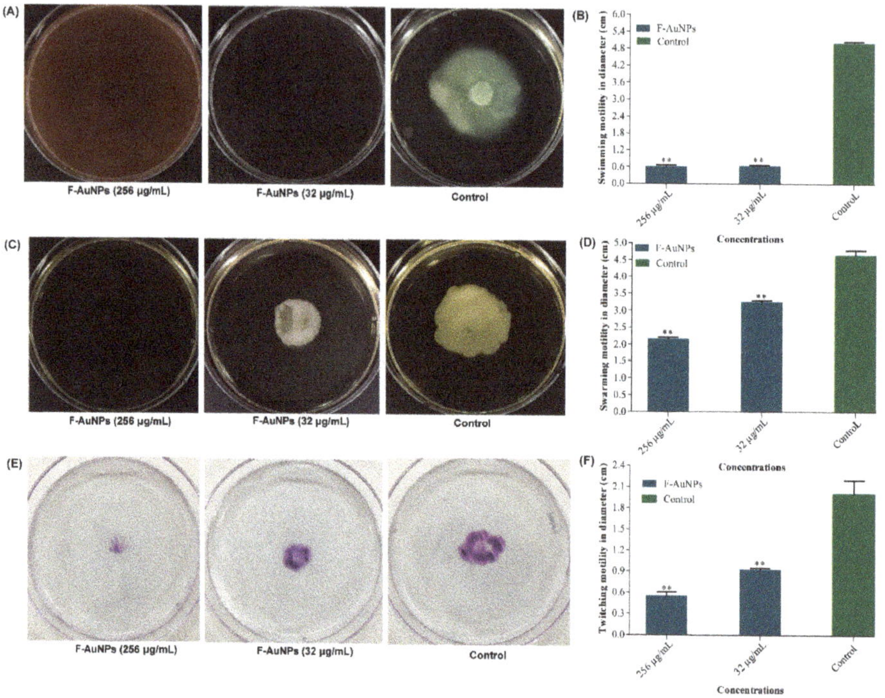

Figure 9. Motility inhibiting properties of F-AuNPs in *P. aeruginosa*. (**A**) Swimming motility image, (**B**) swimming motility values, (**C**) swarming motility image, (**D**) swarming motility values, (**E**) twitching motility image, and (**F**) twitching motility values. All the experiments were performed in triplicate. ** $p < 0.01$ versus the control (not treated by F-AuNPs).

Similarly, another type of flagellar motility known as swarming was investigated on the surface of Bacto agar (0.4%) plates in LB broth supplemented with glucose (0.5%) and casamino acids (0.5%). As shown in Figure 9C,D, swarming motility was also inhibited in a concentration-dependent manner, with values of approximately 30% and 53% at concentrations of 32 and 256 μg/mL, respectively. Furthermore, the present study also monitored type IV pili-mediated twitching motility using solid Bacto agar (1.5%) prepared in LB broth containing glucose (30 mM) and casamino acids (0.2%). In contrast to swarming and swimming, the twitching assay was monitored by staining with crystal violet (0.1%). The results showed that twitching motility was found to be significantly inhibited in a concentration-dependent manner (Figure 9E,F). The results revealed twitching motility inhibition of almost 72% at 256 μg/mL, and almost 54% at 32 μg/mL concentration of F-AuNPs (Figure 9F).

Collectively, the present results indicated that F-AuNPs effectively controlled the different motility modes of *P. aeruginosa*.

4. Discussion

Several strategies have been developed in order to combat antibiotic resistance and related infections caused by pathogenic bacteria [44–47]. Besides targeting resistance enzyme synthesis and efflux pump function, these strategies also aim for inhibition of biofilm formation and attenuation of virulence factors produced by pathogenic bacteria, hence reducing selection pressure and preventing future risk of resistance [6,48,49]. With the recent development of nanotechnology, noble metal-based nanoparticles such as AuNPs in a size range of 1–100 nm, with easy surface modifications, high compatibility, and low toxicity have been recognized as a promising antibiofilm agent, as well as an effective drug delivery system [50–54]. Modern synthesis techniques of AuNPs have shifted from physical and chemical methods to biological approaches, which are mediated by plants, algae, and microorganisms for improvements in modification, stability, economic benefit, production scale-up, and environmental friendliness [55–57]. In fact, it is those biocompatible, biodegradable, and non-toxic active compounds such as polysaccharides, proteins, and phenolics enriched in these biomaterials that initiate both the bio-reduction of metallic ions to NPs and their stabilization [58–60]. Specifically, in AuNPs, biopolymer-based biosynthesis has even been found to be more efficient than other methods [61]. In the present study, fucoidan, which is a sulfonated polysaccharide sourced from various brown seaweed species with significant bioactivities, including antimicrobial, antioxidant, anti-inflammatory, and anti-cancer roles, was used to synthesize stabilized-AuNPs [25,26]. Owing to the availability and relatively high purity of fucoidan ($\geq$95%), the use of commercial fucoidan products, which are extracted from *Fucus vesiculosus*, is recommended as an economically beneficial approach in nanoparticle biosynthesis [62,63]. Several crucial characterization analyses involving UV-vis spectrophotometry, FTIR, DLS, FE-TEM, EDX, and XRD were carried out involving the synthesized F-AuNPs, and the results are presented in Figures 1 and 2. The prepared F-AuNPs were spherical in shape and approximately 15 to 119 nm in size (with an average size of ~53 nm), with high stability and high water solubility, and can be used for subsequent experiments involving anti-biofilm functions.

The resultant F-AuNPs were examined for functional potential in inhibiting biofilm formation and virulence factor production by *P. aeruginosa*. The MIC value was first determined to be 512 μg/mL. High concentrations (i.e., MIC and > MIC) of F-AuNPs exhibited bactericidal activity, while lower concentrations (i.e., sub-MICs) were effective in preventing biofilm establishment, virulence factor production, and eradicating pre-existing mature biofilm. The antibacterial effect of high concentrations of F-AuNPs was also found in several other biogenic NPs derived from either fucoidan or Au. For example, fucoidan was previously used to prepare silver NPs (AgNPs), and results showed that F-AgNPs exhibited significant antibacterial activity against *Klebsiella pneumoniae* [27]. Meanwhile, AuNPs synthesized from *Lignosus rhinocerotis* sclerotial extract and chitosan also induced growth inhibition of a wide range of foodborne bacteria such as *Bacillus* sp., *Escherichia coli*, *P. aeruginosa*, and *Staphylococcus aureus* [64]. Studies have also found that several Gram-negative bacterial species are more susceptible to antibacterial agents than their Gram-positive counterparts due to the lack of a thick peptidoglycan wall, which allows higher uptake of these agents [65,66]. Collectively, the bactericidal effects of F-AuNPs at high concentration have added to the potential use of F-AuNPs as an effective antibacterial agent against *P. aeruginosa*.

The inhibition of formation and eradication of biofilm, as well as the production of other virulence factors by biosynthesized F-AuNPs, were mainly identified at sub-MIC levels. In attempts to lower the selection pressure for resistance, targeting biofilm formation and genetic expression of other important virulence factors are considered to be approaches with the most potential, and which are commonly involved in the application of nanotechnology. NPs of nano-scale sizes and high stability are capable of inhibiting biofilm formation and damaging pre-existing mature biofilm structures mostly formed on infected living tissues and nosocomial systems [12]. In the present study, F-AuNPs exhibited antibacterial activity at a concentration of 512 μg/mL, while exhibiting antibiofilm activity and biofilm eradication activity at 128 μg/mL. Microscopic observations by SEM and fluorescence microscopy also confirmed the effectiveness of F-AuNP treatment, in which the presence of F-AuNPs significantly disrupted 24 h old biofilm thickness and architecture, in comparison with the control without F-AuNPs. Similar results were obtained when AuNPs prepared from baicalein and from apple extract were applied to *P. aeruginosa* biofilms [54,67]. Moreover, crystal violet assays and microscopic observations clearly confirmed the inhibitory and eradicating efficacy of F-AuNPs at sub-MIC levels against *P. aeruginosa* biofilm.

Along with biofilm formation, *P. aeruginosa* is known to produce a wide array of virulence factors actively engaged in chronic infections [68]. Of all of these factors, rhamnolipid, pyocyanin, pyoverdine, hemolysins, protease, and cell motilities were selected to examine their production under sub-MIC levels of F-AuNPs. Results showed that production of pyoverdine, pyocyanin, and rhamnolipid were significantly reduced in the presence of F-AuNPs at sub-MIC levels. With equal amounts of F-AuNP, hemolytic activity was reduced in a concentration-dependent manner. Green-blue pigmented pyocyanin essentially causes oxidative stress and cytotoxicity to the host tissues; pyoverdine maintains the iron requirement for bacterial survival and growth; rhamnolipid is essential for motility and biofilm formation; hemolysins cause rupture of host RBCs; and proteases damage host immune systems. Therefore, reduction of these crucial virulence factors can be considered to effectively attenuate the pathogenesis and colonization of *P. aeruginosa* without affecting bacterial growth or initiating resistance selection [69–73].

To the best of our knowledge, the inhibitory effects of F-AuNPs towards *P. aeruginosa* virulence factors at both the phenotypic and genetic levels have remained unknown. So far, only AuNPs synthesized from ectomycorrhizal fungi were found to completely inhibit pyocyanin production by *P. aeruginosa* [74]. Therefore, the finding of anti-virulence activity of F-AuNPs against bacteria, as obtained in the present study, has provided essential insights for the future application of F-AuNPs in controlling *P. aeruginosa* pathogenesis, as well as against biofilm-related infections.

Motility and attachment of bacterial planktonic cells to biotic or abiotic surfaces are known to set the primary platform for subsequent stages of biofilm formation. Therefore, this transition phase is also considered to be a common target in preventing biofilm formation [75]. In *P. aeruginosa*, swimming, swarming, and twitching motilities are largely mediated by pili IV and flagellae. Here, in the present study, compared to the control, sub-MIC levels of F-AuNPs were able to impair all types of motilities, with the most significant inhibitory effect being observed in swimming and twitching. Likewise, sub-MICs of AuNPs prepared from cinnamon oil, betulinic acid, baicalein, and curcumin have also been reported to target the motility of planktonic *P. aeruginosa* cells, causing a notable reduction in biofilm biomass up to 89% [10,60,75,76].

5. Conclusions and Future Perspectives

Biofilm formation emerged in numerous bacteria as a drug resistance mechanism, and has remained a great threat to the global population to date. Among current novel treatments, noble NPs, such as AuNPs, have been recognized for their significant anti-biofilm efficacy. However, studies on the efficacy of AuNPs synthesized from biological sources have been limited. For this reason, the present study employed fucoidan, a sulfonated polymer sourced from marine seaweed, as a stabilizing and reducing agent to synthesize AuNPs. As the biosynthesized F-AuNPs were characterized as stable and water-soluble, they were further evaluated for anti-biofilm potential against *P. aeruginosa*. F-AuNPs at high concentration killed the bacterial cells, whereas F-AuNPs at sub-MIC inhibited biofilm formation and eradicated mature, established, 24 h old biofilm. The sub-MICs of F-AuNPs also suppressed the production of several virulence factors by *P. aeruginosa*. Inhibition of *P. aeruginosa* hemolytic activity by F-AuNPs was in a concentration-dependent manner. Furthermore, additional activities of the F-AuNPs extended towards different motility properties of *P. aeruginosa*. The results showed that F-AuNPs impaired the swarming, swimming, and twitching motilities at the sub-MIC level. Thus, it can be concluded that the present biosynthesized F-AuNPs constitute a stable, water-soluble anti-biofilm and anti-virulence drug against *P. aeruginosa*. In the long term, future studies are required for more in-depth understanding regarding F-AuNPs' inhibitory mechanisms towards bacterial biofilm, virulence factors, and motility at the molecular level. The antibacterial activity of F-AuNPs should also be researched for its mode of action, because the negatively-charged F-AuNPs might exhibit bactericidal effects differently in comparison with positively-charged NPs such as chitosan NPs. In addition, biocompatibility and efficacy of F-AuNPs should be examined in animal models such as *Caenorhabditis elegans* for potential clinical use. Furthermore, as *P. aeruginosa* biofilm formation is associated with a wide variety of nosocomial infections, the application of F-AuNP treatment in biomedical settings could be a promising solution. Consequently, further investigation regarding to F-AuNP efficacy and multi-species biofilm formation is required.

Author Contributions: The idea of the present study was conceived, designed the experiment, analyzed the data and wrote the paper by F.K., D.T.N.P., P.M., J.O. and Y.-M.K. The experiment was carried out by F.K., J.-W.L., P.M. and D.T.N.P.

Funding: The present research work financially supported by Marine Biotechnology Program (Grant number 20150220) funded by Ministry of Oceans and Fisheries, Republic of Korea.

Conflicts of Interest: Authors declare no conflict of interest.

References

1. Oglesby-Sherrouse, A.G.; Djapgne, L.; Nguyen, A.T.; Vasil, A.I.; Vasil, M.L. The complex interplay of iron, biofilm formation, and mucoidy affecting antimicrobial resistance of *Pseudomonas aeruginosa*. *Pathog. Dis.* **2014**, *70*, 307–320. [CrossRef]
2. Chatterjee, M.; Anju, C.P.; Biswas, L.; Anil Kumar, V.; Gopi Mohan, C.; Biswas, R. Antibiotic resistance in *Pseudomonas aeruginosa* and alternative therapeutic options. *Int. J. Med. Microbiol.* **2016**, *306*, 48–58. [CrossRef]
3. Potron, A.; Poirel, L.; Nordmann, P. Emerging broad-spectrum resistance in *Pseudomonas aeruginosa* and *Acinetobacter baumannii*: Mechanisms and epidemiology. *Int. J. Antimicrob. Agents* **2015**, *45*, 568–585. [CrossRef] [PubMed]
4. Ramirez-Estrada, S.; Borgatta, B.; Rello, J. *Pseudomonas aeruginosa* ventilator-associated pneumonia management. *Infect. Drug Resist.* **2016**, *9*, 7–18. [CrossRef] [PubMed]
5. Gellatly, S.L.; Hancock, R.E. *Pseudomonas aeruginosa*: New insights into pathogenesis and host defenses. *Pathog. Dis.* **2013**, *67*, 159–173. [CrossRef] [PubMed]
6. Roy, R.; Tiwari, M.; Donelli, G.; Tiwari, V. Strategies for combating bacterial biofilms: A focus on anti-biofilm agents and their mechanisms of action. *Virulence* **2018**, *9*, 522–554. [CrossRef]
7. Parrino, B.; Schillaci, D.; Carnevale, I.; Giovannetti, E.; Diana, P.; Cirrincione, G.; Cascioferro, S. Synthetic small molecules as anti-biofilm agents in the struggle against antibiotic resistance. *Eur. J. Med. Chem.* **2019**, *161*, 154–178. [CrossRef]
8. Khan, F.; Manivasagan, P.; Pham, D.T.N.; Oh, J.; Kim, S.K.; Kim, Y.M. Antibiofilm and antivirulence properties of chitosan-polypyrrole nanocomposites to *Pseudomonas aeruginosa*. *Microb. Pathog.* **2019**, *128*, 363–373. [CrossRef]
9. Khan, F.; Khan, M.M.; Kim, Y.M. Recent Progress and Future Perspectives of Antibiofilm Drugs Immobilized on Nanomaterials. *Curr. Pharm. Biotechnol.* **2018**, *19*, 631–643. [CrossRef]
10. Packiavathy, I.A.; Priya, S.; Pandian, S.K.; Ravi, A.V. Inhibition of biofilm development of uropathogens by curcumin—An anti-quorum sensing agent from *Curcuma longa*. *Food Chem.* **2014**, *148*, 453–460. [CrossRef] [PubMed]
11. Wagner, S.; Sommer, R.; Hinsberger, S.; Lu, C.; Hartmann, R.W.; Empting, M.; Titz, A. Novel Strategies for the Treatment of *Pseudomonas aeruginosa* Infections. *J. Med. Chem.* **2016**, *59*, 5929–5969. [CrossRef]
12. Neethirajan, S.; Clond, M.A.; Vogt, A. Medical biofilms—Nanotechnology approaches. *J. Biomed. Nanotechnol.* **2014**, *10*, 2806–2827. [CrossRef] [PubMed]
13. Javaid, A.; Oloketuyi, S.F.; Khan, M.M.; Khan, F.J.B. Diversity of Bacterial Synthesis of Silver Nanoparticles. *BioNanoScience* **2018**, *8*, 43–59. [CrossRef]

14. Cabuzu, D.; Cirja, A.; Puiu, R.; Grumezescu, A.M. Biomedical applications of gold nanoparticles. *Curr. Top. Med. Chem.* **2015**, *15*, 1605–1613. [CrossRef] [PubMed]
15. Elahi, N.; Kamali, M.; Baghersad, M.H. Recent biomedical applications of gold nanoparticles: A review. *Talanta* **2018**, *184*, 537–556. [CrossRef] [PubMed]
16. Baruah, D.; Goswami, M.; Yadav, R.N.S.; Yadav, A.; Das, A.M. Biogenic synthesis of gold nanoparticles and their application in photocatalytic degradation of toxic dyes. *J. Photochem. Photobiol. B* **2018**, *186*, 51–58. [CrossRef] [PubMed]
17. Vimalraj, S.; Ashokkumar, T.; Saravanan, S. Biogenic gold nanoparticles synthesis mediated by *Mangifera indica* seed aqueous extracts exhibits antibacterial, anticancer and anti-angiogenic properties. *Biomed. Pharmacother.* **2018**, *105*, 440–448. [CrossRef]
18. Khan, Z.U.H.; Khan, A.; Chen, Y.; Shah, N.S.; Muhammad, N.; Khan, A.U.; Tahir, K.; Khan, F.U.; Murtaza, B.; Hassan, S.U.; et al. Biomedical applications of green synthesized Nobel metal nanoparticles. *J. Photochem. Photobiol. B* **2017**, *173*, 150–164. [CrossRef]
19. Bankar, A.; Joshi, B.; Kumar, A.R.; Zinjarde, S. Banana peel extract mediated synthesis of gold nanoparticles. *Colloids Surf. B Biointerfaces* **2010**, *80*, 45–50. [CrossRef]
20. Roopan, S.M.; Surendra, T.V.; Elango, G.; Kumar, S.H. Biosynthetic trends and future aspects of bimetallic nanoparticles and its medicinal applications. *Appl. Microbiol. Biotechnol.* **2014**, *98*, 5289–5300. [CrossRef]
21. Gupta, A.; Moyano, D.F.; Parnsubsakul, A.; Papadopoulos, A.; Wang, L.S.; Landis, R.F.; Das, R.; Rotello, V.M. Ultrastable and Biofunctionalizable Gold Nanoparticles. *ACS Appl. Mater. Interfaces* **2016**, *8*, 14096–14101. [CrossRef] [PubMed]
22. Cai, F.; Li, J.; Sun, J.; Ji, Y. Biosynthesis of gold nanoparticles by biosorption using *Magnetospirillum gryphiswaldense* MSR-1. *Chem. Eng. J.* **2011**, *175*, 70–75. [CrossRef]
23. Sharma, D.; Kanchi, S.; Bisetty, K. Biogenic synthesis of nanoparticles: A review. *Arab. J. Chem.* **2015**. [CrossRef]
24. Castro, L.; Blazquez, M.L.; Munoz, J.A.; Gonzalez, F.; Ballester, A. Biological synthesis of metallic nanoparticles using algae. *IET Nanobiotechnol.* **2013**, *7*, 109–116. [CrossRef]
25. Fitton, J.H.; Stringer, D.N.; Karpiniec, S.S. Therapies from Fucoidan: An Update. *Mar. Drugs* **2015**, *13*, 5920–5946. [CrossRef]
26. Zhao, Y.; Zheng, Y.; Wang, J.; Ma, S.; Yu, Y.; White, W.L.; Yang, S.; Yang, F.; Lu, J. Fucoidan Extracted from *Undaria pinnatifida*: Source for Nutraceuticals/Functional Foods. *Mar. Drugs* **2018**, *16*. [CrossRef]
27. Ravichandran, A.; Subramanian, P.; Manoharan, V.; Muthu, T.; Periyannan, R.; Thangapandi, M.; Ponnuchamy, K.; Pandi, B.; Marimuthu, P.N. Phyto-mediated synthesis of silver nanoparticles using fucoidan isolated from *Spatoglossum asperum* and assessment of antibacterial activities. *J. Photochem. Photobiol. B* **2018**, *185*, 117–125. [CrossRef]
28. Aljabali, A.A.A.; Akkam, Y.; Al Zoubi, M.S.; Al-Batayneh, K.M.; Al-Trad, B.; Abo Alrob, O.; Alkilany, A.M.; Benamara, M.; Evans, D.J. Synthesis of Gold Nanoparticles Using Leaf Extract of *Ziziphus zizyphus* and their Antimicrobial Activity. *Nanomaterials* **2018**, *8*, 174. [CrossRef]
29. Tripathi, R.M.; Shrivastav, B.R.; Shrivastav, A. Antibacterial and catalytic activity of biogenic gold nanoparticles synthesised by Trichoderma harzianum. *IET Nanobiotechnol.* **2018**, *12*, 509–513. [CrossRef] [PubMed]
30. Manivasagan, P.; Bharathiraja, S.; Bui, N.Q.; Jang, B.; Oh, Y.O.; Lim, I.G.; Oh, J. Doxorubicin-loaded fucoidan capped gold nanoparticles for drug delivery and photoacoustic imaging. *Int. J. Biol. Macromol.* **2016**, *91*, 578–588. [CrossRef]
31. Clinical and Laboratory Standards Institute. *Performance Standards for Antimicrobial Susceptibility Testing*; Clinical and Laboratory Standards Institute: Wayne, PA, USA, 2016.
32. Lee, J.H.; Cho, M.H.; Lee, J. 3-indolylacetonitrile decreases Escherichia coli O157:H7 biofilm formation and *Pseudomonas aeruginosa* virulence. *Environ. Microbiol.* **2011**, *13*, 62–73. [CrossRef]
33. Lee, J.H.; Kim, Y.G.; Cho, M.H.; Kim, J.A.; Lee, J. 7-fluoroindole as an antivirulence compound against *Pseudomonas aeruginosa*. *FEMS Microbiol. Lett.* **2012**, *329*, 36–44. [CrossRef]
34. Essar, D.W.; Eberly, L.; Hadero, A.; Crawford, I.P. Identification and characterization of genes for a second anthranilate synthase in *Pseudomonas aeruginosa*: Interchangeability of the two anthranilate synthases and evolutionary implications. *J. Bacteriol.* **1990**, *172*, 884–900. [CrossRef]

35. Wilhelm, S.; Gdynia, A.; Tielen, P.; Rosenau, F.; Jaeger, K.E. The autotransporter esterase EstA of *Pseudomonas aeruginosa* is required for rhamnolipid production, cell motility, and biofilm formation. *J. Bacteriol.* **2007**, *189*, 6695–6703. [CrossRef]
36. Stintzi, A.; Evans, K.; Meyer, J.M.; Poole, K. Quorum-sensing and siderophore biosynthesis in *Pseudomonas aeruginosa*: lasR/lasI mutants exhibit reduced pyoverdine biosynthesis. *FEMS Microbiol. Lett.* **1998**, *166*, 341–345. [CrossRef]
37. Luo, J.; Dong, B.; Wang, K.; Cai, S.; Liu, T.; Cheng, X.; Lei, D.; Chen, Y.; Li, Y.; Kong, J.; et al. Baicalin inhibits biofilm formation, attenuates the quorum sensing-controlled virulence and enhances *Pseudomonas aeruginosa* clearance in a mouse peritoneal implant infection model. *PLoS ONE* **2017**, *12*, e0176883. [CrossRef] [PubMed]
38. Manivasagan, P.; Oh, J. Production of a Novel Fucoidanase for the Green Synthesis of Gold Nanoparticles by *Streptomyces* sp. and Its Cytotoxic Effect on HeLa Cells. *Mar. Drugs* **2015**, *13*, 6818–6837. [CrossRef] [PubMed]
39. Saint-Criq, V.; Villeret, B.; Bastaert, F.; Kheir, S.; Hatton, A.; Cazes, A.; Xing, Z.; Sermet-Gaudelus, I.; Garcia-Verdugo, I.; Edelman, A.; et al. *Pseudomonas aeruginosa* LasB protease impairs innate immunity in mice and humans by targeting a lung epithelial cystic fibrosis transmembrane regulator-IL-6-antimicrobial-repair pathway. *Thorax* **2018**, *73*, 49–61. [CrossRef] [PubMed]
40. Bradshaw, J.L.; Caballero, A.R.; Bierdeman, M.A.; Adams, K.V.; Pipkins, H.R.; Tang, A.; O'Callaghan, R.J.; McDaniel, L.S. *Pseudomonas aeruginosa* Protease IV Exacerbates Pneumococcal Pneumonia and Systemic Disease. *mSphere* **2018**, *3*. [CrossRef] [PubMed]
41. O'Toole, G.A.; Kolter, R. Flagellar and twitching motility are necessary for *Pseudomonas aeruginosa* biofilm development. *Mol. Microbiol.* **1998**, *30*, 295–304. [CrossRef]
42. Klausen, M.; Heydorn, A.; Ragas, P.; Lambertsen, L.; Aaes-Jorgensen, A.; Molin, S.; Tolker-Nielsen, T. Biofilm formation by *Pseudomonas aeruginosa* wild type, flagella and type IV pili mutants. *Mol. Microbiol.* **2003**, *48*, 1511–1524. [CrossRef] [PubMed]
43. Chiang, P.; Burrows, L.L. Biofilm formation by hyperpiliated mutants of *Pseudomonas aeruginosa*. *J. Bacteriol.* **2003**, *185*, 2374–2378. [CrossRef] [PubMed]
44. Defoirdt, T. Quorum-Sensing Systems as Targets for Antivirulence Therapy. *Trends Microbiol.* **2018**, *26*, 313–328. [CrossRef] [PubMed]
45. Defraine, V.; Fauvart, M.; Michiels, J. Fighting bacterial persistence: Current and emerging anti-persister strategies and therapeutics. *Drug Resist. Updat.* **2018**, *38*, 12–26. [CrossRef] [PubMed]
46. Tyers, M.; Wright, G.D. Drug combinations: A strategy to extend the life of antibiotics in the 21st century. *Nat. Rev. Microbiol.* **2019**, *17*, 141–155. [CrossRef] [PubMed]
47. Khan, F.; Javaid, A.; Kim, Y.M. Functional diversity of quorum sensing receptors in pathogenic bacteria: Interspecies, intraspecies and interkingdom level. *Curr. Drug Targets* **2019**, *20*, 655–667. [CrossRef]
48. Reuter, K.; Steinbach, A.; Helms, V. Interfering with Bacterial Quorum Sensing. *Perspect. Med. Chem.* **2016**, *8*, 1–15. [CrossRef]
49. Schillaci, D.; Spano, V.; Parrino, B.; Carbone, A.; Montalbano, A.; Barraja, P.; Diana, P.; Cirrincione, G.; Cascioferro, S. Pharmaceutical Approaches to Target Antibiotic Resistance Mechanisms. *J. Med. Chem.* **2017**, *60*, 8268–8297. [CrossRef]
50. Hajipour, M.J.; Fromm, K.M.; Ashkarran, A.A.; Jimenez de Aberasturi, D.; de Larramendi, I.R.; Rojo, T.; Serpooshan, V.; Parak, W.J.; Mahmoudi, M. Antibacterial properties of nanoparticles. *Trends Biotechnol.* **2012**, *30*, 499–511. [CrossRef]
51. Pooja, D.; Panyaram, S.; Kulhari, H.; Reddy, B.; Rachamalla, S.S.; Sistla, R. Natural polysaccharide functionalized gold nanoparticles as biocompatible drug delivery carrier. *Int. J. Biol. Macromol.* **2015**, *80*, 48–56. [CrossRef]
52. Lu, B.; Lu, F.; Ran, L.; Yu, K.; Xiao, Y.; Li, Z.; Dai, F.; Wu, D.; Lan, G. Imidazole-molecule-capped chitosan-gold nanocomposites with enhanced antimicrobial activity for treating biofilm-related infections. *J. Colloid Interface Sci.* **2018**, *531*, 269–281. [CrossRef] [PubMed]
53. Singh, P.; Pandit, S.; Garnaes, J.; Tunjic, S.; Mokkapati, V.R.; Sultan, A.; Thygesen, A.; Mackevica, A.; Mateiu, R.V.; Daugaard, A.E.; et al. Green synthesis of gold and silver nanoparticles from *Cannabis sativa* (industrial hemp) and their capacity for biofilm inhibition. *Int. J. Nanomed.* **2018**, *13*, 3571–3591. [CrossRef] [PubMed]

54. Yu, Q.; Li, J.; Zhang, Y.; Wang, Y.; Liu, L.; Li, M. Inhibition of gold nanoparticles (AuNPs) on pathogenic biofilm formation and invasion to host cells. *Sci. Rep.* **2016**, *6*, 26667. [CrossRef] [PubMed]
55. Hussain, I.; Singh, N.B.; Singh, A.; Singh, H.; Singh, S.C. Green synthesis of nanoparticles and its potential application. *Biotechnol. Lett.* **2016**, *38*, 545–560. [CrossRef] [PubMed]
56. Ahmed, S.; Ahmad, M.; Swami, B.L.; Ikram, S. A review on plants extract mediated synthesis of silver nanoparticles for antimicrobial applications: A green expertise. *J. Adv. Res.* **2016**, *7*, 17–28. [CrossRef]
57. Singh, P.; Kim, Y.J.; Zhang, D.; Yang, D.C. Biological Synthesis of Nanoparticles from Plants and Microorganisms. *Trends Biotechnol.* **2016**, *34*, 588–599. [CrossRef] [PubMed]
58. Nadeem, M.; Abbasi, B.H.; Younas, M.; Ahmad, W.; Khan, T. A review of the green syntheses and anti-microbial applications of gold nanoparticles. *Green Chem. Lett. Rev.* **2017**, *10*, 216–227. [CrossRef]
59. Thakkar, K.N.; Mhatre, S.S.; Parikh, R.Y. Biological synthesis of metallic nanoparticles. *Nanomedicine* **2010**, *6*, 257–262. [CrossRef]
60. Rajkumari, J.; Busi, S.; Vasu, A.C.; Reddy, P. Facile green synthesis of baicalein fabricated gold nanoparticles and their antibiofilm activity against *Pseudomonas aeruginosa* PAO1. *Microb. Pathog.* **2017**, *107*, 261–269. [CrossRef] [PubMed]
61. Shankar, P.D.; Shobana, S.; Karuppusamy, I.; Pugazhendhi, A.; Ramkumar, V.S.; Arvindnarayan, S.; Kumar, G. A review on the biosynthesis of metallic nanoparticles (gold and silver) using bio-components of microalgae: Formation mechanism and applications. *Enzym. Microb. Technol.* **2016**, *95*, 28–44. [CrossRef]
62. Li, B.; Lu, F.; Wei, X.; Zhao, R. Fucoidan: Structure and Bioactivity. *Molecules* **2008**, *13*, 1671–1695. [CrossRef] [PubMed]
63. Wijesekara, I.; Pangestuti, R.; Kim, S.-K. Biological activities and potential health benefits of sulfated polysaccharides derived from marine algae. *Carbohydr. Polym.* **2011**, *84*, 14–21. [CrossRef]
64. Katas, H.; Lim, C.S.; Nor Azlan, A.Y.H.; Buang, F.; Mh Busra, M.F. Antibacterial activity of biosynthesized gold nanoparticles using biomolecules from *Lignosus rhinocerotis* and chitosan. *Saudi Pharm. J.* **2019**, *27*, 283–292. [CrossRef]
65. Richter, M.F.; Hergenrother, P.J. The challenge of converting Gram-positive-only compounds into broad-spectrum antibiotics. *Ann. N. Y. Acad. Sci.* **2019**, *1435*, 18–38. [CrossRef]
66. Slavin, Y.N.; Asnis, J.; Hafeli, U.O.; Bach, H. Metal nanoparticles: Understanding the mechanisms behind antibacterial activity. *J. Nanobiotechnol.* **2017**, *15*, 65. [CrossRef]
67. Ahmed, A.; Khan, A.K.; Anwar, A.; Ali, S.A.; Shah, M.R. Biofilm inhibitory effect of chlorhexidine conjugated gold nanoparticles against Klebsiella pneumoniae. *Microb. Pathog.* **2016**, *98*, 50–56. [CrossRef] [PubMed]
68. Sandri, A.; Ortombina, A.; Boschi, F.; Cremonini, E.; Boaretti, M.; Sorio, C.; Melotti, P.; Bergamini, G.; Lleo, M. Inhibition of *Pseudomonas aeruginosa* secreted virulence factors reduces lung inflammation in CF mice. *Virulence* **2018**, *9*, 1008–1018. [CrossRef] [PubMed]
69. Gloyne, L.S.; Grant, G.D.; Perkins, A.V.; Powell, K.L.; McDermott, C.M.; Johnson, P.V.; Anderson, G.J.; Kiefel, M.; Anoopkumar-Dukie, S. Pyocyanin-induced toxicity in A549 respiratory cells is causally linked to oxidative stress. *Toxicol. In Vitro* **2011**, *25*, 1353–1358. [CrossRef]
70. Hall, S.; McDermott, C.; Anoopkumar-Dukie, S.; McFarland, A.J.; Forbes, A.; Perkins, A.V.; Davey, A.K.; Chess-Williams, R.; Kiefel, M.J.; Arora, D.; et al. Cellular Effects of Pyocyanin, a Secreted Virulence Factor of *Pseudomonas aeruginosa*. *Toxins* **2016**, *8*, 236. [CrossRef] [PubMed]
71. Oldak, E.; Trafny, E.A. Secretion of proteases by *Pseudomonas aeruginosa* biofilms exposed to ciprofloxacin. *Antimicrob. Agents Chemother.* **2005**, *49*, 3281–3288. [CrossRef] [PubMed]
72. Huang, H.; Lai, W.; Cui, M.; Liang, L.; Lin, Y.; Fang, Q.; Liu, Y.; Xie, L. An Evaluation of Blood Compatibility of Silver Nanoparticles. *Sci. Rep.* **2016**, *6*, 25518. [CrossRef]
73. Chrzanowski, L.; Lawniczak, L.; Czaczyk, K. Why do microorganisms produce rhamnolipids? *World J. Microbiol. Biotechnol.* **2012**, *28*, 401–419. [CrossRef] [PubMed]
74. Samanta, S.; Singh, B.R.; Adholeya, A. Intracellular Synthesis of Gold Nanoparticles Using an Ectomycorrhizal Strain EM-1083 of *Laccaria fraterna* and Its Nanoanti-quorum Sensing Potential Against *Pseudomonas aeruginosa*. *Indian J. Microbiol.* **2017**, *57*, 448–460. [CrossRef] [PubMed]

75. Kalia, M.; Yadav, V.K.; Singh, P.K.; Sharma, D.; Pandey, H.; Narvi, S.S.; Agarwal, V. Effect of Cinnamon Oil on Quorum Sensing-Controlled Virulence Factors and Biofilm Formation in *Pseudomonas aeruginosa*. *PLoS ONE* **2015**, *10*, e0135495. [CrossRef] [PubMed]
76. Rajkumari, J.; Borkotoky, S.; Murali, A.; Suchiang, K.; Mohanty, S.K.; Busi, S. Attenuation of quorum sensing controlled virulence factors and biofilm formation in *Pseudomonas aeruginosa* by pentacyclic triterpenes, betulin and betulinic acid. *Microb. Pathog.* **2018**, *118*, 48–60. [CrossRef] [PubMed]

© 2019 by the authors. Licensee MDPI, Basel, Switzerland. This article is an open access article distributed under the terms and conditions of the Creative Commons Attribution (CC BY) license (http://creativecommons.org/licenses/by/4.0/).

marine drugs

MDPI

Article

Trichormus variabilis (Cyanobacteria) Biomass: From the Nutraceutical Products to Novel EPS-Cell/Protein Carrier Systems

Erika Bellini [1], Matteo Ciocci [2], Saverio Savio [1], Simonetta Antonaroli [2], Dror Seliktar [3], Sonia Melino [2,4,*,†] and Roberta Congestri [1,*,†]

[1] Laboratory of Biology of Algae, Department of Biology, University of Rome Tor Vergata, 00133 Rome, Italy; erikabellini1990@gmail.com (E.B.); saverio.savio@gmail.com (S.S.)
[2] Department of Chemical Science and Technologies, University of Rome Tor Vergata, 00133 Rome, Italy; ciocci.matteo@gmail.com (M.C.); simonetta.antonaroli@uniroma2.it (S.A.)
[3] Department of Biomedical Engineering, Technion Israel Institute of Technology, 3200003 Haifa, Israel; dror@bm.technion.ac.il
[4] CIMER, Center of Regenerative Medicine, University of Rome Tor Vergata, via Montpelier 1, 00133 Rome, Italy
* Correspondence: melinos@uniroma2.it (S.M.); roberta.congestri@uniroma2.it (R.C.); Tel.: +39-06-7259-4410 (S.M.); +39-06-7259-5989 (R.C.)
† These authors contributed equally to the work.

Received: 28 July 2018; Accepted: 24 August 2018; Published: 27 August 2018

Abstract: A native strain of the heterocytous cyanobacterium *Trichormus variabilis* VRUC 168 was mass cultivated in a low-cost photobioreactor for a combined production of Polyunsaturated Fatty Acids (PUFA) and Exopolymeric Substances (EPS) from the same cyanobacterial biomass. A sequential extraction protocol was optimized leading to high yields of Released EPS (REPS) and PUFA, useful for nutraceutical products and biomaterials. REPS were extracted and characterized by chemical staining, Reversed Phase-High-Performance Liquid Chromatography (RP-HPLC), Fourier Transform Infrared Spectroscopy (FT-IR) and other spectroscopic techniques. Due to their gelation property, REPS were used to produce a photo-polymerizable hybrid hydrogel (REPS-Hy) with addition of polyethylene glycol diacrylated (PEGDa). REPS-Hy was stable over time and resistant to dehydration and spontaneous hydrolysis. The rheological and functional properties of REPS-Hy were studied. The enzyme carrier ability of REPS-Hy was assessed using the detoxification enzyme thiosulfate:cyanide sulfur transferase (TST), suggesting the possibility to use REPS-Hy as an enzymatic hydrogel system. Finally, REPS-Hy was used as a scaffold for culturing human mesenchymal stem cells (hMSCs). The cell seeding onto the REPS-Hy and the cell embedding into 3D-REPS-Hy demonstrated a scaffolding property of REPS-Hy with non-cytotoxic effect, suggesting potential applications of cyanobacteria REPS for producing enzyme- and cell-carrier systems.

Keywords: Extracellular Polymeric Substances; hydrogel; mesenchymal stem cells; biomaterials; enzyme; omega 3; PUFA; *Trichormus variabilis*; Cyanobacteria

---

1. Introduction

Cyanobacteria are known as the most abundant phototrophic organisms in the Ocean. They are versatile and successfully colonize a wide range of aquatic and terrestrial habitats also thriving in strongly fluctuating environments, including the most extreme habitats on Earth [1]. Cyanobacterial diversity is enormous and represents a source of biotechnologically important organisms for new products and applications [2,3]. Commercial exploitation of cyanobacteria relies on intensive cultivation of biomass for the production of high-value compounds useful not only in nutraceutics, therapeutics and cosmetics but also for the production of advanced bio-material [4–10]. In this context, we focused on a strain of *Trichormus variabilis* (Kützing ex Bornet & Flahault) Komárek & Anagnostidis, isolated from sediment biofilms of a dystrophic coastal lagoon [11]. *T. variabilis* VRUC168 was selected based on prior studies that showed ease of growth in a range of photobioreactors (PBRs), even in suspension, self-flocculation, and interesting productivity of nutraceutical products, such as Polyunsaturated fatty acids (PUFA) and Exopolymeric Substances (EPS) [12,13].

EPS may constitute up to 60% of the dry biomass (as in the case of *Nostoc commune* and *Trichocoleus sociatus*) [14,15] and can be tightly bound (cell-attached or capsular), loosely adhere (slime type) to cells or exist as free dissolved matter called Released EPS (REPS). We focused on REPS that are usually recovered from the liquid growth media of cyanobacterial cultures with a green, environmentally safe process without using chemicals [16,17].

In the past few years, several studies have demonstrated a high potential application of cyanobacterial EPS that consist of various organic substances: mainly extracellular polysaccharides, uronic acids, proteins, nucleic acids and lipids [16]. Generally, they are characterized by a high complexity in terms of monosaccharidic composition. EPS can contain up to 15 sugar moieties, organized in complex repeating units and are often characterized by a high molecular weight, of up to 1–2 MDa [18]. The presence of hydrophilic moieties on one side (sulfated sugars, uronic acids and ketal-linked pyruvyl groups, among others), and hydrophobic on the other (acetyl groups, dehoxysugars and peptides) confers an amphiphilic character to the macromolecules and hence provides greater plasticity in organisms' response to surrounding environment [19]. While sulfate groups and uronic acids contribute to the anionic nature of the EPS, conferring a negative charge and a "sticky" behavior to the overall macromolecule [20–22], hydrophobic compounds are responsible for their emulsifying and rheological properties [23,24]. Due to these features, EPS are also used for the production of emulsifiers, viscosifiers, soil conditioners, biosorbants and bioflocculants [18]. Cyanobacterial EPS can play diverse roles in vivo; they form a three-dimensional network holding cells together and mediating their attachment to exposed surfaces [12,25,26]. A recent application of EPS-rich cyanobacteria, related to the physiological role of the EPS, is their use as nutrient supplements and physical soil amendments for the recovery of eroded soils [27–29]. EPS hydration and rheological properties are important to prevent cell desiccation and to confer pseudoplastic behavior of the extra-cellular environment [18,19,30]. These polymers are also involved in other relevant physiological roles from the UV protection and antibiotic resistance, to the mechanical strength and exo-enzymatic degradation activity [18,31,32], which could be of interest for biomedical applications. Although these substances are widely studied, in fact, the potential applications of the EPS and REPS are not completely understood. Due to their high content of polysaccharides, these polymers are highly promising materials for applications in biomedicine and tissue engineering [33,34]. Indeed, the ability of natural polysaccharides to form hydrogels, in which three-dimensional (3D) cross-linked network structures retain a large amount of water, makes them very useful for the production of drug- or cell-carrier systems and scaffolds. In particular, therapeutic molecules or macromolecules (proteins and nucleic acids) can be entrapped into the inner structure of these hydrogels or adsorbed onto their external surface, to facilitate better targeting to organs and tissues. The embedding of active molecules into polysaccharide gels usually increases their availability, also permitting for the drug administration at lower doses and, consequently, the reduction of the toxicity for the patient [35]. Moreover, hydrogels have become important as cell-carrier systems [36,37] for the transplantation of cells in the therapy of a variety of diseases (e.g., liver failure and diabetes) [38]. In our study, a novel photo-polymerizable REPS hydrogel was produced, combining the properties of natural REPS from *T. variabilis* with those of the synthetic polyethylene-glycol diacrylated (PEGDa). Here, we investigated the chemico-physical and mechanical properties of this hybrid hydrogel and its potential applications in production of detoxification enzyme- and stem cell-carrier systems. Therefore, the feasibility of an integrated approach that combines the cyanobacterial biomass production with the extraction of unsaturated FA and the fabrication of EPS hydrogels for enzyme- and cell-carrier systems are demonstrated.

2. Results and Discussion

2.1. *T. variabilis Growth and Biomass Yields in the PBR*

T. variabilis VRUC168 showed the ability to grow intensively and in suspension in the low-cost, 10 L polyethylene vertical bags used in this study (Figure 1). These growth systems allowed optimization of the space occupied by the culture and of the illumination provided. Although biofilm growth systems have recently proved more productive [14,39] to investigate potential employment of REPS as advanced bioactive material, the selected PBR configuration and material appeared satisfactory. Indeed, in our experiment, nutrient provision occurred only at the start of the PBR growth to test further reduction in biomass costs and open the path to a scale-up of *T. variabilis* biomass production for extraction of valued products [7,9]. Growth curves showed that the exponential growth reached its maximum after 20 days of culture (Figure 2A), when the maximum production of 0.787 ± 0.010 gDW L^{-1} was also measured.

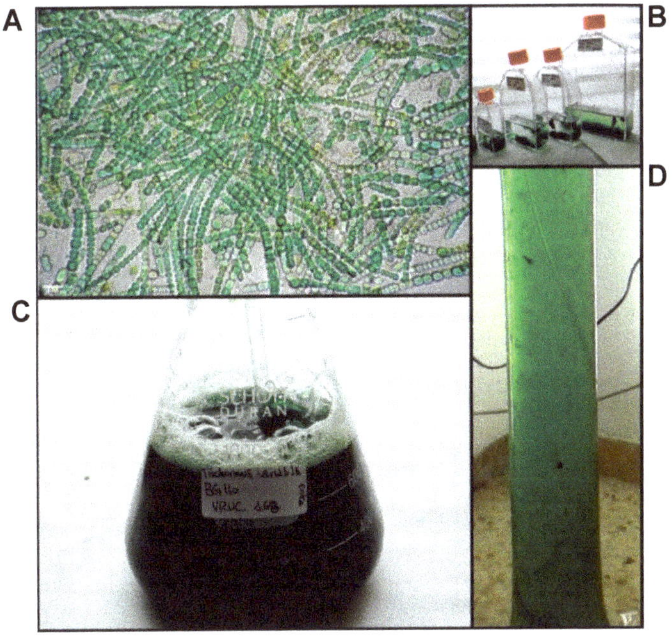

Figure 1. Biomass production. Light micrograph of *T. variabilis* trichomes in: culture (**A**); bench-scale growth system used (**B**,**C**); and pilot-scale growth system used (**D**).

Data obtained for the filamentous, non-heterocytous, cyanobacterium *Arthrospira* sp. grown in a 5 L reactor with air mixing show lower biomass production (0.67 ± 0.03 g L^{-1}), but higher rates, reaching exponential phase after only four days [40]. Studies conducted on mass cultivation of other filamentous forms report lower biomass and daily productivity values, as in the case of *Limnothrix* sp., grown in a 3.5 L PBR system (0.02 gDW L^{-1} d^{-1}; 0.29 gDW L^{-1}) [41] and *Oscillatoria* sp. in suspension, with 0.26 gDW L^{-1} produced after 20 days [42]. Our results show the ability of *T. variabilis* to grow in a simple intensive growth system and to produce rapidly a sufficient amount of biomass to be exploited for biotechnological applications.

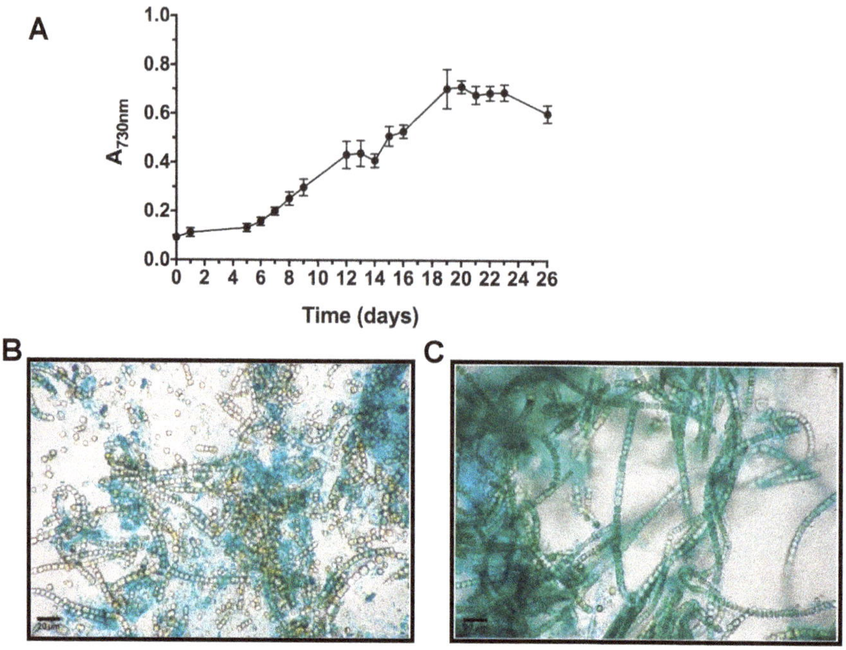

Figure 2. Growth curve recorded in polyethylene bag growth experiment (**A**). Light micrographs of cultures after Alcian Blue staining at pH 0.5 (**B**) and 2.5 (**C**) for sulfated and carboxylic EPS residues, respectively. Sulfated EPS were diffluent and less abundant (**B**), while carboxylic groups were observed in more bound matrix material (**C**).

2.2. FA Extraction and Characterization

Among several metabolites produced from cyanobacteria, PUFA have gained much consideration due to their nutritional importance. Particularly, single FA are valued in food and pharmaceutical production due to their antioxidant, anti-inflammatory and anti-microbial activities [43,44]. With the aim of combining EPS production with that of FA from the same biomass, Fatty Acid Methyl Esters (FAME) were extracted and characterized as co-products. The total FAME content rather than its pattern is known to be dependent on the species and growth conditions, and is often considered as the most important factor for industrial applications [45,46]. In this study, no culture stress to induce lipid production was applied and 63.44 ± 0.46 mg/gDW (6.34% *w*/*w*) of FAME were obtained from *T. variabilis* biomass. Our results were comparable to those obtained by Gayathri and colleagues [47] for the same species (reported as its synonym *Anabaena variabilis*) while were higher than those reported by the same authors for other heterocytous cyanobacteria, *Nostoc commune* (about 1.49% *w*/*w*) and *Nostoc muscorum* (about 5% *w*/*w*), grown without stress. The FAME composition of *T. variabilis* is shown in Table 1, with higher amounts of PUFA (57.45 ± 4.77%) obtained as compared to both monounsaturated FA (MUFA) (18.29 ± 0.02%) and saturated FA (SAFA) (24.25 ± 4.76%). The MUFA and PUFA, here produced in high yields were hexadecanoic acid (16:1) (15.25 ± 1.34%), octadecanoic acid (18:1; 3.05 ± 1.36%), octadecadienoic acid (18:2; 24.46 ± 1.91%), and octadecatrienoic acid (18:3, 27.71 ± 2.33%), which are also relevant FA for industrial production [48,49]. These yields were higher than those obtained without stress in *Anabaena cylindrica*, *Aphanizomenon gracile* and *Nostoc muscorum* [50]. Moreover, linoleic acid (C18:2 (n-6)) and α-linolenic acid (C18:3 (n-6)) were the most abundant FA in the *T. variabilis* FAME profile. From the biological activity point of view, ω-3 and ω-6 FA are essential nutritional components that display important functions in the human metabolism [51], such as in the regulation of oxygen and electron transport and membrane fluidity [52,53]. Therefore, they can be effective in cardiac protection [54,55] and cancer prevention [56–59], type 2 diabetes, inflammation and obesity [53,60,61]. These results suggest the possibility to use *T. variabilis* biomass as a low-cost source of PUFA for nutraceutical applications and to integrate the production of REPS with that of PUFA. This allows reducing operational costs and making the exploitation of the studied cyanobacterial strain economically more advantageous.

Table 1. Fatty acid methyl esters pattern (FAME % *w/w*) obtained from *T. variabilis* biomass.

Fatty Acids			% FAME *w/w*		
Systematic name	**Common name**	**Number of carbon atoms:double bond(s)**	**Family**	**Mean ***	**SEM [1]**
Decanoic acid	Capric acid	C10:0	Saturated	0.61	0.03
Tetradecanoic acid	Myristic acid	C14:0	Saturated	0.70	0.01
Hexadecenoic acid	Palmitoleic acid	C16:1 (n-7)	Monounsaturated	15.25	1.34
Hexadecadienoic acid		C16:2 (n-4)	Polyunsaturated	5.28	0.54
Octadecanoic acid	Stearic acid	C18:0	Saturated	0.83	0.19
Octadecenoic acid	Oleic acid	C18:1 (n-7)	Monounsaturated	3.05	1.36
Octadecadienoic acid	Linoleic acid	C18:2 (n-6)	Polyunsaturated	24.46	1.91
Octadecatrienoic acid	α-Linolenic acid	C18:3 (n-3)	Polyunsaturated	27.71	2.33
Eicosanoic acid	Arachidic acid	C20:0	Saturated	22.11	4.60
SAFA				24.25	4.76
MUFA				18.29	0.02
PUFA				57.45	4.77

[1] SEM refers to standard error; * Mean of three replicates.

2.3. EPS Extraction and REPS Characterization

The ability to synthesize relevant amounts of highly heterogeneous, hydrated and charged EPS plays critical roles in cyanobacterial cellular cohesion, protection and metabolic integrity. In response to water availability, EPS undergo striking changes in their rheological properties [62]. A first insight into their variable composition can be obtained by microscopic observations of cyanobacterial biomass after specific staining. Cytochemical characterization was performed using Alcian Blue (AB) at two pH values (Figure 2B,C). AB staining at 2.5 pH revealed the presence of carboxylic groups in the EPS material adherent to *T. variabilis* cell surface (bound EPS), while AB at 0.5 pH reacted with sulfated residues evidencing a lower amount in the released material, confirming what was previously observed for the same strain in our laboratory [12].

The obtained REPS after 20 days of growth were 465 mg/gDW and the plot of REPS production over growth is shown in Figure S1. Previous data on the same strain grown at bench-scale, without air mixing, showed lower REPS content, of about 86.7 mg/gDW [12]. Therefore, our data, in agreement with Pereira and colleagues [18], would evidence that the culture turbulence, due to the aeration, may facilitate the release of EPS from the cell surface and stimulate their synthesis. The REPS produced by *T. variabilis* in this study were about 46.5% of the dried biomass, a value comparable to that recently obtained from *Trichocoleus sociatus* (60%) grown in an aerosol-based emerse photobioreactor (ePBR) to simulate this terrestrial cyanobacterium natural environment [14]. It has to be noted that that the proportion and composition of released and bound EPS can show high variability depending on external environmental/cultivation factors and on the strain itself. Indeed, a combination of drought and salt stress was successfully used to increase EPS production in *Trichocoleus sociatus* [14,63]. Previous data on the studied strain cultivated at smaller scale without any aeration showed a complex monosaccharide composition of its exopolysaccharides that were composed of ten different residues whose glucose and xylose were the most abundant and uronic acids, such as galacturonic acid and glucuronic acid, that contributed to their anionic nature and sticky character [12]. Figure 3A shows the RP-HPLC and the spectrophotometric data of the REPS solution demonstrating the absence of both hydrophobic compounds and chromophores. The low peptide or protein content was also confirmed by bicinchoninic acid (BCA) assay resulting in a protein concentration of 0.39 ± 0.02 mg/mL, corresponding to 3.6% *w*/*w* of REPS dry weight. Sugar content was assessed using phenol method, showing 10.2% *w*/*w* of REPS dry weight. Infrared spectroscopic analysis of the REPS powder, obtained after freeze-drying, was also performed (Figure 3B).

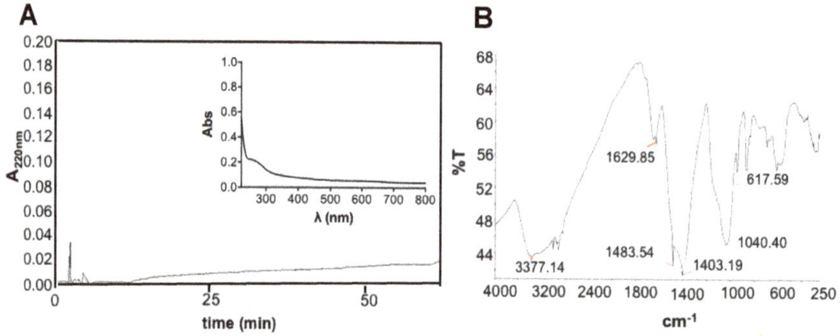

Figure 3. Characterization of REPS: (**A**) RP-HPLC chromatogram of REPS solution (10 mg/mL) using C_{18} column at 0.8 mL/min flow rate and the following gradient: 0–5 min, 0%; 5–50 min, 60%; 50–55 min, 60%; 55–60 min, 90%; and 60–65 min, 90% of solvent B (80% *v*/*v* CH_3CN and 0.1% *v*/*v* TFA). Inset: UV-vis absorption spectrum of REPS solution. (**B**) FT-IR spectrum of REPS showing signals within 4000 to 250 cm^{-1}; the measurements were consistent among three replicates.

The FT-IR spectrum confirmed the presence of polysaccharides showing the presence of specific absorption bands. The observed bands were characteristic of carbohydrates (1403 cm^{-1} and 1040 cm^{-1}) and polymeric substances (3377 cm^{-1}) with –OH, –COOH, phenolic and –CH_2 groups [64–67]. In particular, the signal around 1040 cm^{-1} suggested the presence of carbohydrates with sulfur functional groups confirming what was observed after cytochemical staining in light microscopy. A peak around 3377 cm^{-1} was attributed to stretching vibration of hydroxyl groups, characteristic of –OH groups into polymeric substances. Furthermore, bands at 2915–2935 cm^{-1} were due to asymmetrical C–H stretching vibration of aliphatic CH_2-group [64,65]. Moreover, a band at 1629 cm^{-1} of the amide I region was observed, probably suggesting the presence of proteins [66]. The presence of several peaks at wavelengths lower than 1000 cm^{-1} may be due to several visible bands attributed to phenolic groups, phosphate functional groups and/or to the occurrence of possible linkages between monosaccharide units [68]. Furthermore, the presence of carboxylic groups suggests, when combined with the other observed bands, the presence of uronic acids (especially with sugar-characteristic bands) and of humic substances (–CH_2 and phenolic groups).

2.4. REPS-Hy Synthesis and Characterization

Generally, many polysaccharides are characterized by gelling property that was investigated by preparing several solutions at different concentrations of REPS and pH values. Although a gelation tendency was observed at 68.67 mg/mL in H_2O, the REPS gel was not stable. Therefore, hybrid hydrogels made of 8.0 mg/mL of REPS solution and 2% or 3% (*w*/*v*) of PEGDa (6 kDa) were prepared by UV photo-polymerization, according to the schematic representation shown in Figure 4A. The presence of REPS was relevant for the gelation process, as shown in Figure 4B, wherein an unstable hydrogel obtained after photo-polymerization of a solution with 2% (*w*/*v*) of PEGDa without REPS (Figure 4B, top) is compared to a stable REPS-Hy with 3% of PEGDa. The stability of the REPS-Hy in PBS was assessed both over two weeks at 4 °C and after 72 h at 37 °C (Figure 4B, bottom); neither condition exhibited spontaneous hydrolysis.

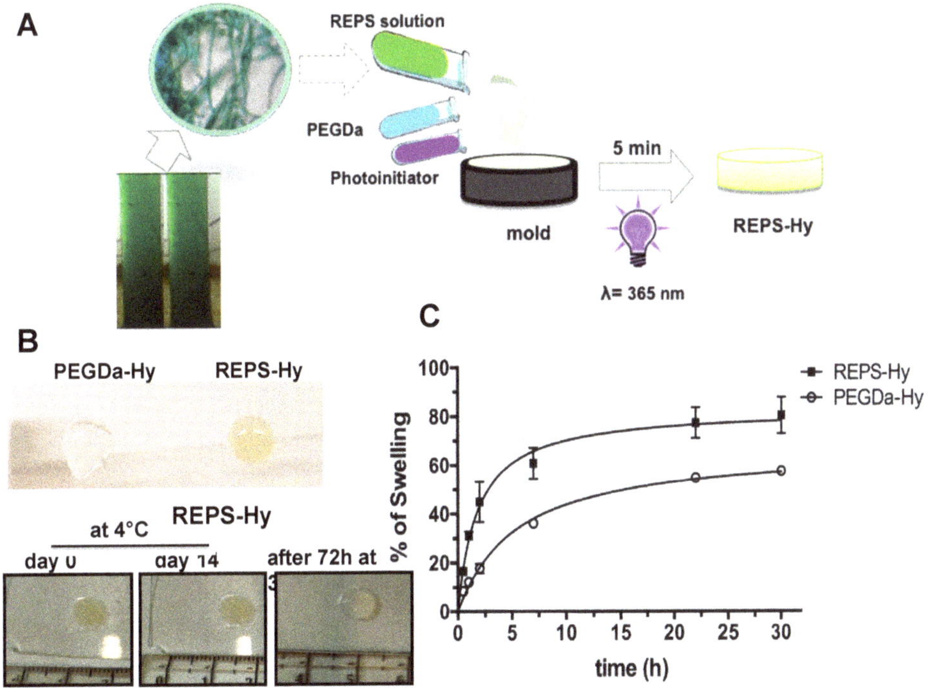

Figure 4. Synthesis and characterization of the REPS-Hy: (**A**) Schematic representation of REPS-Hy production: the gelling of the solution of 8.83 mg/mL of REPS with 3% of PEGDa (6 kDa) (*w*/*v*), and 0.1% of Irgacure®2959 (*w*/*v*) was obtained after 5 min of UV light (365 nm) exposition. (**B**) Resistance of REPS-Hy to dehydration and spontaneous hydrolysis. Digital macro-photographs of: PEGDa-Hy with 2% of PEGDa without REPS and REPS-Hy with 2% of PEGDa (*w*/*v*) (**top**); REPS-Hy with 3% of PEGDa-Hy (*w*/*v*) at Day 0 and Day 14 after storage at 4 °C, and after 72 h of incubation at 37 °C in PBS (**bottom**). (**C**) Swelling rate curves of REPS-Hy and PEGDa-Hy in PBS up to the equilibrium swelling (30 h). The R^2 of the hyperbolic fits of the swelling trend of REPS-Hy and PEGDa-Hy are 0.9284 and 0.9912, respectively.

Moreover, REPS-Hy was resistant to dehydration and morphological changes were not detectable also after long incubation times (Figure 4B). The REPS-Hy degree of swelling was analyzed over time (Figure 4C) and compared to that of PEGDa-Hy, which was obtained using 3% of PEGDa (6 kDa). The percentage of water-uptake (%WU) at the "equilibrium swelling" (% S_{eq}), was corresponding to 80.20 ± 7.5% WU for REPS-Hy in PBS after 22 h of hydration. Moreover, the swelling of REPS-Hy was about 22.8 ± 6.5% more than that observed for PEGDa-Hy. These results agree with the natural hydration properties of the EPS from cyanobacteria and such properties are crucial for the survival of these organisms. Important physiological properties, in fact, have been attributed to EPS including the physical barrier to the environment and the desiccation tolerance, as well as the subsequent rehydration [62,69]. These properties highly stabilize cells during long-term storage in the air-dried state [62]. The rheological properties of EPS are strictly related to their 3D supramolecular structure, which changes in response to environmental variables regulating the mass transfer and other biophysical properties that modulate cell activity. Therefore, the intrinsic EPS properties preserved in our REPS-Hy could be important in biomedical applications as well as in the emerging field of 3D-bioprinting.

Rheological analysis of REPS-Hy and PEGDa-Hy (without REPS) reveals differences in the shear storage modulus (G′) that are likely associated with additional crosslinking in the REPS-Hy (Figure 5). The plateau storage moduli of the REPS-Hy and PEGDa-Hy were 2778 Pa and 1785 Pa, respectively (Figure 5A). The average shear loss modulus of the REPS-Hy was also higher than that of the PEGDa-Hy. This order of magnitude increase in shear loss modulus is likely attributed to higher viscosity associated with high molecular weight REPS macromolecules. The frequency and strain sweep rheological analysis confirms that the REPS-Hy and PEGDa-Hy both display similar viscoelastic behavior, notably that both show a uniform stress response to alternations in strain or frequency of oscillatory deformation (Figure 5B,C). Therefore, it is assumed that the REPS do not alter the polymer network structure beyond those attributes associated with the additional cross-linking and increased macromolecular chain length of the REPS.

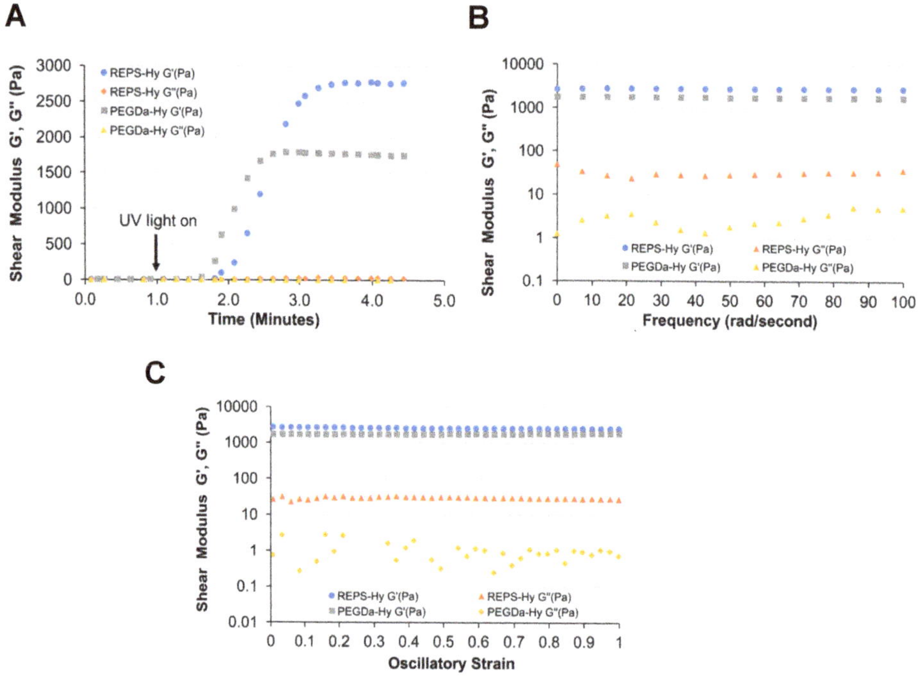

Figure 5. REPS improve hydrogel mechanical properties. Rheological measurement of REPS-Hy and PEGDa-Hy as evaluated by: time-sweep tests (**A**); frequency-sweep tests (**B**); and strain-sweep tests (**C**). The shear storage modulus (G′) and shear loss modulus (G″) are shown for both hydrogels. (**A**) The time sweep data reveal an increase in G′ upon the light-activated free-radical polymerization reaction of the REPS-Hy and PEGDa-Hy liquid precursors. The plateau G′ of the REPS-Hy was 55% higher as compared to the plateau G′ of the PEGDa-Hy, indicating that the REPS improves the elastic mechanical properties of the hydrogels. Following the chemical cross-linking of the hydrogels, the frequency-sweep (**B**) and strain-sweep (**C**) data confirmed a linear relationship between the shear modulus in the range of the applied frequency and strain.

2.5. REPS-Hy as Enzyme-Carrier System

REPS-Hy was studied as a potential enzyme-carrier system and the detoxification enzyme thiosulfate:cyanide sulfurtranferase (TST) was used as enzymatic model. The recombinant TST from *Azotobacter vinelandii* used herein is characterized by the presence of only one Cys residue, which is also the catalytic residue present in the active site. Figure 6A shows the scheme of its enzymatic activity. First, the TST activity was assessed in the presence and in the absence of REPS solution (8.0 mg/mL REPS, 8 mM $CaCl_2$ in PBS) at room temperature at different times of incubation (0 min, 30 min and 20 h) (Figure 6B). The REPS solution did not significantly affect the TST activity, even after many hours of incubation (Figure 6B). These results suggested us the possibility to embed the TST into REPS-Hy. The TST enzyme solution was mixed with REPS-Hy precursor solution and, after photo-polymerization, the TST activity was evaluated using the Sörbo assay at different incubation times in the presence of the substrates (1, 5, 15, 30 and 60 min) at 37 °C (Figure 6C).

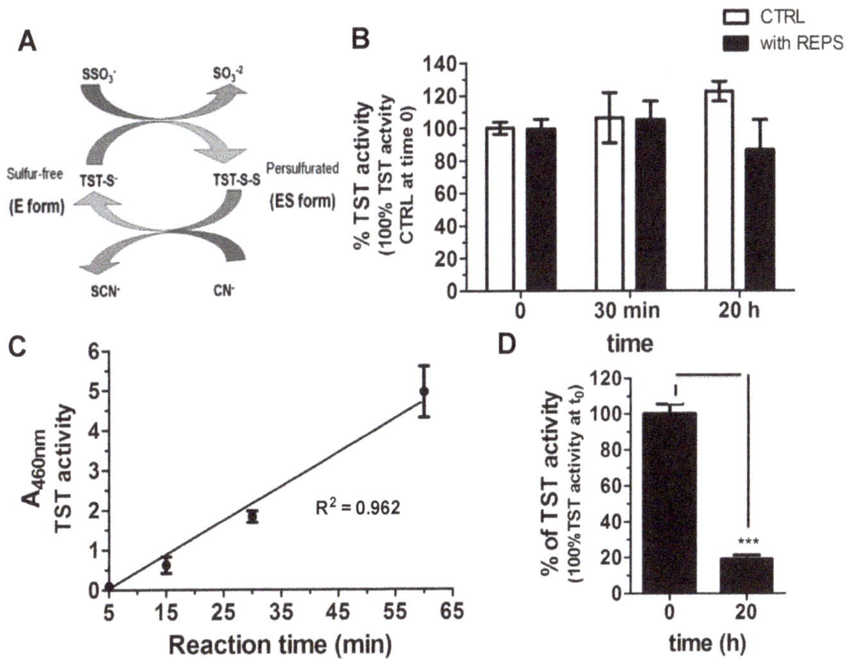

Figure 6. REPS-Hy as detoxification enzyme-encapsulating hydrogel: (**A**) Scheme of the catalytic cycle of the TST enzyme. (**B**) Percentage of TST activity over time of 3.12 μM of TST in presence of 50 μL of PBS (white) or of REPS solution (8 mg/mL of REPS and 8 mM of $CaCl_2$ in PBS, pH 7.4) (black) (100% is the activity in PBS at time 0). The Sörbo assay was performed at 23 °C. (**C**) TST activity of TSTREPS-Hy at different incubation times (5, 15, 30 and 60 min) at 37 °C. The reaction was stopped after incubation and the absorbance of the solutions measured after dilution. The line equation is $y = 0.07611x$ and R^2 is 0.9621. (**D**) TST activity of TSTREPS-Hy at time 0 and after 20 h at room temperature (23 °C) in 200 μL of 50 mM Tris-HCl, pH 8.0, buffer (100% is the TSTREPS-Hy activity at time 0). *** $p < 0.001$, $n = 3$ or 5.

TSTREPS-Hy showed enzymatic activity (Figure 6D), although a statistically significant decrease of the enzymatic activity of the embedded TST in the gel with respect to the TST in solution was observed. This was probably due to both the photo-polymerization process and to the diffusion rates of the substrates and the final product.

A linear increase of the TST activity of the TSTREPS-Hy in a time-dependent manner was observed, likely owing to the diffusion phenomena in the gel (Figure 6C). Accordingly, the selected time to perform the activity assay of TSTREPS-Hy was 30 min, which was a good compromise to have a detectable TST activity, minimizing the effect due to diffusion of the substrates and products in and out the gel and at least avoid the dilution for the measure of the absorbance. The enzymatic activity of TSTREPS-Hy was assessed over time (Figure 6D), and after 20 h of incubation into 200 μL of 50 mM

Tris-HCl buffer, pH 8.0, at 37 °C only the 20% of the TST activity was recovered. The decrease of the enzymatic activity could be due to the release of the enzyme from the gel considering that the REPS solution did not induce a statistically significant inhibition of the enzymatic activity. The RP-HPLC analysis of the soluble fraction was performed, but unfortunately the TST release was not detectable for the overlapping of the retention times of TST peak with PEGDa-derivative molecules that were released from the gel (Figure S2). These preliminary results suggest the possibility to use the REPS-Hy as TST carrier system for the cyanide detoxification. A rapidly growing class of modern therapeutics is constituted by proteins and peptides, which often show a better efficiency than small drugs for the therapy and diagnosis of serious and deadly diseases. However, their administration is often difficult due to the loss of the native structure and rapid cleavage in the liver or other body tissues. Their instability could be diminished by biocompatible and biodegradable hydrogels useful as carriers able to improve their bioavailability and to provide other routes of administration [70]. Several proteins including insulin, growth hormones, and interferons at other proteins have been already encapsulated in microbial exopolysaccharide hydrogel particles [71–74] and the improving their administration has been demonstrated. In this context, the results herein proved activity of the detoxification enzyme either in the presence of REPS solution from *T. variabilis* or into REPS-Hy. They suggest the possibility to use EPS for the production of hydrogel carrier systems of enzymes characterized by the presence of cysteine at the catalytic site, although other experiments, using different enzymes, are necessary to support this hypothesis. Moreover, the enzyme-REPS-Hy could represent a good opportunity to combine the EPS natural properties, such as antibacterial, anti-oxidative and anti-inflammatory properties [75], with a specific enzymatic activity.

2.6. REPSHy as Stem Cell Carrier for Tissue Engineering

The biocompatibility of REPS-Hy was also evaluated by analysis of the cell adhesion of human mesenchymal stem cells (hMSCs) seeded onto REPS-Hy and cultured for two weeks in the presence of DMEM medium. Figure 7 shows the confocal laser scanning micrographs of hMSCs after two weeks of growing on REPS-Hy.

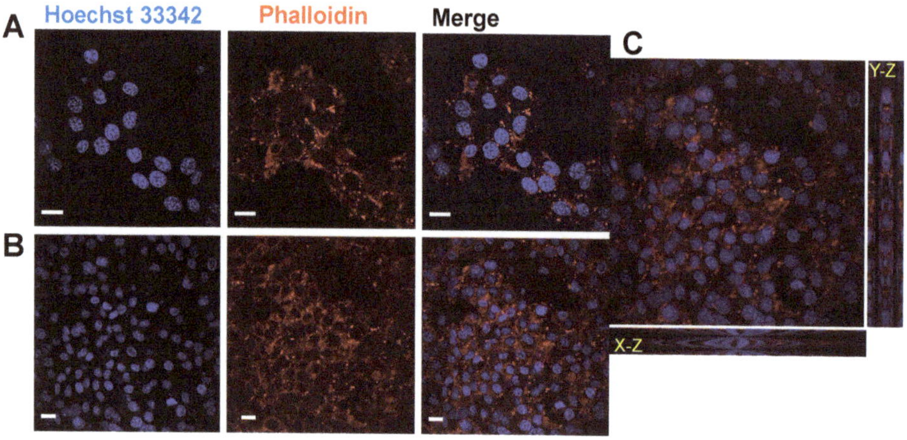

Figure 7. hMSCs cultures using REPS-Hy as scaffold. Confocal laser scanning micrographs of hMSCs cultured for two weeks on REPS-Hy: (**A**) at 60× magnificantion; (**B**) at 40× magnification; and (**C**) micrographs with Y–Z and X–Z projections. F-actin was stained with Alexa-fluor 568 phalloidin-conjugate (in red) and the nuclei were stained using Hoechst 33342 (in blue). Scale bars = 10 μm.

The nuclei were stained with Hoechst 33342 and F-actin with Alexa-fluor 568 phalloidin-conjugate and it was notably the presence of multicellular networks. The presence of many cells with elongated morphology demonstrated a good adhesion of the hMSCs to the material and not cytotoxicity. Moreover, hMSCs were embedded into the REPS-Hy during the photo-polymerization, thus producing a 3D-stem cell culture system. The scheme of the 3D-stem cell culture system preparation is shown in Figure 8A. The cell viability was evaluated after zero and three days of growth (Figure 8B,C) and 82.43 ± 0.01% cell proliferation was observed.

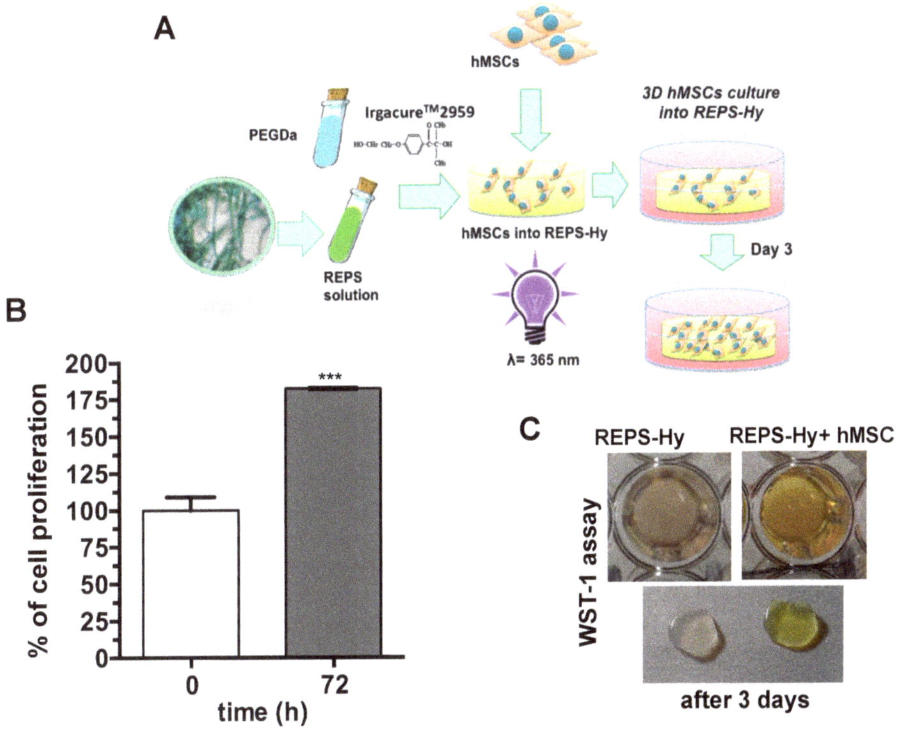

Figure 8. REPS-Hy as stem cell-carrier system: (**A**) Schematic representation of the production of REPS-Hy scaffolds for 3D hMSC cultures. (**B**) Cell viability of hMSCs embedded into the REPS-Hy, immediately after photo-polymerization (time 0) and after 72 h of 3D cell culture (100% is the cell viability at time 0). (**C**) Digital macro-photographs of REPS-Hy with and without embedded hMSCs after colorimetric WST-1 cell viability assay. *** $p < 0.001$.

These preliminary results confirm the cytocompatibility of the REPS-Hy and open the way to produce new 3D-hybrid scaffolds for tissue engineering, where the physiological role of the EPS to protect the cell from unfavorable stress and to increase the cell–cell interaction [75] could be exploited for improving the tissue formation.

Moreover, an emerging technological and biomedical field is represented by 3D-bioprinting [76,77] of tissues and organs using stem cells and biomaterials. Photo-polymerizable hydrogels represent optimal biomaterials for this new technology for generating injectable cell/drug carrier systems.

The preparation of an appropriate bio-ink represents in 3D-bioprinting one of the main challenges. The printable biomaterials should have optimal structural and mechanical properties to drive the fate of the stem cell, while also protecting the cells from damage during printing. The peculiar intrinsic characteristics of the EPS such as the high water-uptake, dehydration resistance and the radical scavenging could be relevant properties of a bio-ink in reduce the cellular damage during the bio-printing process. Indeed, EPS can naturally inhibit the desiccation stress of the cyanobacteria, reducing the damage to cell membranes, nucleic acids and proteins induced by reactive oxygen species (ROS) under high light and UV irradiation [78]. Accordingly, with the radical scavenging property of the cyanobacterial EPS, the REPS presence in the hydrogel could reduce oxidative damages due to photo-polymerization process for 3D-bioprinting technologies.

3. Materials and Methods

3.1. *Trichormus Variabilis Biomass Cultivation*

A strain of the heterocytous cyanobacterium *T. variabilis* (Kützing ex Bornet & Flahault) Komárek & Anagnostidis (VRUC168) was isolated from microphytobenthos of a Mediterranean shallow coastal lagoon (Cabras lagoon, Sardinia, Italy) [11] and maintained in standard Blue Green Medium (BG11) [79] at 18–20 °C, irradiance of 30 μmol photons m^{-2} s^{-1} and 12:12 hs L/D cycle. A polyphasic approach was used for strain circumscription elsewhere [12]. The stock culture was acclimated at higher irradiance and temperature conditions (80 μmol photons m^{-2} s^{-1}, 25 °C) and used as inoculum for biomass production. Three culture replicates were set up in 400 mL flasks in batch and the growth curves recorded by measuring the optical density (OD) at 730 nm (BECKMAN DU-65 spectrophotometer, BECKMAN COULTER, High Wycombe, UK) and the dry weight (T = 60 °C) at 24 h intervals. At the stationary phase, Day 35, each culture was used as inoculum to mass cultivate *T. variabilis* in three low-cost polyethylene bags (PBRs), of 10 L each. BG11 medium was supplied only at the beginning of the growth experiments. The PBRs were kept, at the optimized growth conditions with air mixing, in a growth cabinet equipped with white fluorescent lamps (OSRAM L 30w/956, Munich, Germany) and thermostated (25 °C). Subsamples (1 mL for OD and 5 mL for dry weight) of each PBR cultures were taken in triplicate every 48 h and the growth estimated as above. The daily biomass productivity was calculated by dividing the difference between the dry weights estimated at the end and at the beginning of the experiments by the experiment duration (days) [80]. Biomass separation was carried out at the stationary phase (Day 20) when air mixing was stopped and biomass settled at the bottom of the PBRs and the total biomass yield was evaluated after centrifuging (5000× *g* for 20 min; Heraeus SEPATECH, Megafuge 1.0, Thermo Fisher Scientific, Waltham, MA, USA) and freeze-drying.

Light microscopy observations of culture samples at the stationary phase were conducted after staining for 10 min using Alcian Blue (AB) 1%, in HCl 0.5 N (pH 0.5), specific for sulfated polysaccharidic residues present in the REPS or in 3% acetic acid (pH 2.5) specific for carboxylic moieties. A light microscope (ZEISS Axioskop, CARL ZEISS, Jena, Germany) equipped with differential interference was used and the micrographs were acquired using a digital camera Coolpix995 (Nikon, Tokyo, Japan).

3.2. *Extraction of REPS*

Released-EPS fraction was obtained according to Ahmed and colleagues procedure [81]. The culture solutions from the PBRs were centrifuged (5000× *g* for 20 min) and the supernatants containing REPS were separated from pellets. The following steps were designed and adapted to the scaling up of REPS production. Thus, the supernatants were evaporated and the REPS concentrated using a Rotavapor Buchi WaterBath B-480 at 45 °C. The concentrated supernatant was precipitated in 96% cold ethanol and the REPS fraction was obtained. The fraction was dialyzed against bi-distilled water at 4 °C for 2–3 days using a dialysis membrane with a cut-off of 18 kDa (Spectrum Laboratories, Inc., Breda, Netherlands), and then freeze-dried and stored at −20 °C for further analysis.

3.3. *REPS Characterization*

Ten milligrams of freeze-dried REPS were dissolved in 1 mL MilliQ water and total sugar content determined by the phenol-sulfuric acid method, using glucose as standard [82] (Figure S3). Total protein concentration was also assessed using BCA colorimetric assay (Sigma-Aldrich, Milan, Italy) and bovine albumin (BSA) as standard protein for calibration curve.

The RP-HPLC analysis of the REPS solutions was performed using LC-10AVP equipment (Shimadzu, Milan, Italy), 0.1% *v/v* trifluoroacetic acid as solvent A and 80% *v/v* acetonitrile and 0.1% *v/v* trifluoroacetic acid as solvent B. The analyses were performed using a C_{18} column (CPS Analitica, 150 mm × 4.6 mm, 5 μm), a loop of 20 μL, flow of 0.8 mL/min and the following solvent B gradient: 0–5 min, 0%; 5–50 min, 60%; 50–55 min, 60%; 55–60 min, 90%; and 60–65 min, 90%. The elution was monitored at 220 nm by a UV detector (Shimadzu, Milan, Italy).

FT-IR Spectroscopy was used for chemical analysis of freeze-dried REPS material, using a Perkin Elmer Spectrum 100 (PerkinElmer Inc., Paris, France). Spectra were acquired in the range 4000–250 cm^{-1}, by averaging 32 scans at a resolution of 4 cm^{-1}, using CsI cells. Data were processed using Spectrum 6.3.5 software (PerkinElmer Inc., Paris, France).

3.4. FAME Extraction and Characterization

FAME extraction from residual biomass and in situ trans-esterification, were carried out as previously described [13,83]. Briefly, the biomass after EPS extraction, was resuspended in a methanol and sulfuric acid (*v/v* 15:1) mixture for 6 h at 60 °C. After filtration, hexane was used to separate the FAME fraction. FAMEs content was estimated as the percentage of esterified lipids per dry biomass (grams). The FAME profile was determined using a gas chromatograph-mass spectrometry (Gas chromatograph GC-2010 Plus mass spectrometer GCMS-QP2010 Ultra; Shimadzu Corp., Kyoto, Japan). Eight microliters of each sample were injected into the column (SLB-5ms Fused Silica Capillary Column; 30 m × 0.25 mm × 0.25 μm film thickness) with a temperature program starting from 170 °C, increasing of 3 °C/min to 240 °C final, hold for 20 min. Split ratio was 1:80 and injection temperature 280 °C, helium was used as carrier gas. The run time for every single sample was 35 min. The identification of FA was performed by comparing the obtained mass spectra with NIST Mass Spectral Data Base (http://webbook.nist.gov/chemistry/). Total lipid concentration refers to the sum of total FAMEs.

3.5. REPS-Hydrogel Preparation

PEGDa 6 kDa MW (Sigma-Aldrich, Milan, Italy) and REPS solution were used for synthesizing highly cross-linked hydrogels (REPS-Hy). REPS (8.83 mg/mL), 10 mM $CaCl_2$ and 2 or 3% (*w/v*) of PEGDa were solubilized in PBS, pH 7.4. The free-radical photo-polymerization of the hydrogels was achieved by addition of 0.1% (*w/v*) Irgacure®2959 (Ciba Specialty Chemicals, Basel, Switzerland) to the precursor solution, followed by 5 min exposure to long-wave UV light (365 nm, 4–5 mW/cm^2). Finally, REPS-Hys were washed with sterile PBS solution to remove non-polymerized material.

3.6. REPS-Hy Characterization

3.6.1. Rheological Analyses of REPS-Hy

The mechanical properties of the REPS-Hy were measured using oscillatory, strain-rate controlled rheometry. The shear storage modulus (G′) of the hydrogels was determined by applying oscillatory strain and measuring the shear response, using a TA Instruments AR-G2 rheometer (ARES, TA Instruments, New Castle, DE, USA) equipped with a 20-mm parallel-plate geometry adapted with an ultraviolet (UV) light-curing assembly. The sample (200 μL) of the liquid hydrogel precursor was pipetted onto the transparent lower plate, and the upper plate was lowered until it reached a gap of ~600 μm. For hydrogel curing, the precursor was exposed from underneath the geometry to long-wave UV light (365 nm, 5 mW/cm^2). Dynamic time sweeps were performed at 25 °C, 2% sinusoidal strain, and 3 rad/s constant frequency, while continuously monitoring the shear response of the materials before, during and after light-activated polymerization (in situ rheometry). The measurements were carried out for one minute without UV, followed by UV light activation until after the maximum value of G′ was reached (approximately 5 min). Frequency sweep measurements were performed on the hydrogels, whereby constant 2% strain at an oscillation frequency of 0.1–100 rad/s was applied while measuring the shear response. Strain sweep measurements were performed on the hydrogels whereby the oscillation frequency was held constant at 3 rad/s and strain was varied from 1% to 100%, while measuring the shear response. The sample rheology measurements were performed on two replicates for each treatment.

3.6.2. Swelling Analysis of REPS-Hy

Swelling behavior of REPS-Hydrogel was investigated over 24 h, at room temperature, until equilibrium swelling as described elsewhere [84,85]. Briefly, three replicas of REPS-Hy and PEGDa-Hy (used as control) were weighted immediately after photo-polymerization and placed into a well with 500 μL of PBS and weighed at different times: 1, 2, 6, 24 and 30 h. The degree of swelling, corresponding to the percentage of water uptake (WU), was calculated following Equation (1):

$$\%WU = (W_t - W_0)/W_0 \times 100 \quad (1)$$

where W_t is the mass of the swollen hydrogel at time t, and W_0 is the mass after gel-polymerization.

3.7. Detoxification Enzyme Synthesis and Encapsulation into the REPS-Hy

Recombinant thiosulfate:cyanide sulfurtransferase (TST, rhodanese EC.2.8.1.1) from *Azotobacter vinelandii* was produced and purified as previously described [86,87]. TST activity of the enzyme was tested using the Sörbo assay [88] obtaining an enzymatic activity of 64.06 U/mg. Briefly, the Sörbo assay was performed as follow: the recombinant TST enzyme was incubated at 37 °C in a reaction mixture (650 μL of 58 mM KCN and 58 mM sodium thiosulfate in 50 mM Tris-HCl buffer, pH 8.0). The reaction was stopped after 1 min by adding 100 μL of 15% formaldehyde and addition of 250 μL Sörbo reagent (100 g of ferric nitrate and 200 mL of 65% nitric acid per 1500 mL). The product was monitored reading the absorbance at 460 nm. The Sörbo assay for evaluating the TST activity in the presence and in the absence of REPS solution (8 mg/mL REPS, 8 mM $CaCl_2$ in PBS) was performed at 23 °C after 1 min of incubation. Then, 10.08 μM of TST in 60 μL of REPS-Hy precursor solution (solution with 6.67 mg/mL REPS, 3% *w*/*v* PEGDa, 1.6% *v*/*v* Irgacure®2959 and PBS) was photo-polymerized for 5 min under UV light at 365 nm. The solution was photo-polymerized into a teflon mold (50 mm inner diameter) and the TST activity of the TSTREPS-Hy was assessed at different times of incubation (1, 5, 15, 30 and 60 min) of the gel at 37 °C with 58 mM KCN and 58 mM sodium thiosulfate in 50 mM Tris-HCl buffer, pH 8.0, the reaction was stopped by addition of formaldehyde and Sörbo reagent and the absorbance evaluated at 460 nm.

3.8. Stem Cell Viability in 2D and 3D Cell Growth Systems

Human cardiac resident Mesenchymal Stem Cells (hMSC) line expressing stem cell marker Sca^-1^+ Lin^-, was obtained as previously described [37,89]. Briefly, the cell line was obtained from cells isolated from human auricular biopsies made during the course of coronary artery bypass surgery of patients undergoing cardiac surgery after signing a written consent form for the research study, according to a joint protocol approved by the Ethic Committees of Ospedale Maggiore della Carita, Novara and University Hospital Le Molinette, Turin 2011. The cells were cultured in Dulbecco's modified Eagle medium (DMEM) (Gibco, Monza, Italy) supplemented with 10% of fetal bovine serum (FBS) (*v*/*v*) (Gibco, Monza, Italy), 2 mM L-Glutamine (Sigma-Aldrich, Milan, Italy), 100 U/mL penicillin and 100 μg/mL streptomycin (Sigma-Aldrich, Milan, Italy) (hereafter referred to as "complete medium") at 37 °C and with 5% CO_2. After trypsinization, the cells were seeded onto the surface of the polymerized REPS-Hy (at a density of 1×10^4 cells/cm^2), or embedded into the hydrogels by re-suspending them in the REPS-Hy precursor solution prior the photo-polymerization procedure (at a density of 0.417×10^6 cells/mL). The cell-seeded hydrogels and the cell-embedded ones were cultivated in 1 mL of complete medium in 24-multiwell plates for 14 and 3 days, respectively. The cell viability was quantified by WST-1 colorimetric assay [90]. Briefly, WST-1 assay (4-[3-(4-Iodophenyl)-2-(4-nitrophenyl)-2*H*-5-tetrazolio]-1,3-benzene disulfonate) (Roche Diagnostics, Sigma Aldrich, Milan, Italy) was performed by incubating the hydrogel samples for 3 h in complete DMEM (without phenol-red) in the presence of 5% (*v*/*v*) cell proliferation Reagent WST-1 at 37 °C and in 5% CO_2. The absorbance of the medium was evaluated using iMark™ Microplate Reader (Bio-Rad, Milan, Italy) at a 450 nm wavelength.

3.9. Immunofluorescence Microscopy Analyses

hMSC phenotype of the cells seeded and cultured on REPS-Hy was analyzed by immunofluorescence microscopy. Gels were washed in PBS, fixed in 4% paraformaldehyde (PFA) (Sigma-Aldrich, Milan, Italy) in PBS for 30 min at room temperature. After that, the cells were permeabilized with 0.3% Triton X-100 (Sigma-Aldrich, Milan, Italy) for 5 min and maintained in a blocking buffer (10% *v*/*v* FBS, 0.1% *v*/*v* Triton X-100 and 1% *w*/*v* glycine in PBS) overnight at 4 °C. Hydrogels were incubated with F-actin 488-Alexa fluorochrome-conjugated phalloidin (Life Technologies, Milan, Italy). Nuclei were stained with 1:25,000 *w*/*v* Hoechst 33342 (Sigma-Aldrich, Milan, Italy) in PBS. Hydrogels were stored at 4 °C in 20 mM Gly PBS under dark conditions. Confocal microscopy was performed using Nikon Eclipse Ti (Nikon, Tokyo, Japan) and the signal was detected using EZ C.1 software (Nikon, Tokyo, Japan).

3.10. Statistical Analysis

GraphPad Prism version 6.0 program (GraphPad Software, San Diego, CA, USA) was used for statistical analysis. Three or five independent experiments were performed for each result and the analysis of the variables was made using ANOVA One-way test or the one-tailed Student's *t*-test. A *p*-value of <0.05 was considered to be statistically significant. Standard deviations (SD) or the standard errors (SEM) of the mean were calculated and reported for each sample.

4. Conclusions

In this work, efficient biomass production by a native brackish strain of the cyanobacterium *T. variabilis* was obtained in a low-cost PBR to optimize a sequential extraction protocol for the EPS and PUFA production. This strain showed suitable productivity in the 10 L bags used, after 20 days without nutrient repletion, allowing us to collect sufficient biomass to be exploited for the target application. The potential to obtain an integrated and economically advantageous production of nutraceuticals and biomaterials was demonstrated. REPS fraction was characterized and used for producing a new photo-polymerizable hybrid-hydrogel. REPS-Hy was characterized for its physical, mechanical and biological properties and for its ability to embed detoxification enzymes with catalytic cysteine residues, such as TST. The results herein presented show the possibility to fabricate new functional non-cytotoxic hydrogels with enzymatic activity for therapeutic and environmental applications. The presence of carboxyl groups in the REPS could also help to produce hydrogels that exhibit pH-sensitive swelling behavior that could increase their pore size at basic pHs and allow the protein release from the matrix in the intestinal environment, significantly improving the absorption of the protein-drugs, as already demonstrated for insulin embedding hydrogels [91,92]. Moreover, in a proof-of-concept experiment, REPS-Hy was also used for fabricating 3D-cell embedding hydrogels, demonstrating the feasibility for the production of cell-carrier systems in cell therapy and of photo-printable bio-inks for tissue engineering applications. This is a first and preliminary study, which combines the multiple inexpensive production of cyanobacteria nutraceutical products with that of photo-polymerizable hydrogels for enzyme- and stem cell-carrier systems. Although the data reported suggest a good potential feasibility, further experiments are necessary to demonstrate the in vivo applicability.

Supplementary Materials: The following are available online at http://www.mdpi.com/1660-3397/16/9/298/s1, Figure S1: REPS production over time; Figure S2: RP-HPLC analysis of the TST solution and of the fraction released from the REPS-Hy; Figure S3: Biochemical analysis of REPS.

Author Contributions: Conceptualization, S.M. and R.C.; Methodology, S.M., M.C., E.B., S.A. and R.C.; Software, S.S., E.B. and M.C.; Formal Analysis, E.B., S.M., S.A., M.C., S.S., D.S. and R.C.; Investigation, S.M., E.B., M.C. and R.C.; Resources, S.M. and R.C.; Data Curation, S.M., E.B., D.S. and S.A.; Writing—Original Draft Preparation, S.M., E.B. and R.C.; Writing—Review and Editing, S.M., E.B., M.C., R.C. and D.S.; Supervision, S.M. and R.C.; Project Administration, S.M. and R.C.; and Funding Acquisition, S.M. and R.C.

Funding: This research received funding from: Italian MAECI with "Rita Levi Montalcini Award".

Acknowledgments: We thank P. Di Nardo for giving us the Lin^- $Sca1^+$ human cardiac resident MSCs cell line for collaborative exchanges. ES1408 Cost Action EUALGAE is also acknowledged for networking and knowledge transfer. The authors are grateful to the association of Italian MAECI, MIUR and CRUI foundation for the Rita Levi Montalcini Award for the financial support to the Italy–Israel collaboration.

Conflicts of Interest: The authors declare no conflict of interest.

Abbreviations

3D	three-dimensional
AB	Alcian Blue
BG11	Blue-Green Medium
BCA	bicinchoninic acid
BSA	Bovine serum albumin
BSCs	Biological Soil Crusts
hMSCs	human $Lin^-Sca\text{-}1^+$ cardiac mesenchymal stem cells
DMEM	Dulbecco's Modified Eagle Medium
EPS	Extracellular Polymeric Substances
ePBR	emerse photobioreactor
FA	fatty acids
FAME	Fatty Acid Methyl Esters
FBS	fetal bovine serum
FT-IR	Fourier Transform Infrared Spectroscopy
Hy	hydrogel
MUFA	monounsaturated FA
PBR	photobioreactor
PUFA	polyunsaturated FA
PEGDa	PEG-diacrylate
PFA	paraformaldehyde
REPS	Released Extracellular Polymeric Substances
REPS-Hy	REPS PEGDa-hydrogel
RP-HPLC	Reversed Phase-High-Performance Liquid Chromatography
SAFA	saturated FA
SD	standard deviations
SEM	standard errors of the mean
TST	thiosulfate: cyanide sulfur transferase
TFA	trifluoroacetic acid
WST-1	4-[3-(4-Iodophenyl)-2-(4-nitrophenyl)-2*H*-5-tetrazolio]-1,3-benzene disulfonate
WU	water uptake

References

1. Seckbach, J. *Algae and Cyanobacteria in Extreme Environments*; Springer Science & Business Media: Berlin, Germany, 2007; ISBN 978-1-4020-6111-0.
2. Grewe, C.B.; Pulz, O. The Biotechnology of Cyanobacteria. In *Ecology of Cyanobacteria II*; Springer: Dordrecht, The Netherlands, 2012; pp. 707–739. ISBN 978-94-007-3854-6.
3. Brodie, J.; Chan, C.X.; De Clerck, O.; Cock, J.M.; Coelho, S.M.; Gachon, C.; Grossman, A.R.; Mock, T.; Raven, J.A.; Smith, A.G.; et al. The Algal Revolution. *Trends Plant Sci.* **2017**, *22*, 726–738. [CrossRef] [PubMed]

4. Shah, S.A.A.; Akhter, N.; Auckloo, B.N.; Khan, I.; Lu, Y.; Wang, K.; Wu, B.; Guo, Y.W. Structural diversity, biological properties and applications of natural products from cyanobacteria. A review. *Mar. Drugs* **2017**, *15*, 354. [CrossRef] [PubMed]
5. Bruno, L.; Di Pippo, F.; Antonaroli, S.; Gismondi, A.; Valentini, C.; Albertano, P. Characterization of biofilm-forming cyanobacteria for biomass and lipid production. *J. Appl. Microbiol.* **2012**, *113*, 1052–1064. [CrossRef] [PubMed]
6. Yen, H.W.; Hu, I.C.; Chen, C.Y.; Ho, S.H.; Lee, D.J.; Chang, J.S. Microalgae-based biorefinery—From biofuels to natural products. *Bioresour. Technol.* **2013**, *135*, 166–174. [CrossRef] [PubMed]
7. Bharathiraja, B.; Chakravarthy, M.; Ranjith Kumar, R.; Yogendran, D.; Yuvaraj, D.; Jayamuthunagai, J.; Praveen Kumar, R.; Palani, S. Aquatic biomass (algae) as a future feed stock for bio-refineries: A review on cultivation, processing and products. *Renew. Sustain. Energy Rev.* **2015**, *47*, 635–653. [CrossRef]
8. Noreen, A.; Zia, K.M.; Zuber, M.; Ali, M.; Mujahid, M. A critical review of algal biomass: A versatile platform of bio-based polyesters from renewable resources. *Int. J. Biol. Macromol.* **2016**, *86*, 937–949. [CrossRef] [PubMed]
9. Wijffels, R.H.; Kruse, O.; Hellingwerf, K.J. Potential of industrial biotechnology with cyanobacteria and eukaryotic microalgae. *Curr. Opin. Biotechnol.* **2013**, *24*, 405–413. [CrossRef] [PubMed]
10. Velu, C.; Cirés, S.; Alvarez-Roa, C.; Heimann, K. First outdoor cultivation of the N2-fixing cyanobacterium *Tolypothrix* sp. in low-cost suspension and biofilm systems in tropical Australia. *J. Appl. Phycol.* **2015**, *27*, 1743–1753. [CrossRef]
11. Di Pippo, F.; Di Gregorio, L.; Congestri, R.; Tandoi, V.; Rossetti, S. Biofilm growth and control in cooling water industrial systems. *FEMS Microbiol. Ecol.* **2018**, *94*, fiy044. [CrossRef] [PubMed]
12. Di Pippo, F.; Ellwood, N.T.W.; Gismondi, A.; Bruno, L.; Rossi, F.; Magni, P.; de Philippis, R. Characterization of exopolysaccharides produced by seven biofilm-forming cyanobacterial strains for biotechnological applications. *J. Appl. Phycol.* **2013**, *25*, 1697–1708. [CrossRef]
13. Gismondi, A.; Di Pippo, F.; Bruno, L.; Antonaroli, S.; Congestri, R. Phosphorus removal coupled to bioenergy production by three cyanobacterial isolates in a biofilm dynamic growth system. *Int. J. Phytoremediation* **2016**, *18*, 869–876. [CrossRef] [PubMed]
14. Strieth, D.; Schwing, J.; Kuhne, S.; Lakatos, M.; Muffler, K.; Ulber, R. A semi-continuous process based on an ePBR for the production of EPS using *Trichocoleus sociatus*. *J. Biotechnol.* **2017**, *256*, 6–12. [CrossRef] [PubMed]
15. Hill, D.R.; Keenan, T.W.; Helm, R.F.; Potts, M.; Crowe, L.M.; Crowe, J.H. Extracellular polysaccharide of *Nostoc commune* (Cyanobacteria) inhibits fusion of membrane vesicles during desiccation. *J. Appl. Phycol.* **1997**, *9*, 237–248. [CrossRef]
16. Delattre, C.; Pierre, G.; Laroche, C.; Michaud, P. Production, extraction and characterization of microalgal and cyanobacterial exopolysaccharides. *Biotechnol. Adv.* **2016**, *34*, 1159–1179. [CrossRef] [PubMed]
17. Ekelhof, A.; Melkonian, M. Microalgal cultivation in porous substrate bioreactor for extracellular polysaccharide production. *J. Appl. Phycol.* **2017**, *29*, 1115–1122. [CrossRef]
18. Pereira, S.; Zille, A.; Micheletti, E.; Moradas-Ferreira, P.; De Philippis, R.; Tamagnini, P. Complexity of cyanobacterial exopolysaccharides: Composition, structures, inducing factors and putative genes involved in their biosynthesis and assembly. *FEMS Microbiol. Rev.* **2009**, *33*, 917–941. [CrossRef] [PubMed]
19. Rossi, F.; De Philippis, R. Exocellular Polysaccharides in Microalgae and Cyanobacteria: Chemical Features, Role and Enzymes and Genes Involved in Their Biosynthesis. In *The Physiology of Microalgae*; Developments in Applied Phycology; Springer Nature: New York, NY, USA, 2016; pp. 565–590. ISBN 978-3-319-24943-8.
20. Arias, S.; del Moral, A.; Ferrer, M.R.; Tallon, R.; Quesada, E.; Béjar, V. Mauran, an exopolysaccharide produced by the halophilic bacterium *Halomonas maura*, with a novel composition and interesting properties for biotechnology. *Extremophiles* **2003**, *7*, 319–326. [CrossRef] [PubMed]
21. De Philippis, R.; Vincenzini, M. Outermost polysaccharidic investments of cyanobacteria: Nature, significance and possible applications. *Recent Res. Dev. Microbiol.* **2003**, *7*, 13–22.
22. Nichols, C.A.M.; Guezennec, J.; Bowman, J.P. Bacterial Exopolysaccharides from Extreme Marine Environments with Special Consideration of the Southern Ocean, Sea Ice, and Deep-Sea Hydrothermal Vents: A Review. *Mar. Biotechnol.* **2005**, *7*, 253–271. [CrossRef] [PubMed]
23. Neu, T.R.; Dengler, T.; Jann, B.; Poralla, K. Structural studies of an emulsion-stabilizing exopolysaccharide produced by an adhesive, hydrophobic *Rhodococcus* strain. *Microbiology* **1992**, *138*, 2531–2537. [CrossRef] [PubMed]

24. Shepherd, R.; Rockey, J.; Sutherland, I.W.; Roller, S. Novel bioemulsifiers from microorganisms for use in foods. *J. Biotechnol.* **1995**, *40*, 207–217. [CrossRef]
25. Di Pippo, F.; Bohn, A.; Congestri, R.; De Philippis, R.; Albertano, P. Capsular polysaccharides of cultured phototrophic biofilms. *Biofouling* **2009**, *25*, 495–504. [CrossRef] [PubMed]
26. Flemming, H.C.; Wingender, J. The biofilm matrix. *Nat. Rev. Microbiol.* **2010**, *8*, 623–633. [CrossRef] [PubMed]
27. Adessi, A.; Cruz de Carvalho, R.; De Philippis, R.; Branquinho, C.; Marques da Silva, J. Microbial extracellular polymeric substances improve water retention in dryland biological soil crusts. *Soil Biol. Biochem.* **2018**, *116*, 67–69. [CrossRef]
28. Gupta, V.; Ratha, S.K.; Sood, A.; Chaudhary, V.; Prasanna, R. New insights into the biodiversity and applications of cyanobacteria (blue-green algae)—Prospects and challenges. *Algal Res.* **2013**, *2*, 79–97. [CrossRef]
29. Rossi, F.; Mugnai, G.; De Philippis, R. Complex role of the polymeric matrix in biological soil crusts. *Plant Soil* **2018**, *429*, 19–34. [CrossRef]
30. Di Pippo, F.; Bohn, A.; Cavalieri, F.; Albertano, P. ^{1}H-NMR analysis of water mobility in cultured phototrophic biofilms. *Biofouling* **2011**, *27*, 327–336. [CrossRef] [PubMed]
31. Wingender, J.; Neu, T.R.; Flemming, H.C. What are Bacterial Extracellular Polymeric Substances? In *Microbial Extracellular Polymeric Substances*; Springer: Berlin, Germany, 1999; pp. 1–19. ISBN 978-3-642-64277-7.
32. Sutherland, I.W. Biofilm exopolysaccharides: A strong and sticky framework. *Microbiology* **2001**, *147*, 3–9. [CrossRef] [PubMed]
33. Caldorera-Moore, M.; Peppas, N.A. Micro- and Nanotechnologies for Intelligent and Responsive Biomaterial-Based Medical Systems. *Adv. Drug Deliv. Rev.* **2009**, *61*, 1391–1401. [CrossRef] [PubMed]
34. Patel, D.M.; Patel, D.K.; Patel, B.K.; Patel, C.N. An overview on intelligent drug delivery systems. *Int. J. Adv. Pharm. Rev.* **2011**, *2*, 57–63.
35. Liu, Z.; Jiao, Y.; Wang, Y.; Zhou, C.; Zhang, Z. Polysaccharides-based nanoparticles as drug delivery system. *Adv. Drug Deliv. Rev.* **2008**, *60*, 1650–1662. [CrossRef] [PubMed]
36. Seliktar, D. Designing cell-compatible hydrogels for biomedical applications. *Science* **2012**, *336*, 1124–1128. [CrossRef] [PubMed]
37. Ciocci, M.; Mochi, F.; Carotenuto, F.; Di Giovanni, E.; Prosposito, P.; Francini, R.; De Matteis, F.; Reshetov, I.; Casalboni, M.; Melino, S.; et al. Scaffold-in-Scaffold Potential to Induce Growth and Differentiation of Cardiac Progenitor Cells. *Stem Cells Dev.* **2017**, *26*, 1438–1447. [CrossRef] [PubMed]
38. Rokstad, A.M.A.; Lacík, I.; de Vos, P.; Strand, B.L. Advances in biocompatibility and physico-chemical characterization of microspheres for cell encapsulation. *Adv. Drug Deliv. Rev.* **2014**, *67*, 111–130. [CrossRef] [PubMed]
39. Podola, B.; Li, T.; Melkonian, M. Porous Substrate Bioreactors: A Paradigm Shift in Microalgal Biotechnology? *Trends Biotechnol.* **2017**, *35*, 121–132. [CrossRef] [PubMed]
40. Chentir, I.; Hamdi, M.; Doumandji, A.; HadjSadok, A.; Ouada, H.B.; Nasri, M.; Jridi, M. Enhancement of extracellular polymeric substances (EPS) production in *Spirulina* (*Arthrospira* sp.) by two-step cultivation process and partial characterization of their polysaccharidic moiety. *Int. J. Biol. Macromol.* **2017**, *105*, 1412–1420. [CrossRef] [PubMed]
41. Economou, C.N.; Marinakis, N.; Moustaka-Gouni, M.; Kehayias, G.; Aggelis, G.; Vayenas, D.V. Lipid production by the filamentous cyanobacterium *Limnothrix* sp. growing in synthetic wastewater in suspended- and attached-growth photobioreactor systems. *Ann. Microbiol.* **2015**, *65*, 1941–1948. [CrossRef]
42. Rodjaroen, S.; Juntawong, N.; Mahakhant, A.; Miyamoto, K. High biomass production and starch accumulation in native green algal strains and cyanobacterial strains of Thailand. *Kasetsart J. Nat. Sci.* **2007**, *41*, 570–575.
43. De Morais, M.G.; Vaz, B.D.S.; De Morais, E.G.; Costa, J.A.V. Biologically Active Metabolites Synthesized by Microalgae. *BioMed Res. Int.* **2015**, *2015*. [CrossRef] [PubMed]
44. Das, U.N. Arachidonic acid and other unsaturated fatty acids and some of their metabolites function as endogenous antimicrobial molecules: A review. *J. Adv. Res.* **2018**, *11*, 57–66. [CrossRef] [PubMed]
45. Stengel, D.B.; Connan, S.; Popper, Z.A. Algal chemodiversity and bioactivity: Sources of natural variability and implications for commercial application. *Biotechnol. Adv.* **2011**, *29*, 483–501. [CrossRef] [PubMed]
46. Bellou, S.; Baeshen, M.N.; Elazzazy, A.M.; Aggeli, D.; Sayegh, F.; Aggelis, G. Microalgal lipids biochemistry and biotechnological perspectives. *Biotechnol. Adv.* **2014**, *32*, 1476–1493. [CrossRef] [PubMed]

47. Gayathri, M.; Shunmugam, S.; Mugasundari, A.V.; Rahman, P.K.S.M.; Muralitharan, G. Growth kinetic and fuel quality parameters as selective criterion for screening biodiesel producing cyanobacterial strains. *Bioresour. Technol.* **2018**, *247*, 453–462. [CrossRef] [PubMed]
48. Plaza, M.; Herrero, M.; Cifuentes, A.; Ibáñez, E. Innovative Natural Functional Ingredients from Microalgae. *J. Agric. Food Chem.* **2009**, *57*, 7159–7170. [CrossRef] [PubMed]
49. Steinhoff, F.S.; Karlberg, M.; Graeve, M.; Wulff, A. Cyanobacteria in Scandinavian coastal waters—A potential source for biofuels and fatty acids? *Algal Res.* **2014**, *5*, 42–51. [CrossRef]
50. Galhano, V.; de Figueiredo, D.R.; Alves, A.; Correia, A.; Pereira, M.J.; Gomes-Laranjo, J.; Peixoto, F. Morphological, biochemical and molecular characterization of *Anabaena*, *Aphanizomenon* and *Nostoc* strains (Cyanobacteria, Nostocales) isolated from Portuguese freshwater habitats. *Hydrobiologia* **2011**, *663*, 187–203. [CrossRef]
51. Koller, M.; Muhr, A.; Braunegg, G. Microalgae as versatile cellular factories for valued products. *Algal Res.* **2014**, *6*, 52–63. [CrossRef]
52. Funk, C.D. Prostaglandins and Leukotrienes: Advances in Eicosanoid Biology. *Science* **2001**, *294*, 1871–1875. [CrossRef] [PubMed]
53. Cardozo, K.H.M.; Guaratini, T.; Barros, M.P.; Falcão, V.R.; Tonon, A.P.; Lopes, N.P.; Campos, S.; Torres, M.A.; Souza, A.O.; Colepicolo, P.; et al. Metabolites from algae with economical impact. *Comp. Biochem. Physiol. Part C Toxicol. Pharmacol.* **2007**, *146*, 60–78. [CrossRef] [PubMed]
54. Judé, S.; Roger, S.; Martel, E.; Besson, P.; Richard, S.; Bougnoux, P.; Champeroux, P.; Le Guennec, J.Y. Dietary long-chain omega-3 fatty acids of marine origin: A comparison of their protective effects on coronary heart disease and breast cancers. *Prog. Biophys. Mol. Biol.* **2006**, *90*, 299–325. [CrossRef] [PubMed]
55. Maehre, H.K.; Jensen, I.J.; Elvevoll, E.O.; Eilertsen, K.E. ω-3 Fatty Acids and Cardiovascular Diseases: Effects, Mechanisms and Dietary Relevance. *Int. J. Mol. Sci.* **2015**, *16*, 22636–22661. [CrossRef] [PubMed]
56. Rose, D.P.; Connolly, J.M. Omega-3 fatty acids as cancer chemopreventive agents. *Pharmacol. Ther.* **1999**, *83*, 217–244. [CrossRef]
57. Xu, Y.; Qian, S.Y. Anti-cancer Activities of ω-6 Polyunsaturated Fatty Acids. *Biomed. J.* **2014**, *37*, 112–119. [CrossRef] [PubMed]
58. Molfino, A.; Amabile, M.I.; Mazzucco, S.; Biolo, G.; Farcomeni, A.; Ramaccini, C.; Antonaroli, S.; Monti, M.; Muscaritoli, M. Effect of Oral Docosahexaenoic Acid (DHA) Supplementation on DHA Levels and Omega-3 Index in Red Blood Cell Membranes of Breast Cancer Patients. *Front. Physiol.* **2017**, *8*, 549. [CrossRef] [PubMed]
59. Ciocci, M.; Iorio, E.; Carotenuto, F.; Khashoggi, H.A.; Nanni, F.; Melino, S. H_2S-releasing nanoemulsions: A new formulation to inhibit tumor cells proliferation and improve tissue repair. *Oncotarget* **2016**, *7*, 84338–84358. [CrossRef] [PubMed]
60. García, J.L.; de Vicente, M.; Galán, B. Microalgae, old sustainable food and fashion nutraceuticals. *Microb. Biotechnol.* **2017**, *10*, 1017–1024. [CrossRef] [PubMed]
61. Lee, J.M.; Lee, H.; Kang, S.; Park, W.J. Fatty Acid Desaturases, Polyunsaturated Fatty Acid Regulation, and Biotechnological Advances. *Nutrients* **2016**, *8*, 23. [CrossRef] [PubMed]
62. Potts, M. Desiccation tolerance of prokaryotes. *Microbiol. Rev.* **1994**, *58*, 755–805. [PubMed]
63. Kuhne, S.; Strieth, D.; Lakatos, M.; Muffler, K.; Ulber, R. A new photobioreactor concept enabling the production of desiccation induced biotechnological products using terrestrial cyanobacteria. *J. Biotechnol.* **2014**, *192*, 28–33. [CrossRef] [PubMed]
64. Comte, S.; Guibaud, G.; Baudu, M. Relations between extraction protocols for activated sludge extracellular polymeric substances (EPS) and complexation properties of Pb and Cd with EPS. *Enzyme Microb. Technol.* **2006**, *38*, 246–252. [CrossRef]
65. Comte, S.; Guibaud, G.; Baudu, M. Biosorption properties of extracellular polymeric substances (EPS) resulting from activated sludge according to their type: Soluble or bound. *Process Biochem.* **2006**, *41*, 815–823. [CrossRef]
66. Guibaud, G.; Comte, S.; Bordas, F.; Dupuy, S.; Baudu, M. Comparison of the complexation potential of extracellular polymeric substances (EPS), extracted from activated sludges and produced by pure bacteria strains, for cadmium, lead and nickel. *Chemosphere* **2005**, *59*, 629–638. [CrossRef] [PubMed]
67. Mishra, A.; Jha, B. Isolation and characterization of extracellular polymeric substances from micro-algae *Dunaliella salina* under salt stress. *Bioresour. Technol.* **2009**, *100*, 3382–3386. [CrossRef] [PubMed]

68. Trabelsi, L.; M'sakni, N.H.; Ouada, H.B.; Bacha, H.; Roudesli, S. Partial characterization of extracellular polysaccharides produced by cyanobacterium *Arthrospira platensis*. *Biotechnol. Bioprocess Eng.* **2009**, *14*, 27–31. [CrossRef]
69. Ophir, T.; Gutnick, D.L. A role for exopolysaccharides in the protection of microorganisms from desiccation. *Appl. Environ. Microbiol.* **1994**, *60*, 740–745. [PubMed]
70. Ganguly, K.; Chaturvedi, K.; More, U.A.; Nadagouda, M.N.; Aminabhavi, T.M. Polysaccharide-based micro/nanohydrogels for delivering macromolecular therapeutics. *J. Control. Release* **2014**, *193*, 162–173. [CrossRef] [PubMed]
71. Akiyoshi, K.; Kobayashi, S.; Shichibe, S.; Mix, D.; Baudys, M.; Wan Kim, S.; Sunamoto, J. Self-assembled hydrogel nanoparticle of cholesterol-bearing pullulan as a carrier of protein drugs: Complexation and stabilization of insulin. *J. Control. Release* **1998**, *54*, 313–320. [CrossRef]
72. Sarmento, B.; Ribeiro, A.; Veiga, F.; Ferreira, D. Development and characterization of new insulin containing polysaccharide nanoparticles. *Colloids Surf. B Biointerfaces* **2006**, *53*, 193–202. [CrossRef] [PubMed]
73. Chalasani, K.B.; Russell-Jones, G.J.; Jain, A.K.; Diwan, P.V.; Jain, S.K. Effective oral delivery of insulin in animal models using vitamin B12-coated dextran nanoparticles. *J. Control. Release* **2007**, *122*, 141–150. [CrossRef] [PubMed]
74. Yuan, W.; Hu, Z.; Su, J.; Wu, F.; Liu, Z.; Jin, T. Preparation and characterization of recombinant human growth hormone–Zn^{2+}-dextran nanoparticles using aqueous phase–aqueous phase emulsion. *Nanomed. Nanotechnol. Biol. Med.* **2012**, *8*, 424–427. [CrossRef] [PubMed]
75. Liu, L.; Pohnert, G.; Wei, D. Extracellular metabolites from industrial microalgae and their biotechnological potential. *Mar. Drugs* **2016**, *14*, 191. [CrossRef] [PubMed]
76. Calvert, P. Materials science. Printing cells. *Science* **2007**, *318*, 208–209. [CrossRef] [PubMed]
77. Mironov, V.; Boland, T.; Trusk, T.; Forgacs, G.; Markwald, R.R. Organ printing: Computer-aided jet-based 3D tissue engineering. *Trends Biotechnol.* **2003**, *21*, 157–161. [CrossRef]
78. Franca, M.B.; Panek, A.D.; Eleutherio, E.C. Oxidative stress and its effects during dehydration. *Comp. Biochem. Physiol. A Mol. Integr. Physiol.* **2007**, *146*, 621–631. [CrossRef] [PubMed]
79. Rippka, R.; Deruelles, J.; Waterbury, J.B.; Herdman, M.; Stanier, R.Y. Generic Assignments, Strain Histories and Properties of Pure Cultures of Cyanobacteria. *J. Gen. Microbiol.* **1979**, *111*, 1–61. [CrossRef]
80. Mata, T.M.; Martins, A.A.; Caetano, N.S. Microalgae for biodiesel production and other applications: A review. *Renew. Sustain. Energy Rev.* **2010**, *14*, 217–232. [CrossRef]
81. Ahmed, M.; Moerdijk-Poortvliet, T.C.W.; Wijnholds, A.; Stal, L.J.; Hasnain, S. Isolation, characterization and localization of extracellular polymeric substances from the cyanobacterium *Arthrospira platensis* strain MMG-9. *Eur. J. Phycol.* **2014**, *49*, 143–150. [CrossRef]
82. Dubois, M.; Gilles, K.A.; Hamilton, J.K.; Rebers, P.A.; Smith, F. Colorimetric Method for Determination of Sugars and Related Substances. *Anal. Chem.* **1956**, *28*, 350–356. [CrossRef]
83. Ehimen, E.A.; Sun, Z.F.; Carrington, C.G. Variables affecting the in situ transesterification of microalgae lipids. *Fuel* **2010**, *89*, 677–684. [CrossRef]
84. Karadağ, E.; Üzüm, Ö.B.; Saraydin, D. Water uptake in chemically crosslinked poly(acrylamide-co-crotonic acid) hydrogels. *Mater. Des.* **2005**, *26*, 265–270. [CrossRef]
85. Ciocci, M.; Cacciotti, I.; Seliktar, D.; Melino, S. Injectable silk fibroin hydrogels functionalized with microspheres as adult stem cells-carrier systems. *Int. J. Biol. Macromol.* **2018**, *108*, 960–971. [CrossRef] [PubMed]
86. Colnaghi, R.; Pagani, S.; Kennedy, C.; Drummond, M. Cloning, sequence analysis and overexpression of the rhodanese gene of Azotobacter vinelandii. *Eur. J. Biochem.* **1996**, *236*, 240–248. [CrossRef] [PubMed]
87. Sabelli, R.; Iorio, E.; Martino, A.D.; Podo, F.; Ricci, A.; Viticchiè, G.; Rotilio, G.; Paci, M.; Melino, S. Rhodanese–thioredoxin system and allyl sulfur compounds. *FEBS J.* **2008**, *275*, 3884–3899. [CrossRef] [PubMed]
88. Sörbo, B.H. Rhodanese. *Acta Chem. Scand.* **1973**, *7*, 1129–1133. [CrossRef]
89. Forte, G.; Pietronave, S.; Nardone, G.; Zamperone, A.; Magnani, E.; Pagliari, S.; Pagliari, F.; Giacinti, C.; Nicoletti, C.; Musaró, A.; et al. Human Cardiac Progenitor Cell Grafts as Unrestricted Source of Supernumerary Cardiac Cells in Healthy Murine Hearts. *Stem Cells* **2011**, *29*, 2051–2061. [CrossRef] [PubMed]
90. Koyanagi, M.; Kawakabe, S.; Arimura, Y. A comparative study of colorimetric cell proliferation assays in immune cells. *Cytotechnology* **2016**, *68*, 1489–1498. [CrossRef] [PubMed]

91. Morishita, M.; Lowman, A.M.; Takayama, K.; Nagai, T.; Peppas, N.A. Elucidation of the mechanism of incorporation of insulin in controlled release systems based on complexation polymers. *J. Control. Release.* **2002**, *81*, 25–32. [CrossRef]
92. Lowman, A.M.; Morishita, M.; Nagai, T.; Peppas, N.A. Method for Oral Delivery of ProteinsA Hydrogel Matrix. U.S. Patent Application WO1998043615 A1, 1998.

© 2018 by the authors. Licensee MDPI, Basel, Switzerland. This article is an open access article distributed under the terms and conditions of the Creative Commons Attribution (CC BY) license (http://creativecommons.org/licenses/by/4.0/).

MDPI
St. Alban-Anlage 66
4052 Basel
Switzerland
Tel. +41 61 683 77 34
Fax +41 61 302 89 18
www.mdpi.com

Marine Drugs Editorial Office
E-mail: marinedrugs@mdpi.com
www.mdpi.com/journal/marinedrugs

www.ingramcontent.com/pod-product-compliance
Lightning Source LLC
LaVergne TN
LVHW070745100526
838202LV00013B/1310
* 9 7 8 3 0 3 9 4 3 1 3 0 4 *